FOURTH EDITION

HANDBOOK OF

Family Planning
and
Reproductive
Healthcare

Anna Glasier
Ailsa Gebbie

Foreword by
Nancy Loudon

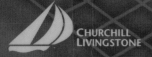
CHURCHILL
LIVINGSTONE

Handbook of Family Planning and Reproductive Healthcare

FOURTH EDITION

Edited by

Anna Glasier BSc MD FRCOG MFFP
Director, Family Planning and Well Woman Services, Lothian Primary Care
NHS Trust and Senior Lecturer, Department of Obstetrics and Gynaecology,
University of Edinburgh

and

Ailsa Gebbie MB ChB DCH MRCOG MFFP
Consultant in Community Gynaecology, Lothian Primary Care NHS Trust,
Edinburgh

Foreword by

Nancy Loudon OBE MB ChB FRCP(Ed) FFFP
Former Medical Co-ordinator, Family Planning and Well Woman Services,
Lothian Health Board, former Vice-Chairman, Health Education Board for
Scotland

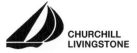
CHURCHILL
LIVINGSTONE

LONDON • EDINBURGH • NEW YORK • PHILADELPHIA • ST LOUIS • SYDNEY • TORONTO 2000

CHURCHILL LIVINGSTONE
An imprint of Harcourt Publishers Limited

© Harcourt Publishers Limited 2000

 is a registered trademark of Harcourt Publishers Limited

The right of Anna Glasier and Ailsa Gebbie to be identified as authors of
this work has been asserted by them in accordance with the Copyright,
Designs and Patents Act 1988

First published 1985
Second edition 1991
Third edition 1995
Fourth edition 2000

ISBN 0 443 06450 4

British Library Cataloguing in Publication Data
A catalogue record for this book is available from the British Library

Library of Congress Cataloging in Publication Data
A catalog record for this book is available from the Library of
Congress

Note
Medical knowledge is constantly changing. As new information
becomes available, changes in treatment, procedures, equipment and
the use of drugs become necessary. The editors/authors/contributors
and the publishers have taken care to ensure that the information given
in this text is accurate and up to date. However, readers are strongly
advised to confirm that the information, especially with regard to
drug usage, complies with the latest legislation and standards of
practice.

The
publisher's
policy is to use
**paper manufactured
from sustainable forests**

Printed in England

Foreword

Family planning has been one of the success stories of the 20th century. Almost 60% of couples of reproductive age worldwide now use contraception. Yet world population has just hit the 6 billion mark and more than 120 million women in developing countries have no way of preventing pregnancy.

The first Birth Control Clinic in the UK was opened nearly 80 years ago but the concept of controlling family size was resisted by society in general, by the church and, with a few notable exceptions, by the medical profession. However, political pressure, particularly from women's groups and the rising number of maternal deaths in the 1930s, fuelled the demand of women to control their own fertility.

In 1930, the National Birth Control Council was formed. In 1939, when the term 'family planning' was accepted as being more appropriate, it became the Family Planning Association (FPA) and for the next 30 years was the main provider of contraceptive services in this country. Family planning services became free in England and Wales in 1967 and a year later in Scotland although contraceptives had to be paid for. It is anomalous that with the Abortion Act of 1967 termination of pregnancy became free under the National Health Service (NHS) yet the majority of women in Scotland still had to pay for contraceptives.

A completely free family planning service from hospitals and clinics came with the reorganization of the NHS in 1974 and was extended to primary care in 1975. From that time, family planning was no longer seen as a service to be provided in isolation but as part of general healthcare. This was recognized by the Royal College of Obstetricians and Gynaecologists in 1993 when the Joint Committee of Contraception was replaced by the Faculty of Family Planning and Reproductive Health Care to set standards of practice and training for doctors working in clinics, hospitals and general practice. Education for nurses became more comprehensive, and they were trained to take responsibility for functions formerly the province of doctors.

The 1960s and 1970s were exciting times in the family planning world. The oral contraceptive pill became available, modern intrauterine devices appeared, and male and female sterilization was an option for those who had completed their families. The Abortion Act of 1967 was a major landmark. Changing attitudes to premarital chastity resulted in a demand for contraception by the unmarried. As this was not official FPA policy until

1970, Brook Clinics were opened in 1964 to meet the need. Counselling was offered to those with difficulties in personal or marital relationships. Sex education programmes for schools and clinics for young people were developed. Cervical screening became available both in clinics and in places of work.

Such was the scene in 1985 when I first edited this *Handbook*. In the second and third editions, chapters on the menopause, sexually transmitted disease, gynaecological problems uncovered during the family planning consultation and contraceptives of the future were added.

Now 5 years later, Dr Anna Glasier and Dr Ailsa Gebbie, both consultant gynaecologists highly experienced in family planning practice and research, have widened the scope of the book yet again to meet changing needs and current practice and to make it more relevant to countries outside the UK. Chapters on adolescent reproductive health and the premenstrual syndrome have been added. Contributors have brought their chapters up to date and five chapters are written by new authors who bring fresh views and approaches to each subject.

Although improvements in many methods of family planning are included throughout the *Handbook* and predicted in the review of new developments, no major breakthrough appears on the horizon. However, a new emergency contraceptive pill containing levonorgestrel has just been licensed for use in the UK. It is as effective as, but has fewer side effects than, the Yuzpe regimen and its launch presents us with a real opportunity to promote emergency contraception and to educate both men and women in its use, effectiveness and availability. The proposal that emergency contraception should be released from prescription and become obtainable from pharmacies is gaining increasing support from family planning workers throughout the country. The potential of such a measure to reduce the number of unwanted pregnancies would be enormous. It may well prove to be the most important advance in family planning in the early years of the 21st century.

It is very fortunate that Anna Glasier, my successor in Edinburgh and an internationally-known expert in family planning, and my daughter-in-law, Ailsa Gebbie, who has wide experience of writing and teaching on the subject, now edit the *Handbook*. I could not leave it in better hands.

Edinburgh 2000   Nancy Loudon OBE

Preface

This, the fourth edition of the *Handbook*, is published in the first year of a new millennium. When the third edition was being planned 6 years ago, we expanded the book to include the broader aspects of reproductive health-care. This change was intended to reflect both the international trends to regard family planning as part of the much larger area of reproductive health and the emergence in the UK of the new specialty of reproductive healthcare. Community gynaecology/reproductive healthcare has expanded significantly as a specialty since 1995 and there are now over 70 consultants in the UK providing specialist reproductive health services. We welcome the increasing tendency to bring genito-urinary medicine and family planning services closer together in an attempt to provide integrated sexual health services. It is still true, however, that the general practice team remains the main provider of reproductive health services in the UK and we hope that this edition of the *Handbook* will be as useful in a general practice setting as it should be in a more specialist clinic.

New developments in contraceptive technology often seem frustratingly slow to appear and the new methods that have become available since the last edition, whilst a useful addition to the range, are not radically different from methods which have been available during the last decade. Advances in other areas of reproductive health have perhaps been more exciting. Whatever the nature of new developments, it is certainly true that the general public is becoming increasingly well informed and, with widespread access to electronic sources of information, can sometimes be better informed than their healthcare advisers!

Perhaps the greatest challenge to those currently working in family planning and reproductive healthcare is to incorporate the recent changes in the practice of clinical medicine which have placed increasing emphasis on evidence-based practice, and the use of nationally developed guidelines to enhance quality of care.

We hope this new edition reflects all these developments. We have kept to the original aim of the book, which is to provide practical and easily accessible information for doctors and nurses in a clinical setting. Our contributors are not only experts in their field but are also actively providing a clinical service. The three new chapters include an international perspective on contraceptive choices and strategies, adolescent sexual health – acknowledging the depressingly high UK teenage pregnancy rates – and premenstrual syndrome, the 'heartsink' of gynaecological consultations, which includes new and effective treatment regimens.

We are deeply indebted to Dr Nancy Loudon OBE for her guidance and support in producing this new edition. Her foreword is, in many ways, a tribute to her own personal contribution to family planning, not just for the women of Lothian but as one of the early pioneers in establishing family planning services in the UK. We thank all the chapter contributors for their hard work and forbearance in coping with our reminders and queries. The swift and efficient assistance received from Sheila Black at Harcourt Health Sciences was an enormous help. Lastly, we thank our families for their support, advice and never-ending tolerance.

Anna Glasier

Edinburgh 2000   Ailsa Gebbie

Contributors

David T. Baird FRCP FRCOG
MRC Clinical Research Professor, University of Edinburgh; Consultant Gynaecologist, Royal Infirmary, Edinburgh

John Bancroft MD FRCP FRCPsych
Director, Kinsey Institute in Research on Sex, Gender, and Reproduction, Indiana University, Bloomington, Indiana

Alan D. G. Brown FRCOG FRCSEd
Consultant Obstetrician and Gynaecologist, Simpson Memorial Maternity Pavilion and Royal Infirmary, Edinburgh; Honorary Senior Lecturer, University of Edinburgh; Consultant to Cases Committee, Medical Protection Society, London; Consultant Gynaecologist and Vice-chair, Lothian Brook Advisory Centre

Audrey H. Brown MBChB MRCOG
Specialist Registrar in Community Gynaecology, Lothian Primary Care NHS Trust, Edinburgh

Charlotte Ellertson MPA PhD
Director of Reproductive Health for Latin America and the Caribbean, Population Council, Mexico City

Ian S. Fraser MD BSc(Hons) FRACOG FRCOG CREI
Professor in Reproductive Medicine, University of Sydney; Visiting Medical Officer, King George V and Royal Prince Alfred Hospitals, Sydney; President, Royal Australian and New Zealand College of Obstetricians and Gynaecologists

Ailsa Gebbie MB ChB DCH MRCOG MFFP
Consultant in Community Gynaecology, Lothian Primary Care NHS Trust, Edinburgh

Anna Glasier BSc MD FRCOG MFFP
Director, Family Planning and Well Woman Services, Lothian Primary Care NHS Trust; Senior Lecturer, Department of Obstetrics and Gynaecology, University of Edinburgh

Lora Green BA (Hons) RGN RM Dip HV FP Cert
Nurse Manager and Senior Nurse, Family Planning and Well Woman
Services, Lothian Primary Care NHS Trust, Edinburgh

John Guillebaud MA FRCSE FRCOG MFFP
Professor of Family Planning and Reproductive Health, Medical Director,
Margaret Pyke Centre for Study and Training in Family Planning, London;
Consultant, Department of Obstetrics and Gynaecology, UCL Medical
School, London

Sally Hope MA (Oxon) FRCGP DRCOG
General Practitioner, Woodstock, Oxford

Meera Kishen MD MFFP Dip Ven
Consultant in Family Planning and Reproductive Health Care, Central
Abacus, North Mersey Community NHS Trust, Liverpool

Alexander McMillan MD FRCP FRCP (Ed)
Consultant Physician, Department of Genito-Urinary Medicine,
Royal Infirmary of Edinburgh and Lothian University Hospitals NHS Trust

P. M. S. O'Brien MB BCH MD FRCOG
Professor of Obstetrics and Gynaecology and Head of Academic
Department of Obstetrics, City General Hospital Maternity Unit, North
Staffordshire NHS Trust

Paul F. A. Van Look MD PhD MFFP
Director, Department of Reproductive Health and Research, World Health
Organization, Geneva

CONTENTS

Foreword **v**

Preface **vii**

Contributors **ix**

1. Contraceptive choice   1
   Charlotte Ellertson

2. Combined oral contraception   29
   John Guillebaud

3. Progestogen-only contraception   77
   Ian S. Fraser

4. Intrauterine contraceptive devices   105
   Meera Kishen

5. Barrier methods   127
   Ailsa Gebbie

6. Natural family planning   161
   Lora Green

7. Sterilization   177
   Anna Glasier

8. Emergency contraception   201
   Anna Glasier

9. Adolescent reproductive health   215
   Audrey H. Brown

10. Legal aspects of family planning   231
    Alan D. G. Brown

11. Therapeutic abortion   249
    David T. Baird

12. Screening and reproductive health promotion   265
    Sally Hope

13. Sexually transmitted infections   281
    Alexander McMillan

14. Sexuality and family planning 313
    John Bancroft

15. Gynaecological problems in the family planning consultation 335
    Anna Glasier

16. Premenstrual syndrome 357
    P. M. S. O'Brien

17. The menopause 371
    Ailsa Gebbie

18. Contraceptives of the future 395
    Paul F. A. Van Look

Index 417

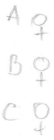

1

Contraceptive choice

Charlotte Ellertson

Fertility regulation strategies
  versus methods 1
  Methods as building blocks 1
  Lifecycle approach 2
  UK and international patterns
    of family planning 2
Effectiveness 4
  Measuring effectiveness 5
  Effectiveness of various
    methods 8
Safety 8
  Measuring safety 8
  Safety of various methods of
    family planning 10
Non-contraceptive benefits 12

Protection against sexually
  transmitted infections 12
Menstrual disorders and bleeding
  control 12
Other non-contraceptive benefits 13
User considerations 13
  Measuring user attitudes 13
  Assessing the user's needs 15
  Back-up options 15
  Interaction with the healthcare
    system 17
  Sexual lifestyle 18
  Plans for future fertility 19
Costs 19
Conclusion 21

FERTILITY REGULATION STRATEGIES VERSUS METHODS

Methods as building blocks

Family planning handbooks have traditionally presented the options for women or couples seeking to limit their fertility as a list of methods or techniques, each with its advantages and disadvantages. Such an approach was appropriate as long as the number of available options remained small and clearly distinct from one another. As the menu of choices grows longer and more intertwined, however, and as the needs of couples who use contraception grow more complex, it may be more useful to think in terms of fertility control strategies rather than methods. A woman who perceives herself to be at risk of sexually transmitted infections (STIs) might choose condoms, even though these have a relatively high contraceptive failure rate, but might opt to back them up with emergency contraception to create a contraceptive strategy that is highly effective and also protective against STIs. Another woman who does not consider herself at any risk of STIs might choose a method with higher contraceptive efficacy such as oral contraception, that offers much less protection against STIs. A woman who has intercourse infrequently but with a mutually monogamous partner, and who does not wish to use a method that requires daily action on her part, might prefer a combination of a diaphragm and spermicide, backed up by abortion (three methods combined, creating a highly effective and acceptable strategy), while another woman who would not like to rely on abortion might prefer the intrauterine device (IUD) in such a situation (a strategy involving just one method).

This chapter presents a brief overview of the various methods of family planning, but with the idea that they are building blocks that women or couples might use singly or in combination to construct a strategy that meets their needs.

Before 1960, the majority of family planning methods used were the so-called 'male' methods (male condoms, withdrawal and vasectomy). Today, with the advent of the oral contraceptive, the modern IUD, and the vastly improved array of female sterilization methods, the mix of methods has shifted so that the 'female' methods are used about three times as often (Segal 1993). Considering also the need for other fertility regulation technologies such as emergency contraception and abortion, it is clear that women shoulder the bulk of the responsibility for family planning today. For that reason, we can think of the 'typical' family planning client as a woman.

The lifecycle approach

Over the course of her life, a woman's needs will vary greatly (Forrest 1993). If she is a composite of modern statistics from industrialized countries, as an adolescent, she may have intercourse sporadically and at unpredictable times, but with partners that place her at risk of STIs. She may feel strongly that her protection must be discreet so that she can keep it private from parents or friends, and her family planning goal may be to protect herself against pregnancy in a way that preserves her options for future fertility, preferably using methods that also offer STI protection. Later, as she enters a more stable relationship, and her sexual activity is more socially sanctioned, she may feel better able to negotiate condom use, or more willing to use a method that requires daily activity on her part. If she wants children, her needs during the next stage may be for methods that help her to space the births appropriately. Finally, she may reach a point where she no longer wants the option of childbearing, and she or her partner may choose a permanent method. A woman who has a large array of family planning options available to her throughout the course of her reproductive life will have an easier time meeting the needs she faces at each one of these stages.

UK and international patterns of family planning

On a population basis, a snapshot of current use patterns will reflect not only the popularity or availability of a given method, but also the population mix of women at different life stages. Two demographic trends in the UK currently influence the method mix in this country. First, the average age of women having their first baby is climbing, and is nearly 30 years today.

Thus women today spend more years requiring contraception options that preserve their fertility and fewer years needing permanent contraceptive methods, such as sterilization. Second, the proportion of couples who opt not to have children at all is rising, and is currently around 25%.

Table 1.1 shows the patterns of contraceptive use found in a nationally representative survey (n = 967) of women aged 15 to 45 at risk of pregnancy, carried out in Britain in 1992 (Oddens et al 1994). The data are presented by age group, since it is clear that the method mix varies dramatically by this variable. Younger women (those under 25) favour the oral contraceptive and barrier methods, often combining the two (around 12% of women report using this dual protection strategy). In the next age category (25 to 34), the IUD and sterilization start to grow in popularity, as couples complete their families, and move toward longer acting methods. Finally, in the older age groups (35 to 45), oral contraceptive use falls to a fraction of its popularity with younger women, and sterilization (most commonly vasectomy) moves into the lead as the most widely used method. The joint use of oral contraceptives and barrier methods drops to zero among women aged 40 to 45. Women in this oldest group are also as likely as women in the very youngest group (15 to 19) to report using no method at all. It is important to note that this method mix implies that the average women in the UK will have at least one contraceptive failure in her lifetime (see below).

In the USA, nationally representative data are available from a large government survey, the National Survey of Family Growth (NSFG), that is repeated every few years. The survey tracks changes in family planning practices over time. Data from 1995 show that, as in 1982 and 1988, female sterilization, the pill and the male condom were the most widely used methods (Piccinino and Mosher 1998). Between 1988 and 1995, however, pill use dropped from 31% to 27% of respondents, while condom use rose from 15% to 20%, with growth in condom use most marked among younger

Table 1.1 Family planning use patterns in Britain, by age group, in 1992 expressed as a percentage (reproduced with permission from Oddens BJ et al 1994 Contraceptive use and attitudes in Great Britain. Contraception 49(1): 73–86.)

Method	Age (years)					
	15–19	20–24	25–29	30–34	35–39	40–45
Oral contraceptives	52.5	57.6	50.5	39.5	16.5	11.7
Oral contraceptives and barrier	11.9	12.1	1.2	0.5	0.6	0.0
Barrier methods	26.6	21.1	20.4	16.3	23.4	20.3
Periodic abstinence	0.0	0.0	1.8	3.1	1.2	1.8
Coitus interruptus	0.0	2.1	1.2	0.5	1.2	0.9
Intrauterine device	0.0	3.0	11.0	6.5	8.2	9.4
Female sterilization	0.0	0.0	5.8	9.5	19.1	18.9
Male sterilization	0.0	3.1	5.5	21.2	28.6	27.7
No method	8.9	1.0	0.6	2.9	1.2	9.2

unmarried women. Clearly, concerns about HIV and other STIs are changing family planning strategies dramatically in the USA.

Worldwide, sterilization is by far the most widely used method. Nearly half of all sterilized men and women of reproductive ages live in China (37%) or India (22%). In Canada, South Korea and the territory of Puerto Rico, over 40% of the population of reproductive age are sterilized. In several other countries, including Brazil, the Dominican Republic, El Salvador, Panama, Sri Lanka, Thailand, Taiwan, the UK and the USA, over 25% of people of reproductive age rely on sterilization. Except in the UK, India and Nepal, where the proportions are roughly equal, far more women than men are sterilized. As sterilization techniques improve, more women are seeking this option, while vasectomy numbers remain constant (Segal 1993).

IUDs are the second most popular method worldwide, driven largely by the popularity of the method in China, where a third of all couples using contraception employ it. Other countries relying heavily on IUD use include Colombia, Cuba, Indonesia, Taiwan and Tunisia in the developing world, and Czechoslovakia, Denmark, Finland, Norway and Sweden among the industrialized countries (Segal 1993).

Hormonal contraceptives as a group rank third in world usage. The bulk of this use (85%) is oral contraception, with implants and injectables accounting for only 15% (Segal 1993). Some countries, however, may rely heavily on one particular method. For example, the South African national programme relies overwhelmingly on injectables.

Condoms are used relatively little in developing countries, although they may grow in popularity as concerns about HIV spread. Japan, where oral contraceptives are only now becoming available, leads the list, with 44% of contraceptive-users relying on the condom. Singapore and the Nordic countries (Denmark, Finland and Sweden) have rates of around 20% condom use. Costa Rica, Hong Kong, Taiwan, and Trinidad and Tobago each have between 10% and 15% condom-users (Segal 1993).

In developed countries as a group, the most popular methods are oral contraception (16%), the male condom (14%) and withdrawal (13%). In developing countries, by contrast, female sterilization (20%), the IUD (13%), oral contraception (6%) and vasectomy (5%) are the most frequently reported methods (Shah 1994).

EFFECTIVENESS

When guiding a new user through the array of contraceptive methods, undoubtedly the single most important question to ask about a method is 'how well does it work?' Unfortunately, the answer is sometimes quite complicated. The following brief guide to interpreting the efficacy literature may be helpful for those readers who do not simply want to trust the authors of handbooks!

Measuring effectiveness

There are several pitfalls to notice when considering the effectiveness of family planning methods. First, not all of the women who use a given method would become pregnant even if the method were completely useless (such as crossed fingers). A certain percentage (perhaps 15%) of couples will not conceive within a year of trying, and for this fraction, 'using' even a useless method would still appear to provide 100% effective contraceptive protection. Second, many users participating in effectiveness studies of various methods do not use the method correctly and consistently every time they have intercourse. Methods that require the woman or couple to follow complex and burdensome instructions will, all things being equal, show a higher failure rate than methods with a similar theoretical effectiveness that demand little from the user. Third, some user characteristics of the participants in the study can have an enormous impact on the failure rates. Studies filled with younger women will tend to have higher failure rates (because younger women are more fecund), as will studies in which the participants have sex very frequently. Good reviews of the literature try to standardize for the population composition of different studies being evaluated. Finally, failure is an observable event (pregnancy) whereas success is typically not. (It would be possible although impractical, for instance, to perform ultrasound every day on each pill-user to see if ovulation really was suppressed each month. Failure of an IUD, correctly placed, however, might be observable only once pregnancy began.)

For these reasons, with most contraceptives, effectiveness based on clinical studies is typically presented in terms of failure rates rather than success rates. Contraceptive clinical trials often include only women of 'proven fertility' and require a minimum frequency of coitus in participants. Usually age requirements are also imposed. Moreover, failure rates are often subdivided into two categories: perfect-use failure rates and typical-use failure rates. A perfect-use failure rate refers to the number of pregnancies observed during cycles when the method was used consistently and correctly at every act of intercourse. Perfect-use failure rates are useful for potential users in that they convey the sense of how well a method can be expected to work for the woman if she uses it consistently and correctly every time. Typical-use failure rates, by contrast, are derived from a mixture of perfect- and imperfect-use failure rates. Pregnancies counted during imperfect use include those that occurred when the user actually did not 'use' the method at all, leaving the diaphragm in the drawer, for instance, or missing her pills for several days in a row. Typical-use failure rates are useful for explaining to women how well the method works for most women who 'use' it. The difference between typical- and perfect-use failure rates can be thought of as a 'hassle factor' for women, penalizing methods that require a lot from the user.

As shown in Figure 1.1, many methods have no or virtually no difference between their perfect- and typical-use failure rates. For instance, sterilization or an IUD requires almost nothing of the user once the method is started. By contrast, some methods have a tremendous gap between perfect- and typical-use failure rates. Abstinence, as one example, has a theoretical failure rate of 0%, but in practice, the method is prone to misuse (couples fail to abstain!), and has a typical-use failure rate of about 25%.

By contrast, effectiveness statistics based on community or population surveys, such as the Oxford Family Planning Association study in the 1970s or the NSFG in the USA, tend to reflect actual use experiences. These types of studies, however, tend to suffer from under-reporting of abortion (and therefore artificially low failure rates of contraceptive methods) and also over-reporting of method 'use'.

There are two exceptions in the family planning literature concerning the way that effectiveness is measured: abortion and emergency contraception. In measuring the effectiveness of various abortion methods, researches can use standard probabilities analogous to the cure rates used in other areas of medicine. This intuitively more straightforward method is possible since, in each case, 100% of the women who use the method start out pregnant and only a few remain pregnant following use of the method. By contrast, since emergency contraception is designed for one-time (or sporadic) use rather than ongoing use month after month, methods to describe how well it works must be calibrated to one-time use, and this makes them difficult to

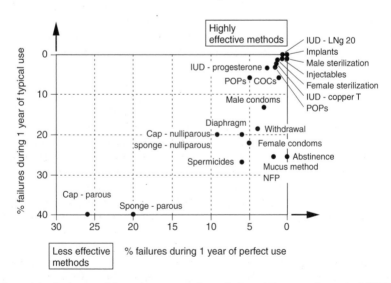

Figure 1.1   Perfect-use failure rates compared to typical-use failure rates, by method. (COC, combined oral contraception; IUD, intrauterine device; NFP, natural family planning; POP, progestogen-only pill.)

compare directly to regular contraceptive methods. Emergency contraception researchers typically present two effectiveness statistics. The first is a straightforward and easily interpretable failure rate. This percentage, around 2% for the Yuzpe regimen, for example, reflects the number of women who use emergency contraception in the trial and end up pregnant anyway. Unfortunately, the failure rate is only partially a reflection of how well the method works. It also reflects the underlying pregnancy risks of the women in the trial. For instance, an emergency contraception trial of extremely cautious women who all took emergency contraception because they had unprotected sex during menses would be expected to have a far lower failure rate than a trial of women who all had unprotected sex during their mid-cycle peak fertility days and took emergency contraception. For this reason, good emergency contraception researchers also present the results that show the number of expected pregnancies (added up by assessing the risk the study participants were facing) that were averted by the use of the method. This figure is also called the 'proportionate reduction in pregnancy.'

Over the past decades, family planning researchers have made great strides in measuring the effectiveness of contraceptives. In many older studies, effectiveness is described in terms of the somewhat misleading Pearl index. Developed by physician Raymond Pearl early last century (Pearl 1932), the Pearl index represents the number of pregnancies observed in a cohort of women using a given method divided by the total number of cycles in which the method was used by all the women put together. It is then usually multiplied by 1300 to standardize the results to reflect the experience of 100 woman-years with each woman contributing 13 cycles per year. The main flaw with the Pearl index is that it is not stable over time, and so researchers can ensure a low Pearl index for whatever method they are studying by running the study for a longer time. For example, in a hypothetical study of the male condom (based on actual data from the 1973 NSFG), the Pearl index would be 7.5 for the first 12 months, but only 4.4 if 60 months of data were analyzed (Hatcher et al 1998). The reason is that the most fecund women will become pregnant first, and for at least a few months, they will not be at risk of falling pregnant again. The remaining women staying in the study will be the less fecund ones. Modern contraceptive researchers rely on life-table techniques that correctly reflect the exposure to pregnancy that each woman contributes starting from the time she joins the trial (Trussell and Kost 1987). The results are presented as the number of pregnancies experienced during 100 woman-years of use of the method (a woman-year is defined as 13 cycles), and are standardized by 1-year, 2-year, 5-year (or much shorter or longer) cut-off points.

Clinical trials themselves have also improved over the decades. Modern clinical trials are stricter about excluding pregnant women and women who are not fertile to begin with. Also, with the advent of superior pregnancy tests, contraceptive failures can be detected sooner and more

accurately. Since a high proportion of very early pregnancies end spontaneously in miscarriage (Wilcox et al 1999), counting each pregnancy that is
chemically, but not yet clinically, confirmed as a failure will give a higher failure rate than will counting only clinically confirmed pregnancies, as was
done in the past.

A final factor to consider is publication bias. Practising physicians who
see the vasectomy failure rates in their clinics as double those in the literature will not rush to publish articles about their techniques. Similarly, a drug
company testing a new pill formulation will abandon the pill formula if the
results look poor compared to most published pill trials.

One difficulty that remains is extrapolating effectiveness rates from the
literature to the typical clinic population. On the one hand, failure rates
might be expected to be higher in 'real life' than in a clinical trial because the
users are perhaps less motivated than they would need to be to endure the
extra burden of participating in a trial. In addition, perhaps they receive less
counselling and special attention than they might in a trial. On the other
hand, participants in clinical trials are often selected because of their
uniquely high risk. Focusing on a high-risk population can dramatically
reduce the number of users needed in a trial, but it will also result in the trial
showing a higher failure rate than would be true in real life. For example, an
emergency contraception study currently underway in Scotland, England
and the USA shows that around half of all women presenting to the study
centres appears to be at negligible risk of pregnancy, and certainly at too low
a risk to justify their enrolment in the study.

Effectiveness of various methods

Table 1.2 shows summary estimates of the 1-year life-table perfect-use and
typical-use failure rates for the ongoing methods of family planning. These
are derived from a combination of population-based studies (wherever
possible) and clinical trials judged to be of good quality. The one-time failure probabilities for the various methods of early abortion and the proportionate reductions in pregnancy for the three most widely available
methods of emergency contraception appear in Chapters 8 and 11.

SAFETY

Measuring safety

The second most common question about a method is likely to concern its
safety. Measuring and comparing the safety of family planning methods is
also difficult, but the reason in this case is that most methods are so safe that
serious adverse events are extremely rare. Less serious ones are often quite
subjective. Moreover, it is difficult to extrapolate side-effect profiles from

Table 1.2   Percentage of women experiencing an unintended pregnancy during the first year of typical use and the first year of perfect use of ongoing methods of contraception (reproduced with permission from Hatcher RA, Trussell J, Stewart F et al 1998 Contraceptive technology, 17th revised edn. Ardent Media, New York.)

Method	% of users experiencing an unintended pregnancy within the first year of use	
	Typical use[1]	Perfect use[2]
Chance[3]	85	85
Spermicides[4]	26	6
Periodic abstinence	25	
Calendar		9
Ovulation method		3
Symptothermal[5]		2
Post-ovulation		1
Cap[6]		
Parous women	40	26
Nulliparous women	20	9
Sponge		
Parous women	40	20
Nulliparous women	20	9
Diaphragm[6]	20	6
Withdrawal	19	4
Condom[7]		
Female (Reality)	21	5
Male	14	3
Oral contraceptives	5	
Progestogen-only		0.5
Combined		0.1
IUD		
Progesterone T	2.0	1.5
Copper T 380A	0.8	0.6
LNg 20	0.1	0.1
Injectable (depot medroxyprogesterone acetate)	0.3	0.3
Implants (Norplant and Norplant-2)	0.05	0.05
Female sterilization	0.5	0.5
Male sterilization	0.15	0.10

Lactational amenorrhea method (LAM) is a highly effective, *temporary* method of contraception.[8]

[1] Among *typical* couples who initiate use of a method (not necessarily for the first time), the percentage who experience an accidental pregnancy during the first year if they do not stop use for any other reason.

[2] Among couples who initiate use of a method (not necessarily for the first time) and who use it *perfectly* (both consistently and correctly), the percentage who experience an accidental pregnancy during the first year if they do not stop use for any other reason.

[3] The percents becoming pregnant in columns 2 and 3 are based on data from populations where contraception is not used and from women who cease using contraception in order to become pregnant. Among such populations, about 89% become pregnant within 1 year. This estimate was lowered slightly (to 85%) to represent the percent who would become pregnant within 1 year among women now relying on reversible methods of contraception if they abandoned contraception altogether.

[4] Foams, creams, gels, vaginal suppositories and vaginal film.

[5] Cervical mucus (ovulation) method supplemented by calendar in the pre-ovulatory and basal body temperature in the post-ovulatory phases.

[6] With spermicidal cream or jelly.

[7] Without spermicides.

[8] To maintain effective protection against pregnancy, another method of contraception must be used as soon as menstruation resumes, the frequency or duration of breast-feeds is reduced, bottle-feeds are introduced, or the baby reaches 6 months of age.

clinical trial populations to real-life clients, in part because the users who join clinical trials often do so because they are not satisfied with any of the existing methods. These 'fussy customers' may be especially sensitive to side effects, and study staff too may prompt them to report side effects that would typically go unreported or unnoticed in a cohort of general users. Finally, safety events often affect only a subset of the users of a given method. For such users, the risks may be too high to justify the benefits, but for the rest of users the risks may be negligible. In choosing methods, however, it is important to bear in mind that the health risks of pregnancy generally far outweigh the health risks of any family planning method mentioned in this book.

Safety of various methods of family planning

Safety may be divided into several categories: the most common side effects (including the medically trivial), any serious dangers that the method might entail (even if rare), and the risks of death. Table 1.3 summarizes safety considerations for each of the methods of fertility regulation currently available. It is important to bear in mind that pregnancy, particularly unwanted pregnancy, is not without health effects and risks of its own. Fully 100% of pregnant women experience 'side effects' and the risk of death from carrying a pregnancy to term is approximately 1/10000.

The likelihood of experiencing side effects, serious or not, can be minimized by strict observance of the contraindications to their use. These are described in the data sheets (summary of product characteristics or labelling) provided by the manufacturers, and in individual chapters in this book. Recognizing that the concept of absolute and relative contraindications is somewhat difficult to understand and to use in clinical settings, the World Health Organization (WHO) has recently reviewed the contraindications for all of the major methods of contraception and developed an alternative system of so-called 'medical eligibility criteria'. For each method, WHO determined whether there were no (graded as '1') or hardly any (graded as '2') medical conditions that would make a given method inadvisable, or whether there are relative (graded as '3') or absolute ('4') contraindications to initiating ('I') or continuing ('C') a method. Methods with just '1' or '2' are not deemed to require any clinical judgements prior to use (World Health Organization 1996).

For hormonal emergency contraception, and for the barrier methods, for example, there are hardly any users who are not eligible ('4'), except for pregnant women who do not need the methods, and in the case of condoms and diaphragms, users with latex allergy (graded as a relative contraindication '3'). Women with a history of toxic shock syndrome should also avoid the sponge and diaphragm ('3'). All other conditions are graded '1' or '2'.

Table 1.3   Chief side effects and dangers, and risks of death of selected family planning methods

Method	Side effects	Serious dangers	Risk of death
Spermicides	Reproductive and urinary tract infections, allergy (causes itching)	None	None measurable
Cervical cap, diaphragm, sponge	Reproductive and urinary tract infections	Toxic shock syndrome	None measurable
Condoms (male latex)	None	Anaphylactic reaction	None measurable
Oral contraceptives (combined)	Nausea, weight gain, dizziness, spotting, breast tenderness, chloasma, decreased libido	Cardiovascular complications, depression, hepatic adenomas, possible increased risk of breast and cervical cancers	Non-smokers aged <35: 1/200 000; non-smokers aged 35+: 1/28 600; heavy smokers <35: 1/5 300; heavy smokers 35+: 1/700
Oral contraceptives (progestogen-only)	Headaches, irregular bleeding, androgenic effects		None measurable
Emergency contraception (Hormonal)	Nausea, vomiting, headaches, breast tenderness	None	None measurable
Abortion (mifepristone-PG in first 9 weeks LMP)	Bleeding, pain, gastrointestinal side effects	Hemorrhage, retained tissue	None measurable
Abortion (surgical)	Pain, bleeding	Anaesthesia complications, uterine perforation, cervical/uterine trauma, infection	<9 weeks: 1/262 800; 9–12 weeks: 1/100 000; 13–15 weeks: 1/34 000; 15+ weeks: 1/10 200
Injectables	Cycle changes, weight gain, headaches, changes in lipid profile, breast tenderness	Depression, allergic reaction, possible bone loss	None measurable
IUD (copper)	Increased menstrual cramping, spotting and bleeding	PID following insertion, uterine perforation, iron deficiency anemia	1:10 000 000
Implants	Tenderness at implant site, cycle changes, alopecia, weight gain, breast tenderness	Infection at implant site, depression, removal complications	None measurable
Female sterilization	Pain at incision site, possible regret that method is permanent	Infection at surgical site, anaesthesia complications, ectopic pregnancy	Laparoscopic tubal ligation: 1/38 500; hysterectomy: 1/1600
Male sterilization	Pain at incision site, possible regret that method is permanent	Infection at surgical site, anaesthesia complications	Vasectomy: 1/1 000 000

LMP, Last menstrual period; PID, pelvic inflammatory disease.
Sources: Medical Economics Company 1999; World Health Organization 1996; other chapters in this book.

A summary of the contraindications (graded '1' to '4') for the most popular hormonal methods and for the copper IUD appears in the Appendix to this chapter. Contraindications for sterilization appear in Chapter 7.

NON-CONTRACEPTIVE BENEFITS

Modern users of contraceptives want more from their methods than just safe and effective contraceptive protection. In one recent study from the USA (Grady et al 1999), for instance, male users, describing the factors important to them in choosing a method of family planning, rated protection from STIs as highly as they did contraceptive protection. Other contraceptive users may be attracted to the help with acne, or the reduction in dysmenorrhoea, offered by certain oral contraceptive formulations. For this reason, family planning providers should be familiar with the non-contraceptive benefits associated with several of the family planning methods. Although, these are covered in detail in the chapters relevant to each individual method, the few most important are covered briefly here.

Protection against sexually transmitted infections

As described more fully in Chapter 13, protection from STIs in the context of family planning is chiefly a function of physical barriers. The male and female condoms, designed to prevent the greatest amount of skin-to-skin contact, offer the best protection. Partial barriers, including the diaphragm and cervical cap, may confer some protection, particularly for the cervical infections chlamydia and gonorrhoea. Chemical barriers of the future (often called 'microbicides') have such protection as an overt goal, and several possibilities are now entering advanced clinical testing. But, in the meantime, nonoxynol-9 spermicides appear to offer limited (perhaps 25%) protection from certain bacterial STIs (Louv et al 1988, Niruthisard et al 1992).

The important point to stress with clients is that while the risk of pregnancy is concentrated during certain times of the menstrual cycle, the risk of transmitting or acquiring an STI is present at all times. In addition, depending on the pathogen, the likelihood of transmission during a single act of unprotected intercourse can far exceed the likelihood of pregnancy during a single act, even at a time in the cycle when the woman is most at risk of pregnancy.

Menstrual disorders and bleeding control

Some hormonal contraceptives can reduce menstrual bleeding, and can help to alleviate the discomfort and inconvenience of irregular or painful periods. For women on honeymoon, women who travel frequently, women who compete in athletic competitions, or women who want, for any other reason, to time their bleeds precisely, combined oral contraceptives can be used continuously (discarding the placebos) during the days the woman does not wish to bleed.

Other non-contraceptive benefits

Several family planning methods offer non-contraceptive benefits, ranging from delays in premature ejaculation (male condoms) to protection against pelvic inflammatory disease (PID) and even certain cancers (several of the hormonal methods) to improvements in acne (oral contraceptives).

USER CONSIDERATIONS

Family planning has advanced farther than perhaps any branch of medicine in user autonomy and responsibility for decision-making. Methods of contraception are relatively safe and effective and the users are typically healthy and expected to use contraception for decades. Information is needed to choose and is typically straightforward. The law and policy governing access to contraception is well developed in the UK. Family planning healthcare providers are able to act as resource persons for information, and to offer counselling, where welcomed, to help the user reach an informed choice. In the equality of this partnership, family planning is a model area of medicine.

Measuring user attitudes

Discontinuation rates. It is difficult to summarize information about the user's role and how well users accept the roles. One indirect measure frequently employed is the discontinuation rate. This measure shows the number of users, from a standardized starting cohort of 100, who have stopped using a method at a certain period in time, typically after 1 year of use. Methods that demand a great deal of the users, or impose a lot on them in terms of the side effects that must be tolerated, tend to have higher discontinuation rates than methods that require little, all other things being equal. Table 1.4 shows the 1-year discontinuation rates associated with the main methods of family planning. Obviously, male and female sterilization has zero discontinuation rates at 1 year. The barrier methods tend to have the highest discontinuation rates, with some 60% of spermicide-users and nearly as many cap-users giving up the method after 1 year. Periodic abstinence also has high discontinuation rates, with nearly 40% stopping after 12 months. About 30% of pill-users discontinue after 12 months. The IUDs tend to have around 20% discontinuation after 1 year, often because of bleeding pattern disturbances that users dislike.

One criticism of the discontinuation rate as a measure is that it fails to reflect that people often choose specific methods for short periods of time

Table 1.4 1-year method-related discontinuation rates of selected family planning methods (reproduced with permission from Hatcher RA, Trussell J, Stewart F et al 1998)

Method	% of users discontinuing use at 1 year[1]
Spermicides	60
Periodic abstinence	37
Calendar	
Ovulation method	
Symptothermal	
Post-ovulation	
Cap	
Parous women	58
Nulliparous women	44
Sponge	
Parous women	58
Nulliparous women	44
Diaphragm	44
Condoms	
Female (Reality)	44
Male	39
Oral contraceptives	29
Progestogen-only	
Combined	
IUD	
Progesterone T	19
Copper T 380A	22
LNg 20	19
Injectable (depot medroxyprogesterone acetate)	30
Implants (Norplant and Norplant-2)	12
Female sterilization	0
Male sterilization	0

[1] Among users attempting to avoid pregnancy.

and use them happily during this time, but with no plans for long-term use. For instance, users might opt for condoms in the first 3 months of a new relationship, but then switch to oral contraceptives if the relationship appears to stabilize into a mutually monogamous one. Similarly, methods typically used by young people have higher discontinuation rates than those preferred by older users. Younger users are more likely to give up contraceptive methods because they stop sexual activity for a while, or because they want to conceive, whereas older users may specifically pick long-acting methods and use them over the long term because their need is for this type of protection.

Other measures of user satisfaction. At least in the clinical trial literature, several measures of user satisfaction are common. These include a user's willingness to use the method again (e.g. in the case of medical abortion methods), and willingness to recommend the method to others. Many studies also inquire directly about satisfaction, asking users to rate the method overall (either numerically or qualitatively) and to rate their satisfaction with specific features of the method (e.g. interference with sexual pleasure, partner's reaction).

Assessing the user's needs

Helping a woman to determine her contraceptive needs and then to find a contraceptive strategy that meets them will make her feel in control of her sexuality and reproductive health generally. As discussed earlier, in family planning, relative to nearly every other area of medicine, the role and responsibility of the user is uniquely important. It is critical that women and men who seek contraceptive advice and assistance feel that the family planning choices they have made are their own.

It is difficult even to generalize about what users want, or even the criteria they consider important. As noted earlier, age, or life stage, is a major determinant of the kinds of factors they will consider. A new study from the USA (Grady et al 1999) also shows that what men and women want can be quite different. In this study, women ranked effectiveness in pregnancy prevention as the single most important factor in selecting a family planning method, with 90% citing it as 'very important'. The health risks of a particular method and its efficacy at preventing STIs were rated the second most important consideration, with each being rated by 77% of women surveyed as 'very important'. Men, however, said that STI prevention was just as important as pregnancy prevention; the two features were mentioned as 'very important' by 84% and 86%, respectively. Women were more interested than men in the ease of use of a method and the need to plan ahead, while men were more concerned with the method's interference with sexual pleasure. Specifically, women reported more favourable perceptions of the pill, and were more likely than men to rate the pill as 'very good' at preventing pregnancy (75% vs 67%). At the same time, women reported generally less favourable perceptions than men about other reversible methods, including the condom. Women were less likely than men to consider the condom very good at preventing pregnancy (29% vs 45%).

In working through a family planning counselling session, Box 1.1 may be helpful. It presents a summary checklist of factors to discuss. There are many factors to consider. These may be grouped into factors related to back-up options the woman is willing to use, factors related to her interaction with the healthcare system, factors related to her sexual lifestyle and factors related to her future fertility plans.

Back-up options

The strength of a user's desire to avoid pregnancy is a critical factor in determining the methods that are right for her. But if she is open to back-up

Box 1.1 Checklist of user considerations

	Implications
Attitude towards back-up options	
✓ Attitude towards abortion	If willing to consider as a back-up, opens a wider range of choices for creating a highly effective family planning strategy.
✓ Attitude towards emergency contraception	Emergency contraception back-up, even without abortion as a safety net, widens options for creating a highly effective strategy involving methods with important collateral benefits, such as sexually transmissible infection protection.
Interaction with the healthcare system	
✓ Regular access to a clinic	Methods that require frequent clinic visits may be inconvenient for busy women, or those with unpredictable schedules.
✓ Provider's role	Provider's personal concerns can influence method selection.
Sexual lifestyle	
✓ Frequency of actions required	Some methods require daily action regardless of sexual frequency; others require action at the time of sex; others require initial or intermittent action only.
✓ Privacy	Particularly for younger users, or others whose sexual activity may not be socially sanctioned, discreet methods may be critical. Methods using bulky commodities, involving storage or disposal problems, are more vulnerable to discovery.
✓ Partner's role	Users may desire or may reject methods that involve a large role for the partner. Many methods can be used in ways that make family planning mutual, although in the UK, women typically bear the majority of the responsibility.
✓ Frequency of intercourse	If intercourse is very infrequent, users may prefer methods that they use only at the time of coitus.
Future fertility	
✓ Wish for future fertility	Some of the most effective methods (male and female sterilization) are only for users who do not wish for any pregnancies in future.
✓ Desired timing of future fertility	Methods have varying standard time horizons, and if a woman plans to conceive soon, her planning would differ from a woman who plans to conceive in 10 years or more.
Cost	
✓ Out-of-pocket costs	Methods impose different cost structures on the user. Time, travel and item costs are all factors.

methods, her choices for creating a highly effective family planning strategy will be greater.

Abortion. Given the length of time that most women in the UK will use contraception, a huge proportion of them will likely experience at least one contraceptive failure. For instance, the woman who starts pill use at age 16, and continues until she is 30, faces a risk of more than 50% that her method will fail (during this 14-year span, if her annual failure rate is 5%, her cumulative risk of pregnancy is $[1.0 - (1.0 - 0.05)^{14}]$ or 51.2%). Even perfect users of most contraceptive methods can expect one or more failures during their lifetimes. For example, the 1-year perfect-use failure rate of the diaphragm is 6%. If we assume for the sake of simplicity that for a given user, this rate stays constant over time, then after 12 years of use (say age 17 to 29), a woman is more likely than not (52.4%) to have experienced a failure. Many women will choose to resolve their unplanned pregnancies by abortion. Modern methods of medical and surgical abortion are exceptionally safe and easy to use, and it is critical that family planning providers do not stigmatize this choice. If a woman is open to using abortion as a back-up, she may also be willing to consider some of the slightly less effective but otherwise very appealing family planning methods available offering non-contraceptive benefits, such as protection from HIV, that may be life-saving in a global context.

Emergency contraception. Even for those women who would not consider using abortion as a back-up method, but who are otherwise highly motivated to prevent pregnancy, emergency contraception (see Ch. 8) can dramatically lower (by around 75% or more) the risk of pregnancy after certain types of contraceptive accidents. If a woman is willing to use emergency contraception as part of her family planning strategy, her choices about a primary method may be wider than if she would not consider this back-up option and still is highly motivated to avoid pregnancy.

Interaction with the healthcare system

Convenience, autonomy, provider attitudes, and (outside the UK) cost, all affect a user's perception of her interaction with the healthcare system. Some methods of contraception require more frequent or intense interaction, while others can be used without setting foot in a clinic.

Regular access to a clinic. The woman who lives in a remote area or who travels extensively may opt for methods that do not require her to consult her family planning provider on a regular basis. For instance, injectable methods (whether monthly or 3-monthly) could pose problems for women with extensive travel responsibilities. Such women might prefer methods that are readily available over the counter, even if greater out-of-pocket costs are involved.

Provider's role. In the case of many methods, the provider has only a one-time role. In the case of others, the provider needs to see the user in person several times each year (monthly or quarterly injectables are not currently marketed for self-administration and therefore require frequent clinic visits by the user). If the user travels extensively, or has pressing work or childcare responsibilities, the prospect of making regular and frequent clinic visits may be daunting. The provider can also influence the method selection process if he or she is biased against one or more methods or is unprofessional enough to put his or her convenience and/or budgetary concerns before the user's needs.

Cost to the user. Given that family planning is free to National Health Service (NHS) users, some relatively inexpensive methods that involve items sold directly in pharmacies (e.g. condoms) may end up costing more to the user than would intrinsically more expensive methods obtained directly from government family planning clinics.

Sexual lifestyle

A user's sexual patterns are an important determinant of the methods that would be suitable for her during a given phase in her reproductive life.

Frequency of actions required. Some users may want a method that requires little or no action on their part. 'Birth control you think about just four times a year' is the slogan for depot medroxyprogesterone acetate (DMPA) 3-monthly injections in the USA. At one extreme are the sterilization methods, the implants and the IUDs. Once action to start use is taken, the user can essentially forget about contraception for at least several years. At the other extreme are the 'coitus-dependent' methods, such as withdrawal, diaphragms, condoms or spermicides, that require action on the user's part with each act of intercourse. Also at this end of the spectrum are the methods that require daily action, such as oral contraception or certain forms of fertility awareness that require daily temperature-taking, or cervical mucus evaluation and charting. Progestogen-only pills require that the pills be taken within a very narrow time interval each day. Some users prefer routine daily actions to those that may be required less often but that can interrupt sexual spontaneity. Other users, particularly if they are sexually active only infrequently, may prefer methods that require action only when needed. A user's daily schedule and ability to stick to a routine are of paramount importance in evaluating her needs along this dimension. If she travels frequently and unexpectedly, has stressful and unpredictable deadlines, or is generally not a creature of habit, then methods requiring strict adherence to a daily regimen might be less desirable.

Partner cooperation. Methods range widely in the role that each member of the couple is required to play. For some methods, such as sterilization, IUD or implants, one of the partners bears the entire responsibility. For others, such as periodic abstinence or withdrawal, both must be willing to co-operate. For some, token responsibility can be shared. For example, a male partner can prepare or insert a diaphragm for a woman, or can even take the placebo pills in her oral contraceptive cycle. A woman can roll the condom onto a man's penis. In choosing a method, the user should consider the role she wants and can reasonably expect her partner to play. If both partners are very committed and cooperative, the range of options is wider than if one partner has strict limitations.

Privacy. Family planning users may attribute the utmost importance to several privacy considerations. In particular, younger women or women who are engaging in sexual relationships that might not be socially sanctioned for them may feel strongly that they need discreet methods. One consideration is storage and disposal of contraceptives. Oral contraceptives, condoms or spermicides kept in a purse or drawer, or thrown in the household rubbish, may be more vulnerable to discovery than injectable methods or IUDs. Another consideration is telltale changes in bleeding patterns, although there are so many causes for cycle disturbance that most changes entailed by contraceptive or abortifacient methods would be unlikely to arouse comment or suspicion.

Frequency of intercourse. The user who engages only seldom in sexual activity may be less interested in methods, such as oral contraceptives, that require daily action. If a mutually monogamous couple is separated during long periods of time, for instance because of labour migration, methods such as period abstinence that may interfere with sexual activity during the short intervals when it is possible for the couple may be undesirable.

Plans for future fertility

It is essential to determine whether and when a user plans to become pregnant in future. Many methods are advisable or cost-effective only if the woman does not have immediate plans to become pregnant. For instance, a woman seeking to conceive within the next few months would be a poor candidate for an implant or an IUD (other things being equal), and certainly any woman who plans on retaining the option of becoming pregnant should not consider sterilization. With the exception of the injectable methods, however, all other methods are considered to offer an immediate return to fertility once use is halted. For norethisterone enanthate (NET-EN) injectables, return to fertility occurs within 6 months of the last injection, and for DMPA, return occurs within 10 months after the last injection (World Health Organization 1996).

COSTS

The cost of a family planning strategy is properly measured by including the cost of the method itself, the costs of the woman's and provider's time, as well as all other indirect costs, including travel to the clinic for visits. Such studies are extremely complicated to undertake, and so are rare. Family planning methods also vary tremendously in the ways in which the costs to the user and provider are spread out over time. In the UK, all methods of contraception, except male and female condoms and Persona are free to the user, who can therefore ignore the costs of the method. Male and female condoms are provided free by most family planning clinics (FPC) but not by general practitioners. The provider, whether general practitioner or FPC, however, is increasingly aware of the cost of contraceptive methods. Indeed, the availability of the newer methods, particularly those with high, one-time up-front costs such as implants or the Levonorgestrel intrauterine system (LNG-IUS) is said to be limited in some parts of the UK because of the price. Although the cost per year of effective contraception provided can be quite low if these methods are used over many years, most NHS drug budgets are set annually and do not make provision for long-term investments.

Another important aspect to cost, at least from the perspective of the NHS or of society as a whole, is the cost of the unintended pregnancies and side effects that result from contraceptive failure. For instance, a year of contraceptive protection using the cervical cap may seem to cost less (counting only the cost of the method) than a year of contraceptive protection from a hormone-releasing IUD. But if the far higher failure rates of the cap and the subsequent costs of the births or abortions are added in, the picture changes. All things considered, the copper IUD is probably the most cost-effective method available.

As a practical matter, however, the clinic manager may be most interested in the accounting costs charged for various contraceptive methods. Some family planning methods, such as vasectomy, abortion under local anaesthetic, and the cervical mucus method of fertility awareness, are cheap (or even free), since most of the cost of the method consists of time and skill. Table 1.5 shows the price of family planning supplies sold to the NHS as of October 1999.

CONCLUSION

Never in history have so many options for planning and regulating fertility been so widely available. The majority are also safer than ever before, as new and improved methods emerge, and better knowledge about how to reduce risks with older methods accumulates. Family planning is also a model area of medicine in terms of advances in user autonomy and responsibility. The challenge for future years will be to develop still better and more

Table 1.5   Price to the National Health Service for selected contraceptive commodities, October 1999

	Unit sold	Months of contraceptive protection	Cost
Oral contraceptives – combined			
Low-dose ethinyloestradiol (≤ 35 µg)			
Cilest	3 × 21	3	£6.42
Microgynon 30	3 × 21	3	£2.13
Loestrin 20	3 × 21	3	£2.58
Mercilon	3 × 21	3	£8.57
Marvelon	3 × 21	3	£7.02
Minulet	3 × 21	3	£5.70
High-dose ethinyloestradiol (50 µg)			
Ovran	3 × 21	1	£1.23
Norinyl-1	3 × 21	3	£1.83
Oral contraceptives – progestogen-only			
Femulen	3 × 28	3	£2.76
Micronor	3 × 28	3	£1.89
Noriday	3 × 28	3	£1.75
Physical barrier methods			
Avanti (polyurethane male condom)*	2	–	£3.49
Durex (latex male condom)*	12	–	£7.69
Femidom (female condom)*	3	–	£4.49
Dumas (cervical cap)	1	12	£5.87
Reflexions (diaphragm)	1	12	£5.49
IUDs			
Nova-T (copper IUD)	1	60	£9.90
Mirena (levonorgestrel IUD)	1	60	£99.25
Gynefix (frameless copper IUD)	1	60	£24.79
Multiload (copper IUD)	1	60	£9.19
Spermicides			
Delfen (foam)	20 g	2	£4.65
Durex Duragel (jelly)	100 g	2	£3.28
Injectables			
Depot medroxyprogesterone acetate	1 mL	3	£4.55
Implants			
Implanon	1	36	£90.00
Natural family planning			
Persona*	Monitor	–	£64.95
	Dipsticks	1	£9.99

* Not available on NHS, typical price from local pharmacist.

diverse methods, and to help users combine the existing methods to build strategies that meet their needs over the decades of use that characterize modern family planning users. Particularly important in this regard will be to reduce the stigma and bias associated with emergency contraception and abortion, just as cultural obstacles to oral contraceptive use, and indeed the barrier methods, were fought earlier last century.

REFERENCES

Forrest JD 1993 Timing of reproductive life stages. Obstetrics and Gynecology 82(1): 105–111
Grady WR, Klepinger DH, Nelson-Wally A 1999 Contraceptive characteristics: The perceptions and priorities of men and women. Family Planning Perspectives 31(4): 168–175
Hatcher RA, Trussell J, Stewart F, et al 1998 Contraceptive Technology, 17th revised edn. Ardent Media, New York
Louv WC, Austin H, Alexander WJ, Stagno S, Cheeks J 1988 A clinical trial of nonoxynol-9 for preventing gonococcal and chlamydial infections. Journal of Infectious Diseases 158(3): 518–523
Medical Economics Company 1999 PDR Physicians' Desk Reference, 53rd edn. Medical Economics Company, Montvale NJ
Niruthisard S, Roddy RE, Chutivongse S 1992 Use of nonoxynol-9 and reduction in rate of gonococcal and chlamydial cervical infections. Lancet 339: 1371–1375
Oddens BJ, Visser AP, Vemer HM, Everaerd WTAM, Lehert P 1994 Contraceptive use and attitudes in Great Britain. Contraception 49(1): 73–86
Pearl R 1932 Contraception and fertility in 2000 women. Human Biology 4: 363–407
Piccinino LJ, Mosher WD 1998 Trends in contraceptive use in the United States: 1982–1995. Family Planning Perspectives 30(1): 4–10, 46
Segal SJ 1993 Trends in population and contraception. Annals of Medicine 25: 51–56
Shah IH 1994 The advance of the contraceptive revolution. World Health Statistics Quarterly 47(1): 9–15
Trussell J, Kost K 1987 Contraceptive failure in the United States: A critical review of the literature. Studies in Family Planning 18(5): 237–283
Wilcox AJ, Baird DD, Weinberg CR 1999 Time of implantation of the conceptus and loss of pregnancy. New England Journal of Medicine 340 (23): 1796–1799
World Health Organization 1996 Improving access to quality care in family planning: Medical eligibility criteria for contraceptive use. World Health Organization, Geneva

Appendix 1
Medical eligibility criteria, according to the World Health Organization, for initiating and continuing selected family planning methods.
Summary tables

Table A1 Medical eligibility criteria, according to the World Health Organization, for initiating and continuing selected family planning methods (reproduced with permission from World Health Organization 2000 *Improving Access to Quality Care in Family Planning*. World Health Organization, Geneva)

Condition	Combined oral	Combined injectable	Progestogen only oral	NET-EN DMPA	Norplant Implants	Copper IUD	LNG
PERSONAL CHARACTERISTICS AND REPRODUCTIVE HISTORY							
PREGNANCY	NA	NA	NA	NA	NA	NA	NA
AGE	Menarche to <40=1 ≥40=2	Menarche to <40=1 ≥40=2	Menarche to 17=1 18–45=1 >45=1	Menarche to 17=2 18–45=1 >45=2	Menarche to 17=1 18–45=1 >45=1	<20=2 ≥20=1	<20=2 ≥20=1
PARITY							
a) Nulliparous	1	1	1	1	1	2	2
b) Parous	1	1	1	1	1	1	1
BREASTFEEDING							
a) <6 weeks postpartum	4	4	3	3	3		
b) 6 weeks to 6 months (primarily breastfeeding)	3	3	1	1	1		
c) ≥ 6 months postpartum	2	2	1	1	1		
POSTPARTUM (in non-breast-feeding women)							
a) 21 days	3	3	1	1	1		
b) ≥ 21 days	1	1	1	1	1		
POSTPARTUM (breastfeeding or non-breast-feeding) including post-caesarian section							
a) <48 hours						2	3
b) 48 hours to 4 weeks						3	3
c) ≥ 4 weeks						1	1[a]
d) Puerperal sepsis						4	4

Condition	Combined oral	Combined injectable	Progestogen only oral	NET-EN DMPA	Norplant Implants	Copper IUD	LNG
POST-ABORTION							
a) First trimester	1	1	1	1	1	1	1
b) Second trimester	1	1	1	1	1	2	2
c) Immediate post-septic abortion	1	1	1	1	1	4	4
PAST ECTOPIC PREGNANCY	1	1	2	1	1	1	1
HISTORY OF PELVIC SURGERY (see also postpartum section including caesarean section)	1	1	1	1	1	1	1
SMOKING							
a) Age <35	2	2	1	1	1	1	1
b) Age ≥ 35							
<15 cigarettes/day	3	2	1	1	1	1	1
≥15 cigarettes/day	4	3	1	1	1	1	1
OBESITY							
≥ 30 kg/m² body mass index (BMI)	2	2	1	2	2	1	2
ANATOMICAL ABNORMALITIES							
a) That distort the uterine cavity						4	4
b) That do not distort the uterine cavity						2	2
BLOOD PRESSURE MEASUREMENT UNAVAILABLE	NA	NA	NA	NA	NA	NA	NA
CARDIOVASCULAR DISEASE							
MULTIPLE RISK FACTORS FOR ARTERIAL CARDIOVASCULAR DISEASE (such as older age, smoking, diabetes and hypertension)	3/4	3/4	2	3	2	1	2
HYPERTENSION							
a) History of hypertension where blood pressure CANNOT be evaluated (including hypertension in pregnancy)	I 3 | C 3	3	3	2	2	2	1	2
b) Adequately controlled hypertension, where blood pressure CAN be evaluated	3	3	1	2	1	1	1
c) Elevated blood pressure levels (properly taken measurements)	I | C						
(i) Systolic 140–159 or diastolic 90–99	3[b] | 3[b]	3	1	2	1	1	1
(ii) Systolic ≥ 160 or diastolic ≥ 100	4 | 4	4	2	3	2	1	2
d) Vascular disease	4 | 4	4	2	3	2	1	2
HISTORY OF HIGH BLOOD PRESSURE DURING PREGNANCY (where current blood pressure is measurable and normal)	2	2	1	1	1	1	1
DEEP VENOUS THROMBOSIS (DVT)/PULMONARY EMBOLISM (PE)							
a) History of DVT/PE	4	4	2	2	2	1	2

	1	2	3	4	5	6	7
b) Current DVT/PE	4	4	3	3	3	1	3
c) Family history (first-degree relatives)	2	2	1	1	1	1	1
d) Major surgery							
With prolonged immobilization	4	4	2	2	2	1	2
Without prolonged immobilization	2	2	1	1	1	1	1
e) Minor surgery without immobilization	1	1	1	1	1	1	1
SUPERFICIAL VENOUS THROMBOSIS							
a) Varicose veins	1	1	1	1	1	1	1
b) Superficial thrombophlebitis	2	2	1	1	1	1	1
CURRENT AND HISTORY OF ISCHEMIC HEART DISEASE	4	4	I 2 | C 3	3	I 2 | C 3	1	I 2 | C 3
STROKE (history of cerebrovascular accident)	4	4	I 2 | C 3	3	I 2 | C 3	1	2
KNOWN HYPERLIPIDAEMIAS (screening is NOT necessary for safe use of contraceptive methods)	2/3c	2/3c	2	2	2	1	2
VALVULAR HEART DISEASE							
a) Uncomplicated	2	2	1	1	1	1	1
b) Complicated (pulmonary hypertension, atrial fibrillation, history of sub-acute bacterial endocarditis)	4	4	1	1	1	2	2

NEUROLOGIC CONDITIONS

	I | C	I | C	I | C	I | C	I | C		I | C
HEADACHES							
a) Non migrainous *Mild or severe*	1 | 2	1 | 2	1 | 1	1 | 1	1 | 1	1	1 | 1
b) Migraine *Without focal neurologic symptoms*							
Age <35	2 | 3	2 | 3	1 | 2	2 | 2	2 | 2	1	2 | 2
Age ≥35	3 | 4	3 | 4	1 | 2	2 | 2	2 | 2	1	2 | 2
With focal neurologic symptoms	4 | 4	4 | 4	2 | 3	2 | 3	2 | 3	1	2 | 3
EPILEPSY	1	1	1	1	1	1	1

REPRODUCTIVE TRACT INFECTIONS AND DISORDERS

			I | C	I | C	I | C		I | C
VAGINAL BLEEDING PATTERNS							
a) Irregular pattern *without* heavy bleeding	1	1	2 | 2	2 | 2	2 | 2	1	1 | 1
b) *With* heavy or prolonged bleeding (includes regular patterns)	1	1	2 | 2d	2 | 2d	2 | 2d	2d	1 | 2d

	I | C	I | C	I | C	I | C	I | C	I | C	I | C
UNEXPLAINED VAGINAL BLEEDING (suspicious for serious condition) Before evaluation	2 | 2	2 | 2	2 | 2	3 | 3	3 | 3	4 | 2	4 | 2

	1	2	3	4	5	6	7
ENDOMETRIOSIS	1	1	1	1	1	2	1
BENIGN OVARIAN TUMOURS (including cysts)	1	1	1	1	1	1	1
SEVERE DYSMENORRHOEA	1	1	1	1	1	2	1
TROPHOBLAST DISEASE							
a) Benign gestational trophoblastic disease	1	1	1	1	1	3	3

Condition	Combined oral	Combined injectable	Progestogen only oral	NET-EN DMPA	Norplant Implants	Copper IUD	LNG
b) Malignant gestational trophoblastic disease	1	1	1	1	1	4	4
CERVICAL ECTROPION	1	1	1	1	1	1	1
CERVICAL INTRAEPITHELIAL NEOPLASIA (CIN)	2	2	1	2	2	1	2
CERVICAL CANCER (awaiting treatment)	2	2	1	2	2	I:4 / C:2	I:4 / C:2
BREAST DISEASE							
a) Undiagnosed mass	2	2	2	2	2	1	2
b) Benign breast disease	1	1	1	1	1	1	1
c) Family history of cancer	1	1	1	1	1	1	1
d) Cancer							
Current	4	4	I:4 / C:4	4	4	1	I:4 / C:4
Past and no evidence of current disease for five years	3	3	3	3	3	1	3
ENDOMETRIAL CANCER	1	1	1	1	1	I:4 / C:2	I:4 / C:2
OVARIAN CANCER	1	1	1	1	1	I:3 / C:2	I:3 / C:2
UTERINE FIBROIDS							
a) Without distortion of the uterine cavity	1	1	1	1	1	2	2
b) With distortion of the uterine cavity	1	1	1	1	1	4	4
PELVIC INFLAMMATORY DISEASE (PID) OR PID RISK							
a) Past PID (assuming no current risk factors of STIs)							
With subsequent pregnancy after past PID	1	1	1	1	1	I:1 / C:1	I:1 / C:1
Without subsequent pregnancy	1	1	1	1	1	I:2 / C:2	I:2 / C:2
b) PID-current or within the last 3 months	1	1	1	1	1	I:4 / C:3	I:4 / C:3
STIs[e]							
a) Current or within 3 months (including purulent cervicitis)	1	1	1	1	1	4	4
b) Vaginitis without purulent cervicitis	1	1	1	1	1	2	2
c) Increased risk of STIs (e.g. multiple partners or partner who has multiple partners)	1	1	1	1	1	3	3
HIV/AIDS[e]							
HIGH RISK OF HIV	1	1	1	1	1	3	3
HIV-POSITIVE	1	1	1	1	1	3	3
AIDS	1	1	1	1	1	3	3

OTHER INFECTIONS

SCHISTOSOMIASIS							
a) Uncomplicated	1	1	1	1	1	1	1
b) Fibrosis of the liver	1	1	1	1	1	1	1

						I	C	I	C
TUBERCULOSIS									
a) Non-pelvic	1	1	1	1	1	1	1	1	1
b) Known pelvic	1	1	1	1	1	4	3	4	3
MALARIA	1	1	1	1	1	1			1

ENDOCRINE CONDITIONS

DIABETES							
a) History of gestational disease	1	1	1	1	1	1	1
b) Non-vascular disease							
Non-insulin dependent	2	2	2	2	2	1	2
Insulin dependent	2	2	2	2	2	1	2
c) Nephropathy/retinopathy/ neuropathy	3/4	3/4	2	3	2	1	2
d) Other vascular disease or diabetes of > 20 years' duration	3/4	3/4	2	3	2	1	2
THYROID							
a) Simple goitre	1	1	1	1	1	1	1
b) Hyperthyroid	1	1	1	1	1	1	1
c) Hypothyroid	1	1	1	1	1	1	1

GASTROINTESTINAL CONDITIONS

GALL BLADDER DISEASE							
a) Symptomatic							
Treated by cholecystectomy	2	2	2	2	2	1	2
Medically treated	3	2	2	2	2	1	2
Current	3	2	2	2	2	1	2
b) Asymptomatic	2	2	2	2	2	1	2
HISTORY OF CHOLESTASIS							
a) Pregnancy-related	2	2	1	1	1	1	1
b) Past COC-related	3	2	2	2	2	1	2
VIRAL HEPATITIS							
a) Active	4	3/4	3	3	3	1	3
c) Carrier	1	1	1	1	1	1	1
CIRRHOSIS							
a) Mild (compensated)	3	2	2	2	2	1	2
b) Severe (decompensated)	4	3	3	3	3	1	3
LIVER TUMOURS							
a) Benign (adenoma)	4	3	3	3	3	1	3
b) Malignant (hepatoma)	4	3/4	3	3	3	1	3

ANAEMIAS

THALASSAEMIA	1	1	1	1	1	2	1
SICKLE CELL DISEASE	2	2	1	1	1	2	1
IRON DEFICIENCY ANAEMIA	1	1	1	1	1	2	1

DRUG INTERACTIONS

COMMONLY USED DRUGS WHICH AFFECT LIVER ENZYMES							
a) certain antibiotics (rifampicin and griseofulvin)	3	3	3	2	3	1	1
b) certain anticonvulsants (phenytoin, carbamezapine, barbiturates, primadone)	3	3	3	2	3	1	1

Condition	Combined oral	Combined injectable	Progestogen only oral	NET-EN DMPA	Norplant Implants	Copper IUD	LNG
OTHER ANTIBIOTICS (excluding rifampicin and griseofulvin)	1	1	1	1	1	1	1

a If the woman is breast-feeding, LNG-IUD becomes a category 3 until 6 weeks postpartum.
b If blood pressure can be monitored periodically, then this situation is a category 2; if not, then it is a category 3.
c Depending on severity of condition.
d This is a category 3 if anaemia is noted clinically. Also, unusually heavy bleeding should raise the suspicion of a serious underlying condition.
e Barrier methods, especially condoms, are always recommended for prevention of STI/HIV/PID.

Key to abbreviations

NET-EN, norethisterone enanthate; DMPA, depot medroxy progesterone acetate; IUD, intrauterine device; LNG, Levonorgestrel; STI, sexually transmitted infection; I, initiation; C, continuation; NA, not applicable.

Classification categories

The suitability of different contraceptive methods were categorized in the presence of specific illnesses or conditions. The categorization was achieved by weighing the health risks and benefits of using a particular contraceptive method when any of these conditions are present:
1. A condition for which there is no restriction for the use of the contraceptive method.
2. A condition where the advantages of using the method generally outweigh the theoretical or proven risks.
3. A condition where the theoretical or proven risks usually outweigh the advantages of using the method.
4. A condition which represents an unacceptable health risk if the contraceptive method is used.
The classification also includes the medical criteria for the *initiation* and *continuation* of use for all methods. Only those instances where the criteria for continuation of a method differed from criteria for initiating the method are included.

2

Combined oral contraception

John Guillebaud

Preparations   30
  Oestrogens   30
  Progestogens   31
  Monophasic pills   31
  Biphasic pills   33
  Triphasic pills   33
Mode of action   34
Practical prescribing   34
Effectiveness   34
Indications   35
  Contraception   35
  Medical conditions   35
Contraindications   36
  Absolute contraindications   36
  Relative contraindications   38
  Intercurrent disease   39
Advantages   41
Disadvantages   41
  Metabolic effects   42
  Cardiovascular system   42
Clinical management   46
  History   46
  Examination   47
  Choice of combined oral
    contraception   47

Practical prescribing since
  April 1999   48
Drug interaction   55
Manipulation of the menstrual
  cycle   56
Follow-up   57
Indications for stopping COC   58
Complications and their
  management   58
  'Minor' side effects   59
  Cardiovascular system   59
  Respiratory system   60
  Central nervous system   60
  Gastrointestinal system   63
  Urinary system   65
  Genital system   65
  Breasts   68
  Musculoskeletal system   70
  Cutaneous system   71
  Infections and inflammations   72
Reversibility   72
Outcome of pregnancy   73
  Exposure during pregnancy   73
Breaks in pill-taking   73
Risks/benefits   73

In 1921, Haberlandt was the first scientist to speculate that extracts from the ovaries and placenta of pregnant animals might be used for fertility control. In 1937, Kurzrok noted that ovulation was inhibited during treatment for dysmenorrhoea with ovarian oestrone, and suggested that this hormone might be of value in contraception. It was only in the 1950s, when potent orally active progestogens (first norethynodrel and then norethisterone) became available, that an oral contraceptive pill became possible. The research chemists chiefly responsible were Russell Marker, who first produced progesterone from diosgenin extracted from the *Dioscorea* plant, George Rosenkranz, Carl Djerassi and Frank Colton (Djerassi 1979).

Encouraged by Mrs Margaret Sanger and Mrs Page McCormick, Gregory Pincus started a screening programme of contraceptive steroids in animals. With Michael Chang and John Rock, Pincus developed the first oral contraceptive pill and reported the first trials in humans in Puerto Rico with Drs Rice-Wray and Garcia in January 1957.

The first pills were thought to contain only progestogen and gave good cycle control. When purified preparations were tried, however, cycle control deteriorated. The impurity had been mestranol, and when this oestrogen was restored to the tablets, the combined pill Enovid (norethynodrel plus mestranol) was created.

Combined oral contraception (COC) was approved for use in America in 1959, and in Britain 2 years later. For several years, its use appeared to be associated with only minor side effects which were acceptable to most women in return for its high effectiveness. Cardiovascular problems, related to the dose of oestrogen, and attributed primarily to venous or arterial thrombosis, first came to light in 1969. Later, some of the earlier synthetic progestogens were thought to be linked to the risk of arterial wall disease, primarily in smokers. Concerns about cancer and COC have intermittently arisen, with some unexpected good news as well as the (always exaggerated) bad. In 1995, a major 'pill-scare' in the UK was precipitated when studies indicated that third-generation progestogens were linked to an increased risk of venous thromboembolism.

The non-contraceptive benefits of COC have taken longer to be established and have always received far less public attention.

Over 200 million women throughout the world have taken the pill since it first became available, and about 65–70 million are current users. In developed countries outside Japan where COC was only finally licensed in 1999, 15–40% of women of reproductive age use it for contraception, rising to 75% of those aged 20 to 30 years. In the UK, it remains one of the most popular methods of fertility control, used by about 3 million women.

PREPARATIONS

COC contains two steroid hormones, oestrogen and a progestogen (a synthetic progesterone). Over the years, the composition of COC has changed markedly. The total dose of steroid has been reduced, the oestrogen by up to a factor of ten, the progestogen by up to twenty. Mestranol has largely been replaced by the more potent ethinyloestradiol (EE). Natural oestrogens, though possibly associated with less thrombotic risk, have so far proved incapable of adequate cycle control or reliable inhibition of ovulation when taken orally.

Oestrogens

Most modern COC contains EE. This affects coagulation factors in such a way as to promote both arterial and venous thrombosis. These changes are dose-dependent. Thus COC in the UK does not contain more than 50 µg of oestrogen and the usual dose is in the 20–35 µg range.

Progestogens

Those in current use are all derivatives of 19-nortestosterone and are, by convention, divided into two groups:

1. Second-generation progestogens: norethisterone (NET); norethisterone acetate; ethynodiol diacetate (both pro-drugs for norethisterone) and levonorgestrel (LNG).
2. Third-generation progestogens: desogestrel (DSG) and gestodene (GSD). Norgestimate has similarities to these but is also metabolized in part to LNG, which makes it difficult to categorize. Cyproterone acetate (as in Dianette) is a progestogenic anti-androgen, making Dianette the most 'oestrogenic' product available. DSG and GSD differ from the second-generation progestogens in that they:
   a. Have a higher affinity for (bind more strongly to) the progesterone receptor thus increasing their effectiveness at inhibiting ovulation and giving good cycle control with low doses
   b. Have a lower affinity for (bind less strongly to) androgen receptors
   c. Appear at a biochemical and somatic level to be less 'anti-oestrogenic'. *Specifically*, COC containing third-generation progestogens produce fewer effects on carbohydrate and lipid metabolism than the earlier formulations. High-density lipoprotein (particularly HDL_2-C) concentrations are increased while low-density lipoproteins (LDL-C) and insulin concentrations are decreased compared with COC containing second-generation progestogens.

These metabolic differences were expected, prior to 1995, to be associated with a reduction in the risk of arterial wall disease and hypertension. As yet, however, there is little epidemiological evidence that third-generation progestogens do confer these clinical advantages over the older, cheaper preparations – and there is no additional benefit for risk of acute myocardial infarction if the woman has no arterial risk factors (Dunn et al 1999).

Currently, there are 18 different combined oral contraceptive formulations available and they are listed in Table 2.1. They can be divided into three groups: monophasic, biphasic and triphasic.

Monophasic pills

Preparations containing 20–35 µg of EE are the most widely used. Only two preparations now contain 50 µg of oestrogen. Of the pills containing 20 µg of

Table 2.1 Currently available preparations of combined oral contraception (UK) (reproduced with the kind permission of MIMS)

Pill type	Preparation	Oestrogen (µg)	Progestogen (mg)	
Monophasic				
Ethinyloestradiol/				
norethisterone type	Loestrin 20	20	1	norethisterone acetate*
	Loestrin 30	30	1.5	norethisterone acetate*
	Brevinor	35	0.5	norethisterone
	Ovysmen	35	0.5	norethisterone
	Norimin	35	1	norethisterone
Ethinyloestradiol/				
levonorgestrel	Microgynon			
	(also ED)	30	0.15	
	Ovranette	30	0.15	
	Eugynon	30	0.25	
	Ovran 30	30	0.25	
	Ovran	50	0.25	
Ethinyloestradiol/				
desogestrel	Mercilon	20	0.15	
	Marvelon	30	0.15	
Ethinyloestradiol/				
gestodene	Femodene (also ED)	30	0.075	
	Femodette	20	0.075	
	Minulet	30	0.075	
Ethinyloestradiol/				
norgestimate	Cilest	35	0.25	
Mestranol/				
norethisterone	Norinyl-1	50	1	
	Ortho-Novin 1/50	50	1	
Biphasic and Triphasic				
Ethinyloestradiol/				
norethisterone	BiNovum	35	0.5	(7 tabs)
		35	1	(14 tabs)
	Synphase	35	0.5	(7 tabs)
		35	1	(9 tabs)
		35	0.5	(5 tabs)
	TriNovum (also ED)	35	0.5	(7 tabs)
		35	0.5	(7 tabs)
		35	1	(7 tabs)
Ethinyloestradiol/				
levonorgestrel	Logynon (also ED)	30	0.05	(6 tabs)
		40	0.075	(5 tabs)
		30	0.125	(10 tabs)
	Trinordiol	30	0.05	(6 tabs)
		40	0.075	(5 tabs)
		30	0.125	(10 tabs)
Ethinyloestradiol/				
gestodene	Tri-Minulet	30	0.05	(6 tabs)
		40	0.07	(5 tabs)
		30	0.1	(10 tabs)
	Triadene	30	0.05	(6 tabs)
		40	0.07	(5 tabs)
		30	0.1	(10 tabs)

**New products
awaited**

Monophasic Ethinyloestradiol/ levonorgestrel	Microgynon 20	20	0.1	
Biphasic Ethinyloestradiol/ desogestrel	Gracial	40	0.025	(7 tabs)
		30	0.125	(15 tabs)

* Converted (> 90%) to norethisterone as the active metabolite.
ED, everyday pills.

oestrogen, Loestrin 20 gives less good cycle control. 15 µg COC preparations containing GSD or LNG are marketed in continental Europe, although they are not yet available in the UK.

Biphasic pills

These are not widely prescribed and there is only one preparation in current use. Gracial (Table 2.1) is a 22-day product already available in some overseas markets, designed to be more 'oestrogenic' during the first 7 days in order to improve cycle control. Having been delayed by the 1995 'pill-scare', it is reportedly due for UK marketing in due course. It appears to be a useful option for women with troublesome breakthrough bleeding (BTB) as well as acne.

Triphasic pills

The triphasic regimen was designed to reduce the total dose of steroids over 21 days, while at the same time mimicking the characteristic fluctuations in oestrogen and progesterone which occur during the menstrual cycle. Although a more normal-looking endometrium develops histologically, there is no good evidence of better cycle control over long-term use (i.e. beyond 6 months). Moreover, while the LNG triphasics do expose the user to a lower total dose of steroids, the newer ones (Tri-Minulet and Triadene) do not as compared with the monophasic alternatives.

Phasic preparations are useful options for early cycle control or as second choices when BTB does not settle. They give a more reliable withdrawal bleed in women unhappy about absent or very scanty withdrawal bleeds. However, they are more complicated to use with respect to advice about missed pills or postponing withdrawal bleeds. They are also expensive for the health service when prescribed by general practitioners as each phase attracts a separate dispensing fee.

MODE OF ACTION

Hormonal contraceptives act both centrally and peripherally by:

1. Inhibition of ovulation – the oestrogen component inhibits pituitary follicle stimulating hormone (FSH) secretion thereby suppressing follicle growth while the progestogen mainly inhibits the luteinizing hormone (LH) surge preventing ovulation.
2. Alteration in cervical mucus – it becomes scanty, viscous and cellular with low spinnbarkeit (stretchiness), thus impairing sperm transport and penetration. This type of cervical mucus is produced by COC at all doses and provides an additional contraceptive action if breakthrough ovulation does occur.
3. Alteration of the endometrium – an atrophic endometrium, unreceptive to implantation, is produced with microtubular glands and a fibroblastic condensation of the stroma. With prolonged COC use, the endometrium becomes progressively thin and atrophic. Development of the vasculature is reduced and less of the uterotonic and vasoactive prostaglandins are produced which explains the scanty, less painful withdrawal bleeding in COC-users.
4. Possible direct effects on the fallopian tubes impairing sperm migration and ovum transport are of doubtful importance.

PRACTICAL PRESCRIBING

Although COC is easy to use, can provide maximum protection from pregnancy, and has many beneficial effects, it is neither suitable for, nor acceptable to, all couples. In the UK, almost 95% of sexually active women under 30 have used it for at least a few months.

Anxiety about adverse effects and possible long-term consequences makes it necessary for all those who prescribe COC to:

1. Form their own opinions based on scrutiny of published work.
2. Keep regularly updated.
3. Prescribe carefully after discussing anxieties, risks and benefits.
4. Reassure women when appropriate, but leave the final decision to them.
5. Supervise follow-up conscientiously.

EFFECTIVENESS

Provided COC is taken correctly and consistently, is absorbed normally, and its metabolism is not increased by interaction with other medication, its reliability is nearly 100%. In practice, the failure rate is 0.2–3 per 100 woman years, or higher, depending mainly on the population studied.

Many more errors in tablet-taking occur than are reported. Detailed questioning – particularly whether any pills might have been missed or not absorbed just before, or just after, the pill-free interval (PFI) – nearly always reveals the reason for any unexpected pregnancy.

Careful teaching of the woman (and sometimes her partner), accompanied by written information, is essential for effective use.

INDICATIONS

Contraception

COC is indicated for young women where maximum protection from pregnancy is required, with menstrual benefits and ready reversibility and where the woman wishes to use a method independent of intercourse.

It is particularly valuable, and associated with lowest circulatory risk and fewest adverse side effects, in healthy young women who do not smoke and who are sufficiently motivated to use it reliably.

Medical conditions

COC is commonly used in the treatment of the following predominantly gynaecological conditions (see Chs. 15, 16 and 17), whether or not contraception is also required:

1. Dysmenorrhoea.
2. Menorrhagia.
3. Premenstrual syndrome (tricycling a monophasic pill is particularly useful).
4. Endometriosis (again, a continuous regimen such as tricycling is usually preferred).
5. To control severe ovulation pain or functional ovarian cysts.
6. Polycystic ovarian syndrome (PCOS): to control the main symptoms.
7. Hypo-oestrogenic amenorrhoea in young women, as a convenient form of oestrogen replacement with contraception.
8. Acne/seborrhoea/hirsutism (using a DSG or GSD product, or Dianette to control more troublesome cases).
9. As hormone replacement therapy in young women with a premature menopause.
10. As prevention, e.g. after a previous ectopic pregnancy. COC is also usable where there is a strong predisposition to/family history of carcinoma of the ovary – or of rheumatoid arthritis (where preventive benefit seems likely to be real).

Notes

a. If the treatment is being used largely to ablate/suppress symptoms of the woman's usual cycle, as in 1–5 above, monophasic are preferable to phasic pills to avoid cyclical fluctuations in hormone levels.
b. In all cases, the additional *therapeutic* benefits may allow use of COC where risks might argue against its use in a standard contraceptive situation. An example might be the use of Marvelon or Dianette to treat PCOS with severe acne in a woman with a body mass index (BMI) above 30 and aged over 35.

CONTRAINDICATIONS

The WHO scheme for classifying contraindications to contraception is a useful recent addition and is outlined in more detail in Chapter 1. It is due for review in 2000 and its application below relates to evidence-based judgement. The useful new feature of the classification is the separation into two categories of relative contraindications.
The four WHO categories as they relate to COC are:

- *WHO* 1 is a condition for which there is no restriction to the use of COC.
- *WHO* 2 is when the advantages of the method generally outweigh the theoretical or proven risks.
- *WHO* 3 is when the theoretical or proven risks usually outweigh the advantages but the method can be used with caution and additional care as 'a method of last choice'.
- *WHO* 4 is a condition which represents an unacceptable health risk and COC should not be used.

Absolute contraindications (WHO 4)

1. Past or present circulatory disease:
    a. Any proven past arterial or venous thrombosis
    b. Ischaemic heart disease, including angina, and cardiomyopathies
    c. Severe or combined risk factors for venous or arterial disease (see Tables 2.2 and 2.3, pp 48 and 49 and also p. 40)
    d. Migraine (pp 61–62) preceded by focal aura; or which is exceptionally severe; or requires ergotamine treatment
    e. Transient ischaemic attacks even without headache
    f. Atherogenic lipid disorders, e.g. cholesterol above 8 mmol/L (COC may be cautiously prescribed if the lipid abnormality is controlled on treatment, following specialist advice.)
    g. Known prothrombotic abnormality of coagulation or fibrinolysis including:
        (i) the inherited thrombophilias

    (ii)   acquired thrombophilias: development of antiphospholipid antibodies such as the lupus anticoagulant; and following splenectomy for any indication if the subsequent platelet count is above $500\,000 \times 10^9/L$

h. Other conditions predisposing to thrombosis including:
    (i)   blood dyscrasias
    (ii)   autoimmune disorders with this risk such as polyarteritis nodosa, scleroderma and severe systemic lupus erythematosus (SLE)
    (iii)   Klippel–Trenaunay syndrome
    (iv)   severe primary or secondary polycythaemia
    (v)   elective major or leg surgery (see below)
    (vi)   during leg immobilization
    (vii)   before and after all varicose vein treatments (medical or surgical) (p. 58)
    (viii)   travel to above 4500 m, which is associated with raised blood viscosity owing to haemoconcentration in the short term (Guillebaud 1998)
    (ix)   severe inflammatory bowel disease during exacerbations (Crohn's disease and ulcerative colitis). In addition, Crohn's disease is sometimes apparently induced by COC (p. 64) and if this is the case, future COC use would be an absolute contraindication

  i. Past cerebral haemorrhage (exceptionally COC may be permitted after successful surgery following a subarachnoid haemorrhage), or cerebral venous thrombosis

  j. Vascular malformations of the brain

  k. Significant structural heart disease, including all known persistent septal defects and complex valve pathology, because of the risk of systemic emboli in the presence of arrhythmias or shunts (Lechat et al 1988). Minor/uncomplicated valve pathology including mitral valve prolapse or after successful surgery: these are WHO 2.

  l. Pulmonary hypertension.

2. Diseases of the liver:
  a. Active liver disease (i.e. currently abnormal liver function tests; infiltrations and severe cirrhosis); past cholestatic jaundice if causally linked with COC (a history of this in pregnancy is WHO 3); Dubin–Johnson or Rotor syndrome. COC can be prescribed after viral hepatitis once liver function tests have returned to normal for at least 3 months
  b. Liver adenoma or carcinoma
  c. Gallstones (although COC used after cholecystectomy is WHO 3)
  d. The acute hepatic porphyrias.

3. History of a serious condition known to be affected by sex-steroids or by previous COC use. This is not necessarily a complete list of examples in the categories given:
   a. Chorea
   b. COC-induced hypertension
   c. Past acute pancreatitis (if linked with hypertriglyceridaemia)
   d. Pemphigoid gestationis (formerly termed herpes gestationis)
   e. Haemolytic uraemic syndrome or thrombotic thrombocytopaenic purpura
   f. Otosclerosis – some authorities permit closely supervised COC use
   g. Stevens–Johnson syndrome (erythema multiforme) if COC-associated
   h. Trophoblastic disease until human chorionic gonadotrophin (hCG) levels are undetectable (p. **67**)
   i. Most cases of SLE – also because of thrombotic risk.
4. Pregnancy.
5. Undiagnosed genital tract bleeding.
6. Oestrogen-dependent neoplasms, e.g. breast cancer. (Selected women in prolonged remission may very occasionally be allowed to take COC, i.e. WHO 3.)
7. If a woman's anxiety about COC safety is not relieved by counselling.

Relative contraindications (WHO 2 and 3)

1. Risk factors for venous disease (see Table 2.2, p. **48**) and arterial disease (see Table 2.3, p. **49**). These are usually WHO 2, provided, normally, that only one is present, and that it is not serious enough to make it an absolute contraindication. In the case of blood pressure (BP), WHO assigns BP in the range 140–159 mmHg systolic and 90–99 mmHg diastolic to category 3 (although in UK practice 95 mmHg diastolic is the usual upper limit).
2. Sex-steroid-dependent cancer. The specialist's advice should be sought. A history of breast cancer is almost invariably considered an absolute contraindication. Breast biopsy showing premalignant epithelial atypia is usually WHO 4.
   Expert opinion is that malignant melanoma, after successful treatment, is no longer a contraindication to starting or continuing with COC.
3. Amenorrhoea or oligomenorrhoea should be investigated but COC may subsequently be prescribed (Ch. 15), and is often positively beneficial (WHO 1).
4. Hyperprolactinaemia is now considered only a relative contraindication for patients under specialist supervision (WHO 2).
5. Very severe depression (WHO 2).
6. Chronic systemic diseases – see below. Crohn's disease is WHO 2 if not COC-induced and not currently severe.

7. Diseases requiring long-term treatment with drugs which might interact with COC (pp **54–56**) (WHO 2).
8. Conditions which impair absorption of COC, such as some operations for obesity. Coeliac disease is *not* a problem, since there is reduced gut wall metabolism leading to improved EE absorption.

Intercurrent disease

There are some conditions in which COC is absolutely contraindicated, but others which are benefited or, at least, unaffected. Persistent myths about conditions such as uncomplicated varicose veins or thrush have often led to women being unnecessarily deprived of COC.

Most medical conditions can be grouped into broad categories:

1. Disorders in which COC is *not known* to have any effect (WHO 2, or even 1 in some cases). Women can be reassured that there is no evidence that COC can affect the progression of the disease itself.

   Lack of conclusive evidence that there is not a problem makes most of them WHO 2; examples only, listed in alphabetical order:

   Asthma (but see p. **60**)

   Carcinoma of the colon
   (indeed a possibility of reduced risk in COC-users, Franceschi and La Vecchia 1998, making this WHO 1)

   Gilbert's disease (WHO 1)

   Hodgkin's disease

   Multiple sclerosis

   Myasthenia gravis

   Neuroblastoma

   Raynaud's syndrome (primary, if no suspicion that it is secondary to arterial disease)

   Renal dialysis (but HDL-C is lowered in some chronic renal disorders)

   Retinitis pigmentosa

   Rheumatoid arthritis

   Sarcoidosis

   Spherocytosis

   Thyrotoxicosis

   Thalassaemia major.

   Note also. Most cancers in current remission are not affected by COC provided hormone-dependency is not suspected and the thrombotic risk is not increased (as it may be in advanced malignancy). COC use should be discussed with the woman's specialist.

2. Disorders of varying degrees of seriousness in which the COC *might have* the potential to interact in a harmful way (mainly WHO 4, sometimes 3).

For many diseases, data are not available or are contradictory. COC is absolutely contraindicated (WHO 4) if the disorder significantly:

a. Increases the risk of arterial or venous thrombosis
b. Predisposes to arterial wall disease
c. Adversely affects liver function
d. Shows a tendency to sex-steroid hormone dependency (e.g. deterioration with previous administration of COC or during pregnancy).

In some cases, the added risks of pregnancy in women with the condition, or the likelihood of deterioration of the disease in pregnancy, may justify COC use and make the disorder only a relative contraindication (i.e. WHO 3): primarily because COC is so effective. Separate therapeutic benefits (e.g. control of heavy or painful menses in someone physically disabled) may also favourably alter the benefit/risk difference (see p. **36**).

3. Conditions treated with drugs which may interact with COC (pp **54–56**) (WHO 2).

For further discussion of contraception and disease, the reader is referred to the excellent chapter with that title in the book by Sapire (1990).

Sickle cell disorders

Sickle cell trait is not a contraindication to COC use although the frank homozygous sickling disease (SS and SC genes) has traditionally been regarded as an absolute contraindication. Both sickle cell disease and COC independently lead to an increased risk of thrombosis, which may be exacerbated during the arterial stasis of a sickling crisis. However, more recent studies suggest that sickle cell disease should be considered only a relative contraindication (WHO 2), especially when the benefits of COC as a very effective contraceptive are balanced against the serious risks of pregnancy. Until this has been confirmed, the injectable depot medroxyprogesterone acetate (DMPA) is considered an even better choice (p. **82**).

Diabetes mellitus

It is well established that COC may decrease glucose tolerance and cause a rise in insulin levels in healthy non-diabetic women. However, COC does not increase the risk of developing clinical diabetes.

Less is known about the effects of COC on existing diabetes. Traditionally, diabetic women have been advised against using COC. However, low-dose COC (DSG/GSD-containing varieties being usually preferred) may certainly be used (WHO 2) in the short term by young non-smoking women in whom diabetic control is good and who neither have other risk factors nor any signs of the complications of the disease (see Table 2.3, p. **49**). If any of the latter provisos are untrue (e.g. *any* diabetic who also smokes), however, the situation changes from WHO 2 straight to WHO 4.

ADVANTAGES

1. Reliable, reversible, convenient method which is independent of intercourse.
2. Periods become more regular. Blood loss is reduced, decreasing the incidence of iron deficiency anaemia.
3. Menstrual and premenstrual symptoms such as dysmenorrhoea and premenstrual tension are often relieved.
4. Ovulation pain is abolished.
5. Unlike most other commonly used drugs, there is no acute toxicity as a result of overdose except withdrawal bleeding (even in prepubertal girls), and vomiting.
6. Decreased incidence while on treatment of:
   a. Benign breast disease
   b. Functional overian cysts
   c. Pelvic inflammatory disease (PID)
   d. Ectopic pregnancy since ovulation is inhibited and PID risk reduced
   e. Seborrhoeic conditions including acne
   f. Endometriosis.
7. Protection against carcinoma of the ovary and endometrium. Numerous studies have shown a reduction in the risk of both ovarian cancer and of endometrial cancer (Vessey 1989). The effect is related to the duration of use and provides a two- to three-fold reduction in the risk of both conditions after 5 years. The protective effect persists for at least 15 years after the pill is stopped.
8. Other possible benefits have been identified in more than one study but have yet to be fully confirmed. These include protection against rheumatoid arthritis, thyroid disease, duodenal ulcer, trichomonal vaginitis and toxic shock syndrome.

DISADVANTAGES

It is hardly surprising that a combination of steroids that proves so effective in controlling reproduction also affects other physiological systems. The safety issue has mainly related to the EE content, since this potent oestrogen with a long half-life is unquestionably prothrombotic. More than 95% of women on the pill now use brands containing only 20–35 μg of oestrogen and 15 μg doses are awaited. With improved assessment and monitoring, this should reduce the already low rate of serious adverse effects.

Clinical experience suggests that modern low-dose preparations are also less likely to cause the so-called 'minor' side effects such as nausea and weight gain.

Metabolic effects

These are numerous and varied. Many are similar to those found in normal pregnancy. Although this may be reassuring, it should be remembered that pregnancy has its own hazards, often not unlike those of COC.

If laboratory investigations are requested in a pill-taker, COC use should be mentioned as it alters many results, e.g. the serum binding of circulating hormones.

The liver

Contraceptive steroids are metabolized by the liver and affect hepatic function. The resultant effects on the metabolism of carbohydrates, lipids, plasma proteins, amino acids, vitamins, enzymes and the factors concerned with coagulation and fibrinolysis explain the majority of adverse effects. Non-oral routes of administration which avoid the first pass of a high-peak dose through the liver are likely to be preferred for the future. Increase in appetite and weight gain, in part the result of fluid retention, which occurs in a small proportion of COC-users must also have a metabolic basis, not as yet fully understood.

Cardiovascular system

The incidence of the conditions discussed below is increased in users of COC. (See Gupta and Harding 1999 and Dunn et al 1999 for further discussion on this major topic.)

Venous disease

This includes: deep venous thrombosis with or without pulmonary embolism, hereafter called venous thromboembolism (VTE); and thrombosis in other veins, e.g. mesenteric, hepatic or retinal.

Influence of oestrogen dose. EE causes an alternation in clotting factor levels, tending to promote coagulation, and also modifies platelet function. There is some evidence of compensatory increased fibrinolytic activity that may partly explain the rarity of overt disease in most COC-users. The pro-thrombotic effects are less marked in COC containing 50 μg of oestrogen or less but they still increase the relative risk of VTE by three- to four-fold compared with women not taking the COC. The evidence does not yet support any further risk reduction with reduced doses below the 50 μg level (WHO

1998). There is no effect of past use (indeed, restoration of clotting factor changes has been shown by 4 weeks).

Possible influence of the progestogen type. In 1995, the Committee on Safety of Medicines (CSM) in the UK alerted all doctors to the findings from a number of studies, unpublished at the time, which demonstrated a differential risk of VTE depending on the type of progestogen in combined pills. COC which contained either GSD or DSG was shown to have a roughly two-fold increased risk of VTE when compared with COC containing first- or second-generation progestogens. As a result, restrictions were placed on the use of COC containing GSD/DSG in the UK, Germany and Norway, although in other countries no regulatory action was taken.

The risk of VTE with all COC is smaller than that associated with pregnancy; which has been estimated at 60 cases per 100 000 pregnancies. The spontaneous incidence of VTE in healthy non-pregnant women (not taking any oral contraception) is about 5 cases per 100 000 women per year. The incidence in users of older second-generation COC is about 15 per 100 000 women per year of use and the incidence in users of GSD/DSG containing COC is about 25 cases per 100 000 women per year of use. The level of all of these risks of VTE increases with age and is likely to increase in women with other known risk factors for VTE such as obesity.

This differential effect on VTE may result from the balance between oestrogens and the newer less androgenic progestogens which antagonize EE less than their predecessors. At the present time, the small excess incidence of VTE with GSD/DSG preparations cannot satisfactorily be explained by bias or confounding and there are some laboratory data demonstrating a differential effect on coagulation tests with COC containing LNG compared with GSD/DSG.

Using the rates given above and assuming an estimated 1–2% mortality for VTE, there is only a 1–2 per million difference in annual VTE mortality between DSG/GSD-containing COC and second-generation COC. In 1999, the CSM in the UK issued a revised statement to the effect that provided women were fully informed of the very small difference in risk of VTE and did not have medical contraindications, then it should be a matter of clinical judgement and personal choice which type of oral contraceptive was prescribed. The practical implication of this statement is that all marketed products are now usable as first line with fully informed verbal consent.

Predisposing factors (in the woman). Hypertension and duration of COC use do not increase the risk of VTE. The risks are enhanced by the factors highlighted in Table 2.2 (p. **48**), particularly:

- marked obesity
- immobility
- tissue damage (including recent major or leg surgery)
- increasing age

- congenital thrombophilias; a predisposition to thrombosis makes an overt event more probable if COCs are used. Examples include deficiency of:
  - —protein C
  - —protein S
  - —antithrombin III
  - —activated protein C. This is due to a gene abnormality named factor V Leiden (Vandenbroucke et al 1994) and around 3–5% of Caucasians are heterozygous for this: meaning an eight-fold increased risk of VTE, rising to 30-fold if the woman also takes COC.

Screening all COC-users for activated protein C deficiency, the commonest predisposition, is not justifiable. Out of every 2 million women screened, 95% would be negative and the current test is complex and costly.

Targeted screening is appropriate, however. A family history of known thrombophilia, or of a thrombotic event (usually venous but occasionally arterial), occurring in a first-degree relative (sibling or parent) under 45, is a valid indication for full investigation. A positive result normally absolutely contraindicates COC (see Table 2.2, p. **48**). With a negative result, the family history would remain a relative contraindication because the woman might still have inherited one of the undiagnosable predispositions.

Acquired predispositions (p. 37), once found, usually in connective tissue disorders and most often after a VTE event, always absolutely contraindicate COC.

Arterial disease

This category includes myocardial infarction (MI), thrombotic stroke, haemorrhagic stroke including subarachnoid haemorrhage, and other arterial events such as thrombosis of mesenteric or retinal arteries.

Myocardial infarction. To quote from the WHO's Scientific Group (WHO 1998):

- The incidence of fatal and non-fatal MI is extremely low in women of reproductive age. Women who do not smoke, who have their BP checked and who do not have hypertension or diabetes, are at no increased risk of MI if they use COC, regardless of their age. (*Note*. In every recent study, this disease has effectively not been reported in a COC-user unless she also smoked or had another arterial risk factor; and importantly, regardless of COC-formulation.)
- There is no increase in the relative risk of MI with increasing duration of use nor through past use of COC.
- The relative risk of MI in current users of COC with hypertension is at least *three times* that in current users without hypertension.
- The increased absolute risk of MI in women who smoke is greatly elevated by use of COC. The relative risk of MI in heavy smokers

who use COC may be as high as *10 times* that in smokers who do not use COC.

- Although the incidence of MI increases exponentially with age, the relative risk of MI in current users of COC does not change with increasing age.
- The suggestion that users of low-dose COC containing GSD/DSG may have a lower risk of MI than users of low-dose formulations containing LNG remains to be substantiated. (*Note.* The most recent study known as the MICA study confirms this statement (Dunn et al 1999) although the Transnational study referenced in the Dunn paper did show a statistically significant relative effect.)

Ischaemic stroke. The same WHO Scientific Group concluded that:

- Ischaemic stroke is very rare in women of reproductive age.
- Among women who do not smoke, who have their BP checked, and who do not have hypertension, the risk of ischaemic stroke is increased about 1.5-fold in current users of low-dose COC compared with non-users.
- There is no detectable effect of increasing duration of use nor of past use of COC.
- The relative risk of ischaemic stroke in current users of COC with hypertension appears to be at least three times that in current users without hypertension.
- The absolute risk of ischaemic stroke in women who smoke is about 1.5–2 times that in non-smokers; this risk is multiplied by a factor of 2–3 if such women are also current COC-users.
- The risk of ischaemic stroke increases with higher oestrogen doses.
- There are insufficient data to assess any effect of type or dose of progestogen.
  (*Note.* Migraine as a risk factor for ischaemic stroke was not evaluated by WHO. It is believed that careful prescribing (pp **61–62**) in relation to migraine headaches and focal neurological symptoms should further reduce the risk of this extremely serious complication, but more data are required.)

Haemorrhagic stroke. The WHO Scientific Group concluded that:

- Haemorrhagic stroke is very rare in women of reproductive age.
- In women aged less than 35 years, who do not smoke, and who do not have hypertension, the relative risk in COC-users is not increased.
- There is no increase in the risk with increasing duration of use nor from past use.
- The relative risk of haemorrhagic stroke in current COC-users with hypertension may be 10 times that in current users without hypertension.

- The risk of haemorrhagic stroke in women who smoke is up to twice that in non-smokers; in women who are current users of COC and who smoke, the relative risk is about 3.
- The incidence of haemorrhagic stroke increases with age, and current use of COC appears to magnify this effect of ageing.

Mortality

There are highly reassuring data available from the Royal College of General Practitioners (RCGP) oral contraception study that 10 years after use of COC ceases, mortality in past users is indistinguishable from that in never-users (Beral et al 1999). The effects of COC on mortality occur mainly in current and recent users and few, if any, effects persist thereafter. Within the study, current and recent COC-users had a significantly decreased risk of death from ovarian cancer (relative risk 0.2) although they had an increased risk of death from both cervical cancer (relative risk 2.5) and stroke (relative risk 1.9).

CLINICAL MANAGEMENT

Current scientific evidence suggests there are only two essential prerequisites for the safe prescribing of COC (Hannaford and Webb 1996):

- A careful personal and family history with particular attention to cardiovascular risk factors.
- An accurate measurement of BP.

Suitability for COC is based on history and physical examination. The concerns of each individual should be discussed, raising the issues relating to circulatory disease and cancer at the appropriate time, even if the woman does not mention them herself.

History

Take a full medical and personal history. Pay particular attention to those conditions which might contraindicate COC use, and the importance for this individual of avoiding pregnancy, including:

1. Past or current illnesses, which might represent possible contraindications.
2. Obstetric history, full menstrual history.
3. Headache or migraine: frequency, site, timing, severity, relation to menstrual cycle, initiating factors, therapy, presence of focal symptoms (pp **61–62**).
4. Current drug therapy.

5. Family history, especially of cardiovascular disease including thrombosis, hypertension, and of breast cancer.
6. Allergies.
7. Social factors, particularly those relating to the risk of sexually transmitted infections (STIs), including HIV and hepatitis B.

Examination

1. Observation on general health.
2. Measure BP.
3. Record baseline weight/height, hence BMI.
4. Although it may be reassuring to establish that the pelvic organs are normal, many women dislike pelvic examination and it is irrelevant to pill-taking. It should not be insisted on at the first visit provided the patient gives a normal menstrual history with a normal last menstrual period, indicating that she is not pregnant.
5. A cervical smear should be taken according to local screening protocols (Ch. 12). This is good preventive medicine, but again a recent smear is not an essential prerequisite for use of the pill or indeed any other method of contraception.
6. Breast examination – a baseline examination is unhelpful unless the woman has any symptom or desires a check-up. Give instruction in breast awareness supplemented with a leaflet.
7. Other investigations are also unnecessary unless suggested by the history. A first-degree relative with venous thrombosis or heart disease under age 45 normally indicates investigation for abnormalities of coagulation or of lipids.

Choice of combined oral contraception

The COC of first (or later) choice should be the one containing the lowest suitable dose of oestrogen and progestogen which:

1. Provides effective contraception.
2. Produces acceptable cycle control.
3. Is also associated with fewest side effects in that woman.

Each doctor needs to be familiar with the composition of a selection of COC. Women may react unpredictably, and several preparations may need to be tried before a suitable one is found. Some women are never suited. This is hardly surprising: individual variation in blood levels, and end-organ response (especially the endometrium), is well recognized (Guillebaud 1999). Thus it is a false expectation that any single COC will suit all women.

Practical prescribing since April 1999

VTE contributes relatively little to the number of COC deaths since mortality is relatively low (1–2%) compared with that from the arterial diseases. Long-term morbidity from non-fatal VTE is also low.

However it remains the most common serious cardiovascular event among young users of COC, so a careful history, prescribing and forewarning (backed by well-worded literature) are essential.

The risk factors for VTE and arterial disease must always be *separately* assessed (Tables 2.2 and 2.3). Thereafter:

- Multiple risk factors, or any one significant arterial or venous factor combined with age above 35 years, mean in general that all COC preparations should be avoided (WHO 4).
- All marketed COC may now be considered 'first line' (see p. **43**). Given the very small, not yet finally established, difference in VTE between the two 'generations', one needs a good reason not to comply with the woman's personal choice if, e.g., a particular preparation suited a friend or relative. The choice may be based on moderate acne or the need for better cycle control.
- In young first-time users, an LNG or NET product should probably remain the *usual* first choice since they will include an unknown subgroup who are predisposed to VTE; VTE is a more relevant consideration than arterial disease at this age. Furthermore, these are cheaper preparations.

Table 2.2 Risk factors for venous thromboembolism

Risk factor	Absolute contraindications	Relative contraindication
Family history (parent or sibling under 45)	Clotting abnormality or tests not done	Clotting factors done, normal
Overweight (high BMI)	BMI > 39	BMI 30–39
Immobility	Confined to bed	Wheelchair life
Varicose veins	Past thrombosis	Extensive varicose veins

Notes
1. A single risk factor in relative contraindication column indicates use of LNG/NET pill, if any COC used.
2. **N.B.** Synergism: more than one factor in the relative contraindication column means COC is absolutely contraindicated plus VTE risk rises with age.
3. The literature on the association of smoking with venous thromboembolic disease offers no consensus (compare arterial disease).
4. There are also important acute VTE risk factors which need to be considered in individual cases: notably long-haul flights and dehydration through any cause.
5. See also p. 37 re antiphospholipid antibodies (acquired thrombophilia).

BMI, body mass index; COC, combined oral contraception; LNG, Levonorgestrel; NET, norethisterone; VTE, venous thromboembolism

- Single risk factor for venous thrombosis: revised Summaries of Product Characteristics (SPC) say that DSG/GSD products are contraindicated. An LNG or NET product would be preferred, if COC is used at all.
- Single definite arterial risk factor such as smoking from the late 20s onwards, *or* if COC is used at all by a healthy and risk-factor-free woman above age 35: a change to the lowest possible dose DSG or GSD product should be discussed as an option, although the relative benefit for the arterial walls of these pills in these circumstances is not proven (see p. **45** and Guillebaud 1999). *The main reason for choosing these remains for the control of side effects.*

Table 2.3 Risk factors for arterial disease

Risk factor	Absolute contraindication	Relative contraindication	Remarks
Family history of arterial CVS disease in parent or sibling <45 years	Known atherogenic lipid profile – or tests not available	Normal blood lipid profile or first attack in relative > 45 years	POP is usually a better choice oral method if contraindications + consider LNG-IUS
Cigarette smoking	30+ cigarettes/day	5–30 cigarettes/day	
Diabetes mellitus	Severe or diabetic complications present (e.g. retinopathy, renal damage)	Not severe/labile, and no complications, young patient with short duration of DM	
Hypertension	BP >160/95 mmHg on repeated testing	BP140–159/90–95 mmHg	These levels are used in the UK (see p. **38**)
Overweight	BMI >39	BMI 30–39	
Migraine	Focal aura symptoms; severe or ergotamine-treated migraine	Migraine without focal aura, sumatriptan treatment	Relates to stroke risk. See pp **60–61**; also Box 2.1

Notes
1. Synergism: if more than one relative contraindication applies or if one only BUT woman now above age 35, in general do not use COC.
2. Smoking: the risk at a given age among smokers is not reached until 10 years later by non-smokers, implying that smoking 'ages the arteries'.
3. Note overweight appears in both Tables 2.2 and 2.3 – if that is the sole risk factor it indicates use of an LNG/NET pill (i.e. Table 2.2 takes precedence). Best choice Loestrin 20 or the new 20 μg EE + LNG pill when available.
4. Some of the numbers selected are arbitrary and perhaps too strict if they are the sole problem (e.g. the COC might actually be allowed, reluctantly, to a currently healthy 25-year-old admitting to two packs of cigarettes a day). They also relate to use for contraception. Use of COC for medical indications often entails a different risk/benefit analysis, i.e. the extra therapeutic benefits may outweigh expected extra risks.

BMI, body mass index; BP, blood pressure; COC, combined oral contraception; CVS, cardiovascular system; DM, diabetes mellitus; EE, ethinyloestradiol; LNG, levonorgestrel; LNG-IUS, levonorgestrel-releasing intrauterine system; NET, norethisterone.

The initial dose of oestrogen should normally be in the range 20–35 μg combined with a low, if not the lowest, dose of progestogen within each group (Table 2.1).

Special circumstances in which a 50 μg EE dose may be required include:

1. Long-term use of an enzyme-inducing drug (see Table 2.5, p. **54**).
2. Past 'true' COC failure, suggesting unusually rapid metabolism or malabsorption. Tricycling (pp **56–57**) to eliminate/shorten the pill-free interval is preferable and usually sufficient.
3. If a lower dose preparation cannot control the cycle after at least 3 months trial, provided no other cause for breakthrough bleeding is found (pp **65–66**).

And, finally:

- This prescribing protocol should be applied flexibly. Psychology in COC prescription may be as important as physiology.

Instructions to patients

Although the pills are dispensed in simple bubble packs, careful teaching and explanation are still essential.

- A user-friendly leaflet, such as the Family Planning Association's 'Choosing and Using COCs', which details symptoms requiring urgent medical advice, should always be given.
- The need for regular pill-taking at a time of day when it is easy to remember, such as when cleaning one's teeth in the morning or evening, must be stressed. Being late in taking pills can lead to BTB, which may then be prolonged over many days and can itself cause compliance problems leading to pregnancy.

Starting the pill

See Table 2.4 for a summary of starting routines.

- The first pill is usually taken on the first day of the next menstrual period. Day 5 starting has been shown to reduce the incidence of BTB in the first cycle.
- Contraceptive protection is immediate if COC is started on day 1. If delayed beyond the second day, there is a very small risk that a follicle will continue to develop, so additional contraceptive precautions are advised for the first 7 days of the first packet.
- The pill labelled for the appropriate day of the week is selected.
- One pill is taken daily for 21 (or 22 days) at approximately the same time.

Table 2.4 COC starting routines

	Start when?	Extra precautions for 7 days?
1. Menstruating	Day 3 or later in cycle Day 1 or 2	Yes (see text) No*
2. Postpartum a. no lactation b. lactation	Day 21 postpartum† Not normally recommended at all (POP or injectable preferred)	No
3. Therapeutic abortion/ miscarriage	Same day/day 2	No
4. Post-trophoblastic disease	1 month after no human chorionic gonadotrophin detected	As 1
5. Post-higher-dose COC	Instant switch	No (see text)
6. Post-lower or same-dose COC	After usual 7-day switch	No (see text)
7. Post-POP	First day of period	No
8. Post-POP or DMPA with secondary amenorrhoea/ following lactation when infant starts solid feeds	Any day, or after last packet of POP	No
9. Other secondary amenorrhoea (pregnancy excluded)	Any day	Yes
10. First cycle after emergency contraception	Day 1 or by day 2 when sure flow is normal	No

* Except in the case of ED pills, since the start-up routine often entails the taking of a variable number of placebos.
† Risk of puerperal CVS thrombosis then minimal except after very severe pregnancy-related hypertension – in which case, delay COC-use until biochemical normality confirmed.
COC, combined oral contraception; CVS, cardiovascular system; DMPA, depot medroxyprogesterone acetate; ED, everyday; POP, progestogen-only pill.

- After the packet is finished, no pills are taken for 7 days (or 6, or even 4 days as instructed for extra efficacy, p. **57**) then a new packet is started. It is important to explain to all COC-users that the start of the next packet must never be delayed (p. **52**).
- Everyday (ED) varieties contain seven placebo tablets which are taken during the 7 days that would otherwise be 'tablet-free'. With this regimen, the next packet of COC is started immediately after the last one is finished.

Postpartum. COC is contraindicated during breast-feeding (Ch. 6). Women who bottle-feed are usually advised to start at 3 weeks postpartum. This delay minimizes the risk of thromboembolism while initiating a reliable method of contraception before ovulation resumes.

After therapeutic abortion or miscarriage. COC should be started immediately (day 1 or 2), without extra precautions. Ovulation can occur within 2 weeks after a first trimester abortion (Ch. 11). COC will not interfere with recovery, nor increase morbidity.

Other starting routines are shown in Table 2.4.

Changing preparations

When changing from one COC to another one of lower dose, the following regimens may be used.

The first pill of the new packet is taken:

- **On the day immediately after the old packet is completed without a PFI**. This way no extra precautions are necessary. This is the preferred advice (Table 2.4).
  Or:
- **On the first day of withdrawal bleeding following completion of the last pack**. No additional precautions are required. Warn the woman that if withdrawal bleeding does not occur, she should not wait longer than 7 days before starting a new packet and should then follow the instructions below.
  Or:
- **After the usual 7 tablet-free days**. Additional precautions are then theoretically required for 7 days if the new pill has a lower dose of either oestrogen or progestogen, or if there is any doubt about its equivalence.

Management of missed pills: importance of the pill-free interval

It is now well established that many women on low-dose COC have a degree of restoration of ovarian function during the PFI shown not only by follicular activity on ultrasound but also by rising concentrations of both gonadotrophins and endogenous oestradiol.

It follows, therefore, that breakthrough ovulation is most likely to occur at the end of any PFI that is lengthened by missing pills either just prior to the 7-day break or immediately following it. 7 pill-free days are acceptable, but in some women anything longer will permit ovulation.

Data reviewed by Korver et al (1995) suggest that when pills have been missed, seven tablets are sufficient after recommencing to return the ovary to full quiescence. This is the basis for the routine advice to use added contraception for 7 days, as in Figure 2.1.

Vomiting, diarrhoea and short-term drug interactions

Similar advice is appropriate when the bio-availability of contraceptive steroids is temporarily reduced by vomiting within 2 hours of ingestion of

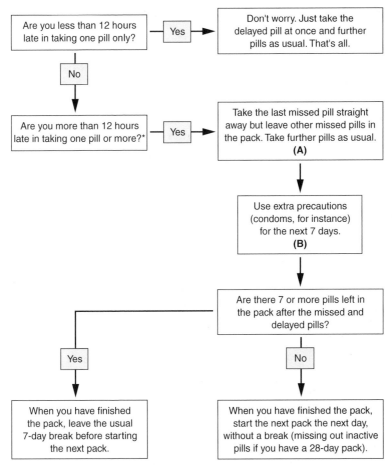

Are you less than 12 hours late in taking one pill only? — **Yes** → Don't worry. Just take the delayed pill at once and further pills as usual. That's all.

No

Are you more than 12 hours late in taking one pill or more?* — **Yes** → Take the last missed pill straight away but leave other missed pills in the pack. Take further pills as usual.
(A)

Use extra precautions (condoms, for instance) for the next 7 days.
(B)

Are there 7 or more pills left in the pack after the missed and delayed pills?

Yes

When you have finished the pack, leave the usual 7-day break before starting the next pack.

No

When you have finished the pack, start the next pack the next day, without a break (missing out inactive pills if you have a 28-day pack).

* If two or more pills are missed **and** they were all from the first 7 of your pack **and** you have had unprotected intercourse since the end of your last pack, talk to your doctor or nurse adviser. You may need emergency contraception **as well** as instructions **(A)** and **(B)** above.

Figure 2.1   Advice for missed pills (21-day packaging).

tablet(s), very severe diarrhoea, or during short-term use of interacting drugs (Table 2.5 and discussion below). 'Stomach upsets' have been shown to be particularly important in this context, accounting for up to 1 in 3 of conceptions occurring in otherwise compliant women.

Extra contraceptive precautions should start from the onset of the illness and continue for 7 days thereafter, with elimination of the PFI as indicated by the advice in Figure 2.1.

Table 2.5 The more important drug interactions with combined oral contraception

Class of drug names of	Approved important examples	Main action	Clinical implications for COC use
Drugs which may reduce COC efficacy			
Anticonvulsants	Barbiturates (esp. phenobarbitone) Phenytoin, Primidone Carbamazepine Topiramate	Induction of liver enzymes increasing their ability to metabolize both COC steroids	Preferably tricycling with shortened PFI. 50 µg oestrogen COC can be used, increasing to 90 µg if BTB occurs. Sodium valproate, clonazepam, vigabactrin and lamotrigine are not enzyme inducers
Antibiotics			
a. antitubercle	Rifampicin Rifabutin	Marked induction of liver enzymes	Use of alternative contraception is preferred, e.g. DMPA with 8-week injection interval
b. antifungal	Griseofulvin	Induction of liver enzymes	Short courses – additional contraception during treatment, and follow 7-day rule. Long courses – as for anticonvulsants
c. other antibiotics	Penicillins Ampicillin and relatives Tetracyclines Cephalosporins	Change in bowel flora, reducing enterohepatic recirculation of EE only, after hydrolysis of its conjugates	Short courses – wisest to use additional contraception during treatment up to 14 days (then resistance develops – see text) plus follow 7-day rule.
Miscellaneous			
a. protease inhibitors	Ritonavir Nelfinavir	Induction of liver enzymes	As for antifungal treatment (see above)
b. others	Lansoprazole Tacrolimus Nevirapine Modafinil	Induction of liver enzymes	As for antifungal treatment (see above) N.B. check with specialists re all new HIV treatments
Drugs which may increase COC efficacy			
	Co-trimoxazole Erythromycin	Inhibit EE metabolism	None if short course given
	Paracetamol	Competition in bowel wall for conjugation to sulphate. Hence more EE available for absorption	Advised: at least 2 hours separation of the analgesic from time of pill-taking. No effect on progestogen

BTB, breakthrough bleeding; COC, combined oral contraception; DMPA, depot medroxyprogesterone acetate; EE, ethinyloestradiol.
St John's Wort (hypericum). This herbal anti-depressant is an enzyme inducer; batch potency varies greatly so CSM has advised (March 2000) that it should not be used by COC takers.

Drug interaction

Reduction in the effectiveness of COC resulting from the simultaneous use of some other medications involves complex mechanisms: induction of liver enzymes, competition for binding sites, and reduced enterohepatic recirculation of oestrogen if the relevant bowel flora are altered by broad-spectrum antibiotics.

Enzyme-inducing drugs can affect both the oestrogen and the progestogen. Broad-spectrum antibiotics have a lesser effect since they only influence the recycling of EE within the bowel.

Table 2.5 shows the more important interactions of this type and their clinical implications and management.

Women show enormous variability in their circulating concentrations of contraceptive steroids and demonstrate different degrees of interaction with other drugs. Many are unaffected, particularly by antibiotics, but the individual response cannot be predicted clinically and it is wise to assume reduced protection in every case.

Long-term use of antibiotics is not a problem because the large bowel flora responsible for recycling oestrogens are reconstituted with resistant organisms by about 2 weeks (Back 1998, personal communication). In practice, therefore, if COC is commenced in a woman who has been taking a tetracycline long term (e.g. for acne), there is no need to advise extra precautions. When a tetracycline is first started by a woman already using COC, extra precautions should be taken for about 3 weeks (i.e. 7 additional days to restore quiescence of the active ovary). If the first 2 weeks of antibiotic use included any of the last 7 days of the pill-taking cycle, the next PFI should be eliminated.

Long-term use of enzyme-inducing drugs

This applies mainly to women suffering from epilepsy and women being treated for tuberculosis. Since rifamycins (rifampicin or rifabutin) are such powerful enzyme inducers, an alternative method of contraception for women taking these drugs is preferable; an intrauterine device (IUD), or the injectable DMPA (with a reduced 8-week injection interval) would be appropriate. An injectable contraceptive is also particularly appropriate for epileptic women, since the frequency of convulsions is often reduced by the maintenance of steady hormone levels.

Otherwise a 50 µg oestrogen preparation should be chosen along with elimination of most of the PFIs by advising the tricycle regimen (pp **56–57**), with a shortened (4-day) gap between each run of packets. If the preferred progestogen for a woman is not marketed as a 50 µg COC, a logical alternative is a combination of tablets, e.g. one Mercilon plus one Marvelon daily. If BTB has no other explanation (see p. **65**), in these circumstances it is permissible to increase the dose further, up to 90 µg of EE daily.

Discontinuing enzyme-inducing drugs

It may take many weeks before liver function reverts to normal after enzyme-inducing drugs are withdrawn (Guillebaud 1999). After long-term use of any drug which induces liver enzymes, a delay of about 4 weeks before the woman returns to a standard low-dose COC regimen is advised. This might reasonably be increased to 8 weeks after very prolonged use.

Effects of COC on other drugs

COC lowers the clearance of cyclosporin, diazepam, prednisolone and other drugs. This may increase the risk of side effects, but except in the case of cyclosporin the effect is unlikely to be clinically significant. COC impairs the metabolism of warfarin, and itself also alters coagulation, but in practice this combination of drugs is rarely indicated.

Manipulation of the menstrual cycle

To postpone a period

COC may be used to postpone menstrual bleeding. Two packets of monophasic pills should be taken consecutively with no break.

Phasic preparations cannot be used in this way. If a woman takes two packets of these pills consecutively, she may bleed since the first pills from the second packet contain a lower dose of progestogen than those she has just finished. Women on phasic preparations may delay menstruation in one of two ways:

1. Continuing to take further tablets from the final phase of another packet of the same brand of the phasic preparation.
2. Transferring directly to a packet of the monophasic brand most similar to the relevant final phase, e.g. Logynon to Microgynon, or Tri-Minulet to Minulet. The original phasic pill can be restarted after the usual PFI.

The tricycle regimen

This is an integral part of the modern management of COC-users who are taking enzyme-inducing drugs. Three (or four) packets of a monophasic COC are taken consecutively followed by the PFI. This leads to a longer COC cycle and means that the woman only has five (or four) withdrawal bleeds per year. This regimen obviously involves a larger annual intake of contraceptive steroids and the majority of women are probably best advised to adhere to the normal cycle. The tricycle regimen should therefore usually be reserved for the specific indications listed in Box 2.1.

Box 2.1 Indications for the tricycle regimen or its variants using a monophasic pill

1. Headaches including migraine without aura and other bothersome symptoms occurring regularly in the withdrawal week.
2. Unacceptably heavy or painful withdrawal bleeds.
3. Paradoxically, to help women who are concerned about absent withdrawal bleeds (this concern and the nuisance of pregnancy testing therefore arising less often!).
4. Pre-menstrual syndrome – tricycling may help if combined oral contraception is used to treat premenstrual syndrome.
5. Epilepsy: this benefits from relatively more sustained levels of the administered hormone (plus increases efficacy if enzyme-inducing drug is in use – see 6).
6. Other enzyme-inducer therapy.
7. Suspicion of decreased efficacy for any other reason.
8. Endometriosis – a monophasic combined oral contraceptive may be tricycled, for maintenance treatment after primary therapy.
9. At the woman's choice.

Note. In view of the possibility that the monthly pill-free interval has health benefits, one of these special indications should normally apply.

Whenever extra efficacy is desired, i.e. in numbers 5, 6 and 7 in Box 2.1, the PFI should also be shortened after each 'run' of packets; usually to 4 days (Guillebaud 1999).

Some women cannot keep postponing uterine bleeding for so long as 63 + days. If unacceptable BTB does not resolve, a shorter duration of continuous pill-taking may be tried (e.g. 'bicycling'), without changing the planned duration for each PFI.

Follow-up

Patients should be seen 3 months after starting the pill (earlier if there are any relative contraindications) and normally 6-monthly thereafter. At each visit, it is important to assess the acceptability of the method and to check that it is being used correctly. Any newly apparent risk factors must be noted. The most clinically significant side effects are rise in BP (pp **59–60**) and change in headache pattern (pp **61–62**).

There should be an 'open-house policy' to return if problems arise, but routine checks should be kept to a minimum, ideally delegated to a family-planning trained nurse:

1. BP should be recorded regularly during the first year and usually 6-monthly thereafter. If this is normal and steady, after 2 years the interval between visits can be increased to annually in women without risk factors or relevant diseases.
2. Measuring weight, though relevant in calculating the initial BMI (see Tables 2.2 and 2.3), is thereafter unhelpful and routine pelvic examinations are also unnecessary.
3. Screening tests should be carried out according to guidelines (Ch. 12).

4. In the presence of symptoms or side effects, the appropriate investigations should be performed, with a change of COC or change of method as required.
5. Women with risk factors for cardiovascular disease, or suffering from any chronic medical condition on which the effect of COC is not definitely known, need to be monitored more closely.

Indications for stopping COC

1. Onset of any of the sudden major symptoms (about which all COC-users should have been informed) listed on page **59**, until a serious cause is excluded.
2. A sustained BP above 160/100 mmHg (or 160/95 mmHg, see p. **38**), or less if other risk factors associated with cardiovascular disease risk are present.
3. Appearance of a new risk factor(s) or disease constituting a risk of cardiovascular disease that is unacceptable for that particular woman. The commonest of these is increasing age to above 35 years in women who smoke.
4. Onset of jaundice, whether or not potentially COC-related.
5. Before *elective surgery* – COC should be stopped at least 2 and preferably 4 weeks before major or leg surgery, or any other surgery known to be associated with an intrinsic increased risk of thrombosis. COC should be re-started no less than 2 weeks after the woman is ambulant. COC should also be stopped for 4 weeks before and 4 weeks after completion of treatment for varicose veins, whether by surgery or sclerotherapy. Injectable progestogens are a good alternative during this period. Urgent major surgery may be carried out under subcutaneous heparin cover. It is not necessary to stop COC before minor surgery, including sterilization.
6. Significant immobilization, including of a limb, e.g. through injury or orthopaedic operation.
7. Erythema multiforme or other severe skin reaction.
8. When pregnancy is desired.
9. When contraception is no longer needed:
   • All women need warning that without another pack following, the next 7 pill-free days will *not* be contraceptively safe.
   • Specific advice needs to be given to an older COC-user who reaches the age of 50 years (see Ch. 17).

COMPLICATIONS AND THEIR MANAGEMENT

Whenever a patient presents with symptoms or signs suggestive of a major side effect relating to COC use, COC should be stopped immediately and appropriate investigation and treatment arranged. COC-users should be warned in advance about the action to take if the following specific symptoms were to occur:

- Painful swelling in the calf (thrombosis).
- Pleuritic pain in the chest (VTE). This is frequently misdiagnosed.
- Breathlessness or cough with blood-stained sputum (VTE).
- Abdominal pain (thrombosis, porphyria, gallstones, liver adenoma).
- A bad fainting attack or collapse, or focal epilepsy (stroke).
- Unusual headache; disturbance of speech or visual field, numbness or weakness of a limb (transient ischaemic attack/incipient stroke – urgent neurological referral if suspected – or migraine with focal aura (pp **61–62**)).

Note. Conditions in parentheses (brackets) above are the most serious possible COC-related diagnoses, though in each case there may well be another explanation. To maintain contraception, switching to any progestogen-only method would always be appropriate.

'Minor' side effects

In general terms, if a change of COC seems appropriate, try empirically:

1. Changing to COC with a lower dose of the same progestogen and/or oestrogen. If appropriate, oestrogen can be removed altogether by trying a progestogen-only pill (POP) (Ch. 3).
2. Changing to a different progestogen, usually starting with the lowest available dose.

Using other drugs to treat COC-induced side effects is almost always bad practice. For example, if a woman complains of headaches, try changing COC or recommending the tricycle regimen rather than prescribing analgesics.

If every brand of COC one tries causes side effects, the POP may prove satisfactory; but bear in mind that emotional and psychological factors may play a part in the inability to find an acceptable preparation.

Cardiovascular system

Hypertension

Hypertension is in itself an important risk factor for heart disease and for both types of stroke. In most women taking COC, there is a slight but not significant increase in both systolic and diastolic BP. Approximately 1% of COC-users become clinically hypertensive with modern formulations. The incidence increases with age and duration of use.

Predisposing factors for COC-induced hypertension include a strong family history and obesity. Pregnancy-induced hypertension does not predispose to hypertension during COC use, though it is linked to risk of a later MI.

Management

- Repeated recordings of BP above 160 mmHg systolic or 100 mmHg diastolic (or in UK practice >95 mmHg, see p. 38) are grounds for stopping COC.

  Even if not that high, repeated elevated BP readings are important as a marker of the risk of cardiovascular disease, particularly if superimposed on other risk factors such as smoking. Patients with a gradual rise in BP should be changed to a lower dose COC or a progestogen-only preparation. BP levels should be rechecked within 3 months in both cases.
- Pill-induced hypertension should not be treated with anti-hypertensive drugs.
- Young women with essential hypertension, which is fully controlled by therapy, may very occasionally be given a low-dose COC under specialist supervision.

Respiratory system

'Pleurisy'

A COC-user is around twice as likely to be given the label of 'pleurisy' as a non-user! If unexplained pleuritic chest pain or dyspnoea occurs in a COC-user, pulmonary embolism must be excluded.

Asthma

A recent study suggests a doubled rate of the diagnosis of VTE in COC-users who have asthma (Farmer 1999, personal communication). This association could be causative, or might be due at least in part to diagnostic bias.

Central nervous system

Depression

This used to be a relatively common complaint among women on high-dose COC but is less frequently reported with modern low-dose preparations. Although depression appears to be more common among women who take COC than among non-users, the cause may be related to general lifestyle factors rather than to COC itself.

Some depressed women find COC relieves them of one of their greatest fears – that of unwanted pregnancy – and they therefore find it very acceptable.

Management. Depression may sometimes be alleviated without necessarily changing methods, by:

1. Lowering the dose of or changing the progestogen.
2. Pyridoxine (vitamin B_6) 50 mg daily. This may take up to 2 months to be effective. See also Chapter 16.

Loss of libido

This is occasionally reported (Ch. 14), particularly among those who are also depressed. Sometimes this is linked to psychological problems associated with using COC, such as anxiety about its dangers, fears about subsequent fertility or guilt about using contraception at all. For other women, libido may be increased because the method is reliable, requires no action related to sexual activity, and often reduces premenstrual syndrome.

Management. Relationship issues and psychosexual aspects of the relationship should be explored (Ch. 14). Any vaginal infection such as thrush should be treated. Use of a vaginal lubricant may help but changing the COC preparation rarely has any effect.

Headaches (including migraine)

In the RCGP study, headache was the second most common reason (after depression) for women stopping COC. Since migraine headaches (even without COC) are linked with an increased risk of ischaemic stroke, any woman reporting headaches on COC must be taken seriously. The headache pattern should be compared with the pattern before starting COC.

The following protocol allows for detailed assessment of the migraine (MacGregor and Guillebaud 1998):

Migraine: absolute contraindications (to commencing or continuing COC):

1. Migraine with aura (previously called 'classical migraine') during which there are focal neurological symptoms (often asymmetrical). True auras precede and usually resolve before the headache itself.
   Focal neurological symptoms comprise:
   - Visual symptoms (occur in 99% of true auras).
   - Loss of sight, or of part or whole of the field of vision, on one side: a scintillating jagged line often surrounds the area of lost vision, a bright scotoma.
   - Other unilateral sensory disturbance (such as marked paraesthesia spreading up from fingers of one arm, or on one side of the tongue).
   - Disturbance of speech.
   - Motor disturbance (unusual, e.g. weakness of a limb).

The main feature that the relevant symptoms share is that they are 'focal' or interpretable as owing to (transient) cerebral ischaemia. Photophobia

or *symmetrical* blurring or 'flashing lights' without any scotoma are not focal symptoms.
2. All other migraines even without aura which are unusually frequent/severe and last more than 72 hours.
3. All migraines treated with ergot derivatives, because of their vasoconstrictor effect.
4. Definite migraines without aura plus significant risk factors or relevant interacting diseases (e.g. connective tissue diseases linked with stroke risk).

Continuing contraception. Any progestogen-only, oestrogen-free hormonal method may be recommended: similar headaches may continue, but now without the potential added risk from the prothrombotic effects of the EE. Particularly useful choices are DMPA (p. **89**) and the levonorgestrel-releasing intrauterine system (LNG-IUS) (p. **108**) or a modern copper IUD.

Migraine: relative contraindications. COC may be used (WHO 2, benefits outweigh risks) but still always with specific instructions regarding the appearance of any focal symptoms.

1. Migraine without focal aura in women under age 35. If these or other 'ordinary' headaches occur particularly in the PFI, tricycling the COC may help (see pp **56–57**).
2. Distant past history during adolescence of migraine with focal aura, before commencing COC. COC may be tried with the caveat above.
3. Occurrence of a woman's first-ever attack of migraine of any type while on COC. It should be stopped if she is seen during the attack, but can be later restarted with the usual forewarning about focal symptoms.
4. Use of a 5-HT$_1$ agonist drug (e.g. sumatriptan) with no other contraindicating factors.

Non-migraine headaches. Though they do not represent a health risk, such headaches are an annoying side effect. If they appear to be COC-induced, try the effect of:

- A different variety of COC. Monophasic preparations are generally preferred to triphasics. The latter are not good for women with any headache tendency, since the extra fluctuations of the hormone levels may act as a trigger.
- The tricycle regimen (p. **56–57**). This is particularly effective in reducing the frequency of headaches (including migraines without aura) which occur during pill-free days.
- Changing to a progestogen-only method.
- Changing to a non-hormonal method.

Epilepsy

This condition is not initiated by COC. In a woman with epilepsy, COC often reduces the frequency of convulsions, especially if hormonal fluctuations are lessened by using a monophasic brand, and reducing the number of PFIs. Rarely, the frequency of convulsions may be increased by COC.

Anti-epileptic therapy with an enzyme-inducing drug is one of the few indications for a relatively high-dose COC (pp **54–55**).

Chorea and benign intracranial hypertension (BICH)

The incidence of these rare and unpleasant conditions may be increased in users of COC. BICH is not always benign, threatening the eyesight in severe cases. COC should be avoided thereafter.

Eyes

Water retention can lead to slight corneal oedema, and result in discomfort or corneal damage in those who wear contact lenses. With modern soft lenses and low-dose COC, this problem is now rare.

The catastrophes of retinal artery or vein thrombosis are extremely rare but may be related to COC use.

Management. If any acute visual disturbance occurs, COC should be stopped at once pending further investigation.

If corneal irritation occurs in wearers of contact lenses, prescribe COC containing the lowest possible dose of both steroids. If symptoms persist, the wearer has to decide whether to give up contact lenses or COC, otherwise corneal ulceration and scarring could result.

Gastrointestinal system

Nausea and vomiting

Nausea may occur in the first few cycles and occasionally recurs with the first few pills of each packet. Vomiting is most unusual.

Both symptoms are related to the oestrogen component and are rare with low-dose preparations. Severe vomiting for any reason may interfere with COC absorption and lead to BTB or spotting (p. **65**).

Management. Nausea and vomiting usually resolve with time; if not, it may be helpful to alter the timing of pill-taking. If nausea occurs in the morning, try taking the pill at night or vice versa. If persistent nausea occurs, try changing to a COC with less oestrogen.

Vomiting starting for the first time after months or years of trouble-free pill-taking should not be attributed to COC. Pregnancy should be excluded.

Weight gain

Increase in weight is unusual with modern COC, although it is frequently and unjustifiably attributed. It is sometimes associated with an increase in appetite on starting COC but is much more likely to be related to lifestyle factors.

Management. The woman should be advised about diet and exercise, and if this does not produce the desired result, COC should be changed to one containing a lower dose of the same progestogen, or to one with a different progestogen. POP can be tried if the problem persists on different brands of COC.

Jaundice

If a user becomes jaundiced, COC must be stopped at once. With a diagnosis of infective hepatitis, COC should not be restarted until 3 months after liver function tests return to normal.

Cholestatic jaundice is a risk for COC-users, as it is in pregnancy – the latter would be WHO 3 for future use of COC. A diagnosis of COC-related cholestatic jaundice, however, means that COC is absolutely contraindicated (WHO 4).

Gallstones

Latest reports imply that the increased risk of gallstones among COC-users is significant only during the early years of pill use. This suggests that the risk applies only to predisposed women.

It is reasonable for a woman who has had a cholecystectomy to take a low-dose COC provided there have been no complications. (WHO 3)

Liver tumours

The relative risk of benign adenoma or hamartoma is increased by COC use. However, the background incidence is so small (1–3 per 1 million women per year) that the COC-attributable risk is minimal. Most reported cases have been in long-term users of relatively high-dose COC.

Three case-control studies support the view that primary hepatocellular carcinoma (without any apparent synergism with cirrhosis or hepatitis B infection) is less rare in COC-users than it is in controls. If the link is causative, the maximum attributable incidence would be about 4 per million users per year (Vessey 1989).

Crohn's disease

There is evidence that this may be more frequent in COC-users. This is usually the non-granulomatous type and resolves if COC is stopped.

If Crohn's disease is severe, there is an added risk of thrombosis, so it is - generally WHO 3 (WHO 4 if COC-induced – and all varieties in severe attacks).

Urinary system

Several studies show that urinary tract infections are more common in COC-users than in controls. Although women taking COC may have more frequent intercourse, predisposing them to 'honeymoon' cystitis, evidence of an increased incidence of symptomless bacteriuria in COC-users does suggest an additional causal link.

Genital system

Breakthrough bleeding/spotting

BTB or spotting may result from circulating concentrations of steroids that are insufficient to maintain the endometrium. It is not usually an indication of increased risk of pregnancy. Most women who become pregnant on COC have no previous BTB just as most women with BTB do not become pregnant.

BTB is common during the first two or three cycles of COC use. Women should be forewarned, and advised to continue regular pill-taking and not to stop in the middle of a packet. Thereafter, a chart may be given on which to record further episodes of bleeding, and the situation reviewed after a further 3 months.

Management. Persistent BTB should be investigated. The following checklist is modified from Sapire (1990):

- **Disease** – examine the cervix. Irregular bleeding from invasive cancer may be wrongly attributed to COC use. Chlamydia can cause a low-grade endometritis with irregular bleeding.
- **Disorder of pregnancy** causing bleeding, e.g. COC after very recent abortion, miscarriage or trophoblastic disease.
- **Default** – poor compliance.
- **Drugs** which interact, primarily enzyme inducers. There is increasing evidence that smoking increases the risk of BTB.
- **Diarrhoea** and/or vomiting. (Diarrhoea alone has to be extremely severe to impair absorption.)
- **Disturbance of absorption**, e.g. after major gut resection. Coeliac disease does not pose a pill-absorption problem. (p. **39**)
- **Diet** – in vegetarians, the gut flora involved in recycling of oestrogen may be reduced although this is an unlikely cause.
- **Duration – too short?** – minimal BTB which is tolerable may resolve after 2 to 3 months.

- **Dose** – after the above causes have been excluded:
  a. Change from a monophasic pill to a phasic type
  b. Increase the dose of progestogen and/or oestrogen
  c. Try a different progestogen
  d. If bleeding during 'tricycling', change to 'bicycling' (p. **57**) or return to normal pill-taking
  e. After rechecking this checklist and following careful discussion, consider using a 50 μg COC preparation.

Absence of withdrawal bleeding

This is not dangerous, does not signify overdosage, nor is it related to 'post-pill amenorrhoea'.
Management. The best management is reassurance:

- Check that the woman is not pregnant, particularly if pills have been missed or where drug interactions may have occurred.
- If a woman misses a single withdrawal bleed, advise her to start the next packet as planned unless the history suggests risk of pregnancy. However, if two withdrawal bleeds have been missed, the woman should not start her next packet of COC until pregnancy has been excluded.
- Absent withdrawal bleeds are less common with triphasic pills.

Vaginal discharge

Low-dose COC usually does not affect vaginal discharge. However, some women may complain of vaginal dryness while others may notice a clear mucoid discharge with or without cervical ectopy. There is no causal link between genital candidiasis and use of COC.
Management. Vaginal discharge (Ch. 13). Cervical erosion (ectopy) (Ch. 15). COC may provide some protection against trichomonal vaginitis (p. **41**) but not against the other common STIs. COC appears to reduce the incidence of ascending PID because of the effect of progestogens on cervical mucus and the endometrium.

Fibroids

Low-dose COC does not appear to increase the size of fibroids and reduces the frequency of the associated symptoms. Patients with fibroids may therefore be given COC with careful monitoring.

Carcinoma of the ovary and the endometrium

A protective effect is well established (p. **41**).

Carcinoma of the cervix

The Oxford/Family Planning Association study demonstrated a significant increase in cervical neoplasia in long-term users of COC compared with IUD users. The UK RCGP Study (Beral et al 1999) found a significantly raised odds ratio for mortality of 2.5 for current and recent COC-users compared with controls. In that study of 46 000 women, the non-users were materially different individuals, however, with a greater use of barrier methods, and differing sexual lifestyles. The association is not in doubt, but causality is less clear.

Studies of cervical cancer lack accurate information on sexual activity, of women and especially their partners. The prime carcinogen is clearly transmitted sexually and is probably a virus or combination of viruses. COC may be acting as a weak co-factor (weaker than cigarette smoking).

Management. Prescribers should ensure that COC-users are screened following agreed guidelines (Ch. 12). The higher mortality of COC-users in the RCGP study ought to be avoidable in future with an effective computerized cervical screening programme, ensuring the inclusion of high-risk groups who were missed before.

COC can be continued during the careful monitoring of any abnormality or after definitive treatment of cervical intraepithelial-neoplasia (CIN).

Choriocarcinoma

There are no data suggesting any increase in the risk of trophoblastic disease in pregnancies following COC use. UK studies (but not others in the USA) have shown that chemotherapy for choriocarcinoma is more often required among women given COC in the presence of active trophoblastic disease (Vessey 1989).

Management
- When any form of trophoblastic disease has been diagnosed, the Regional Centres in the UK, which monitor all cases, still strongly recommend that all sex hormones (including progestogen-only methods, but excluding emergency contraception) should be avoided – though *only* while hCG levels are raised. (Although WHO and all the relevant specialists in the USA permit COC use from the outset.)
- An alternative form of contraception should be recommended. While hCG levels are above 5000 iu/L, ovulation is unlikely so barrier methods will be highly effective.
- Copper IUDs can be used, if there is no invasive damage to the uterine wall from the cancer.

Breasts

Enlargement and discomfort

While some women find that the COC improves cyclical breast symptoms, others complain of breast tenderness and/or swelling. These symptoms seem to be particularly associated with the last phase of triphasic and biphasic brands.

Management:
- Sudden enlargement of the breasts may be the first sign of pregnancy.
- Galactorrhoea among pill-takers is rare and needs investigation.

Carcinoma of the breast

Breast cancer is a common disease and therefore it will inevitably develop in some women whether they take COC or not. In assessing a possible aetiological link between COC and breast cancer, many factors have to be taken into account including:

1. A potentially long latent period between COC use and the diagnosis of breast cancer.
2. That different effects are possible according to the age of COC use.
3. The effects of early menarche and late first delivery, and if these might be compounded by COC use.
4. The influence of a family history of breast cancer or personal history of benign breast disease.
5. Changes in pill formulation – both the oestrogen and progestogen content of COC have changed and reduced in dosage over the years.

The data from the Collaborative Group on Hormonal Factors in Breast Cancer (CGHFBC) (Collaborative Group 1996) are now widely accepted as representing the present state of knowledge. The group re-analysed original data from over 53 000 women with breast cancer and over 100 000 controls from 54 studies in 25 countries. This represents 90% of the worldwide epidemiological data.

The CGHFBC's model shows *current or recent use of COC* as the most important factor and is summarized in Box 2.2.

Box 2.2	
User status	**Percentage increase in annual risk**
● Current user	24%
● 1 to 4 years after stopping	16%
● 5 to 9 years after stopping	7%
● 10+ years an ex-user	No significant increase

From this large meta-analysis, COC-users can be reassured that:

- Use of COC by young women will fortunately lead to very few attributable cases as the background incidence of breast cancer is so low at their age.
- The cancers diagnosed in women who use or have ever used COC are clinically less advanced than those who have never used COC, and are less likely to have spread beyond the breast.
- No excess mortality has been shown (confirmed also in the more recent RCGP study, Beral et al 1999).
- The risk is not associated with duration of use or the dose or type of hormone in COC, and there is no synergism with other risk factors for breast cancer (e.g. family history).
- The risk of breast cancer appears unaffected by age of initiation or discontinuation, use before or after first full-term pregnancy, or duration of use.

Clinical implications. The UK CSM advised that COC-users should be informed and counselled on the basis of the CGHFBC findings, but that there need be no fundamental change in prescribing practice.

In routine clinical practice:

- Breast cancer risks should be discussed in a proactive but sensitive way, as part of routine COC counselling for all women.
- This discussion should be initiated opportunely – not at the very first visit by a teenager who has no concerns about cancer – along with encouragement to report promptly any unusual changes in the breasts in the future ('breast awareness').
- The protective effects against malignancy of the ovary and endometrium should also be mentioned. The benefits of COC may seem so great to many (but not to all), as to compensate for almost any likely lifetime excess risk of breast cancer.

Older women may use COC to age 50 provided they are healthy, migraine-free non-smokers. The cumulative risk of breast cancer in young women is very small – 1 in 500 in women up to age 35. The percentage increment in risk (24%) during current COC use does not increase with age but the cumulative background risk of breast cancer rises steeply after age 35 years (Fig. 2.2) to 1 in 100 at age 45 and 1 in 12 by age 75. The CGHFBC data give three extra cases of breast cancer for COC-use until age 45, added to the background risk of 23/1000 for the same age.

Other higher risk groups for breast cancer are specifically: (a) women with a family history of a young (under 40) first-degree relative with breast cancer and (b) women with benign breast disease. These are WHO 3 categories, but past epithelial atypia on histology is an absolute contraindication (p. **38**). As with increasing age, the percentage increment in risk (24%)

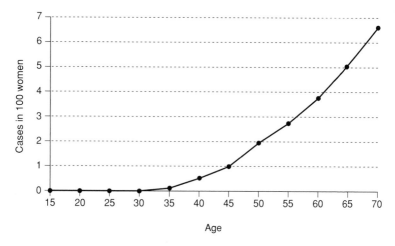

Figure 2.2 Background risk: cumulative number of breast cancers per 100 women, by age.

during current COC use does not increase in women with a family history of breast cancer although it is obviously applied to a bigger background risk.

In discussion, family history and benign breast disease should be seen as relative contraindications requiring careful explanation. If a woman chooses COC, a low-dose preparation should be given with specific counselling.

If carcinoma of the breast develops, the prognosis is good in pill-takers; however, COC should be stopped. During remission, progestogen-only methods are often acceptable, preferably after specialist consultation.

Musculoskeletal system

Oestrogen given in high doses to young female animals can lead to premature closure of the epiphyses. There is no evidence that a daily dose of 30 μg or even 50 μg of EE has any such effect in post-pubertal girls.

Carpal tunnel syndrome

More frequent in pill-takers.

Leg pains and cramps

Careful examination and assessment of women presenting with these symptoms is important. If bilateral, note any altered physical activity, fluid retention, weight increase, varicose veins, chilblains or Raynaud's disease.

If unilateral, venous thrombosis must be excluded. Superficial, as well as deep venous, thrombosis is of relevance to a thrombotic tendency.

If there is any doubt about the diagnosis, COC should be stopped and the woman referred for appropriate imaging. Her contraceptive future depends on an accurate diagnosis being made.

Cutaneous system

Chloasma/melasma

'Pregnancy mask' may develop in women taking COC, after excessive exposure to sunlight, irrespective of whether or not it occurred in a previous pregnancy. It appears that both oestrogen and progestogen can be contributory. The condition may be slow to fade after COC is stopped.

Management. Mild degrees of chloasma can be masked by carefully applied cosmetics. If it is causing distress, a different COC can be tried but often no benefit is gained by changing. A POP benefits some women although many will have to stop all hormonal contraception. Even then the pigmentation may be slow to fade. Depigmenting creams and lotions should be avoided.

Photosensitivity

This may occur on its own or, rarely, be the first manifestation of one of the porphyrias and hence requires referral for assessment as to whether to avoid future use of steroidal contraception.

Acne, greasy skin, hirsutism

These androgenic effects are more commonly associated with pills containing second-generation progestogens (NET and LNG).

Management. Change to a different pill. Good results have been reported with Marvelon and may be expected from Gracial (p. **33**).

Dianette, which contains an anti-androgen (cyproterone acetate) in combination with 35 μg EE, is marketed for the treatment of acne, particularly in association with PCOS. It is an effective contraceptive, giving good cycle control. It has similar 'rules' to other COC for missed tablets, drug interactions, contraindications and similar requirements, also, for monitoring.

Duration of treatment with Dianette. This needs to be individualized. In the data sheet/SPC it is 'recommended that treatment is withdrawn when the acne or hirsutism is completely resolved', but 'repeat courses may be given if the condition recurs'. There are some concerns about hepatic effects including benign and malignant liver tumour risk in long-term use – mostly based on animal work and much higher doses of the cyproterone acetate. So it is usual to advise women to switch to another COC preparation after about 1 to 2 years, at which stage their condition has usually improved and will be maintained by a normal preparation. A COC containing a less androgenic progestogen (DSG/GSD) would be a logical choice. If symptoms recur when Dianette is stopped, it may then be used for much longer.

If the patient is given a prescription for Dianette, she will be charged for the pills unless the prescription states that it is being used for contraception (a female symbol will suffice).

Malignant melanoma

There is no longer any concern among epidemiologists about a causative association between pill use and malignant melanoma.

Other skin conditions

Telangiectasia, rosacea, eczema, erythema nodosum, erythema multiforme and herpes gestationis (now termed pemphigoid gestationis) have all been associated with, or allegedly exacerbated by, COC.

Infections and inflammations

Some studies suggest that COC-users are more likely to suffer from infections such as chickenpox, 'gastric flu', respiratory and urinary tract infections, and also inflammations such as tenosynovitis and a form of allergic polyarthritis.

The effects on Crohn's disease (p. **64**) and the apparent beneficial effect on rheumatoid arthritis and thyroid disease suggest that the pill can modify immune mechanisms.

REVERSIBILITY

When women stop COC they regain, after a delay of about 1 to 3 months, the fertility that they would have had at that age if they had never used the method. Vessey et al (1986) showed that about half of his population who stopped using COC above the age of 30 took up to a year longer to conceive than a control group who stopped using barrier methods. But his study also confirmed that COC does not cause any permanent loss of fertility.

The first period after stopping COC is often delayed. Secondary amenorrhoea after stopping COC is not uncommon and is unrelated to the type of pill or duration of use. It may occur particularly in women who have had a late menarche, previous episodes of amenorrhoea or very irregular cycles and they should be investigated in the same way as any other case of secondary amenorrhoea (Ch. 15). Abnormalities that would normally lead to amenorrhoea are masked by regular withdrawal bleeds while taking COC.

OUTCOME OF PREGNANCY

Some authorities advise that women should discontinue COC and use a barrier method of contraception for two to three cycles before a planned conception. There is no real evidence that this advice is of any benefit. With universal obstetric diagnostic ultrasound, accurate identification of the last menstrual period has become less important for calculating gestation. Any woman who does find herself pregnant less than 3 months after stopping COC should be strongly reassured about any risk to the fetus (WHO 1981). After discontinuing COC, there is no increased risk of miscarriage, ectopic pregnancy or stillbirth, and no alteration in the sex ratio or birth weight.

Exposure during pregnancy

The incidence of birth defects following COC exposure is no higher than expected among any group of women having a planned baby (Bracken 1990). The advice that a pregnant woman should avoid all drugs, especially in the first trimester, remains the ideal. Exposure to COC during pregnancy should never be used as grounds for recommending therapeutic abortion.

BREAKS IN PILL-TAKING

Most risks such as VTE, and benefits such as relief from menstrual symptoms, apply only while COC is being used. There is no evidence that by taking breaks any risk is reduced unless these are long enough to have a real impact on total accumulated years of COC use. Taking breaks will certainly increase the risk of unplanned pregnancy.

The benefits of long-term use tend to balance the risks. Of great potential relevance to this whole discussion is the fact that any woman who has been on the pill for 10 years has in fact taken 130 breaks, each lasting a week.

Future fertility is not enhanced by breaks in pill-taking.

RISKS/BENEFITS

For many women COC provides highly acceptable and reliable contraception as well as many benefits to general health. It is not possible to enjoy these advantages without some disadvantages and, although the risks

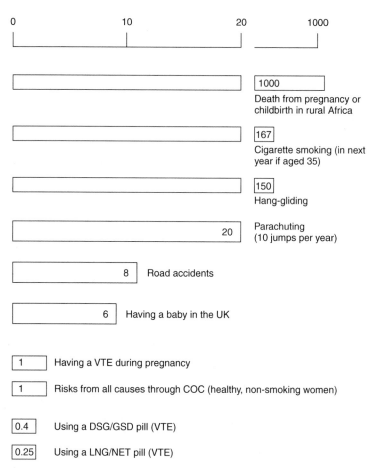

Figure 2.3 Combined oral contraception risks compared with other risks in life; annual numbers of deaths per 100 000 exposed. With regard to cancer, here excess cancer mortality is assumed to be zero, i.e. benefits balancing risks (p. 41, pp 66–70). COC, combined oral contraception; DSG, desogestrel; GSD, gestodene; LNG, levonorgestrel; NET, norethisterone; VTE, venous thromboembolism. (Sources: Anonymous 1991 British Medical Journal 302:743; Dinman BD 1980 The reality and acceptance of risk. Journal of the American Medical Association 244: 1226–1228; Mills AM, Wilkinson CL, Bromham DR et al 1996 Guidelines for prescribing combined oral contraceptives. British Medical Journal 312: 121–122; Singh AD, Paling J 1997 Informed consent: putting risks into perspective. Survey of Ophthalmology 42:83–86; Smith AF 1996 Mad cows and ecstasy: chance and choice in an evidence-based society. Journal of the Royal Statistical Society 159: 367–383; Strom B 1994 Pharmacoepidemiology, 2nd edn. Wiley, Chichester, p 57–65.)

associated with COC are real and should not be denied, their incidence is small. It is important to put these risks into perspective, comparing them with the risks of other methods of contraception and with pregnancy should a less effective method fail – and also with the general risks that we all may run in daily living (Fig. 2.3).

The safety of COC can be further increased by:

1. Prescribing it primarily for healthy women.
2. Ensuring extra care and supervision for women with risk factors or chronic diseases.
3. Using COC containing the lowest suitable dose of both oestrogen and progestogen.
4. Careful monitoring of:
   a. New medical diagnoses or any change in risk factors
   b. New circumstances of risk, e.g. elective surgery
   c. Blood pressure
   d. Headache pattern.
5. Appropriate well-woman screening (Ch. 12).

Even more important than following such a scheme is the attitude of the doctor and the nurse, who should be ready to advise and counsel a woman taking COC in a non-directive way. They must be not only conscientious and up to date in their knowledge, but also able to relate this successfully to the individual woman's needs.

REFERENCES

Beral V, Hermon C, Kay C, Hannaford P, Darby S, Reeves G 1999 Mortality associated with oral contraceptive use: 25 year follow up of cohort of 46 000 women from Royal College of General Practitioners' oral contraception study. British Medical Journal 318: 96–100

Bracken M 1990 Oral contraception and congenital malformations in offspring: a review and meta-analysis of the prospective studies. Obstetrics and Gynaecology 76: 552–557

Collaborative Group on Hormonal Factors in Breast Cancer 1996 Breast cancer and hormonal contraceptives: collaborative reanalysis of individual data of 53 297 women with breast cancer and 100 239 women without breast cancer from 54 epidemiological studies. Lancet 347: 1713–1727

Djerassi C 1979 The chemical history of the pill. In: Djerassi C The Politics of contraception. W W Norton, New York, p 227–255

Dunn N, Thorogood M, Faragher B et al 1999 Oral contraceptives and myocardial infarction: results of the MICA case-control study. British Medical Journal 318: 1579–1584

Franceschi S, La Vecchia C 1998 Oral contraceptives and colorectal tumours. Contraception 58: 3 35–343

Guillebaud J 1998 The Newsletter of the International Society for Mountain Medicine 8(2): 12–13

Guillebaud J 1999 Contraception: your questions answered, 4th edn. Churchill Livingstone, Edinburgh

Gupta S, Harding K 1988 Contraception and cardiovascular disorders. British Journal of Family Planning 25: 13–17

Hannaford P, Webb A 1996 Evidence-guided prescribing of combined oral contraceptives: consensus statement. Contraception 54: 125–129

Korver T, Goorissen E, Guillebaud J 1995 The combined oral contraceptive pill: what advice should we give when tablets are missed? British Journal of Obstetrics and Gynaecology 102: 601–607

Lechat P, Mas J, Lascault G et al 1988 Prevalence of patent foramen ovale in patients with stroke. New England Journal of Medicine 318: 1148–1152

MacGregor A, Guillebaud J 1998 Recommendations for clinical practice – combined oral contraceptives, migraine and ischaemic stroke. British Journal of Family Planning 24: 55–60

Sapire K E (adapted Belfield T, Guillebaud J) 1990 Combined oral contraceptives. Contraception and sexuality in health and disease. McGraw Hill, London

Vandenbroucke J P, Koster T, Reitsma P H, Bertina R M, Rosendaal F R 1994 Increased risk of venous thrombosis in oral contraceptive users who are carriers of factor V Leiden mutation. Lancet 344: 1453–1457

Vessey M P, Smith M A, Yeates D 1986 Return of fertility after discontinuation of oral contraceptives. British Journal of Family Planning 11: 120–124

Vessey M P 1989 Oral contraception and cancer. In: Filshie M, Guillebaud J (eds) Contraception – science and practice. Butterworths, London

World Health Organization (WHO) 1981 The effect of female sex hormones on fetal development and infant health: report of a WHO scientific group. Technical report series 657. WHO, Geneva

World Health Organization (WHO) 1998 Cardiovascular disease and steroid hormone contraception. Report of a scientific group. Technical report series WHO, Geneva 877

3

Progestogen-only contraception

Ian S. Fraser

Advantages 78
  Non-contraceptive health
    benefits 78
  Breast-feeding 79
  Drug interactions 79
  Metabolic effects 79
  Hypertension 79
  Coagulation factors 79
  Major surgery 80
  Overdosage 80
Disadvantages 80
Modes of action 80
**Assessment for
  use 81**
  History 81
  Examination 81
Choice of method 81
Indications 82
Contraindications 82
  Absolute 83
  Relative 83
Side effects 84
  Disturbances of
    the menstrual
    pattern 84

  Persistent ovarian follicles or
    follicular cysts 85
  Other side effects 85
**Management of clinical
  problems 86**
Individual methods 87
  Progestogen-only pills 87
  Injectables 89
  Subdermal implants 94
  Intrauterine systems 98
Special considerations 98
  Adolescents 98
  Older women and the
    perimenopause 98
  Women with pre-existing medical
    disorders 98
  Drug interactions 101
  Future fertility and
    pregnancy 101
  Interpretation of laboratory
    tests 102
  Indications for stopping
    progestogen-only
    contraception 102
Conclusion 102

Progestogen-only methods were originally introduced to avoid the side effects of oestrogen and to reduce total exposure to steroids. With modern, low-dose, oestrogen–progestogen regimens these reasons have become less of an issue, but the progestogen-only approach has encouraged the development of a range of useful methods allowing very prolonged duration of action and low-dose steroid exposure (Table 3.1), while maintaining high contraceptive efficacy.

Progestogen-only contraception has had considerable promise for many years but has only begun to achieve its full potential in the last 15 years. The use of injectable contraceptives has until very recently only accounted for 1–2% of contraceptive use worldwide, although in a few individual countries it has been used more extensively.

Individual progestogen-only methods exhibit considerable differences in their attributes and have varying appeal to different women. These specific attributes are discussed in detail in the section describing each method

Table 3.1   Choices of progestogen-only delivery systems

High dose	Low dose	Very low dose		
Injectables	*Subcutaneous implants*	*Oral*	*Vaginal rings*	*Intrauterine*
Once-a-month	Norplant	Several POPs	Several under development	Levonorgestrel Progesterone
2-monthly	Implanon			
3-monthly	Jadelle			

(pp 87–98); the general characteristics common to each method are described below.

ADVANTAGES
Non-contraceptive health benefits

Combined oral contraception (COC) offers high efficacy and confers a number of substantial non-contraceptive benefits for long-term users (Ch. 2). The evidence for similar benefits for progestogen-only users is limited, and such benefits will probably vary with dosage and route of administration.

There is *strong* evidence for a major degree of protection against endometrial cancer, especially with depot medroxyprogesterone acetate (DMPA).

DMPA also appears to protect against the development of acute pelvic inflammatory disease and vaginal candidiasis.

All progestogen methods probably exert some benefit on symptoms of dysmenorrhoea, premenstrual syndrome, mittelschmerz and mastalgia.

Diseases, for which a moderate or high degree of protection is likely but unconfirmed, include endometriosis, uterine myomas, benign breast disease and ovarian cancer.

There are some medical conditions which are occasionally caused or exacerbated by COC, but which progestogen-only methods do not usually influence. One of the most important of these is venous thromboembolic disease. Others include chloasma, hypertension, systemic lupus erythematosus and other autoimmune diseases, and migraine. Conditions for which we have limited data on long-term interactions during or after progestogen use but where some progestogens may have an advantage include most cardiovascular diseases, obesity, cigarette smoking, contact lens use, epilepsy, non-granulomatous Crohn's disease, obstetric cholestasis, gallstones and possible immunological interactions.

Final answers on these points will require careful case-control studies once there is extensive usage of these methods in specific populations.

Breast-feeding

One of the most useful advantages of progestogen-only methods over COC is the lack of any adverse effect on breast-feeding, with no evidence of reduction in milk volume or quality and no effect on infant growth and development.

Drug interactions

A substantial number of drug interactions with the combined pill have been described. Much less information is available for progestogens alone. Hepatic enzyme-inducing drugs, such as rifampicin and several anti-epileptic drugs, may sometimes reduce the efficacy of low-dose progestogens such as Norplant, vaginal rings and progestogen-only pills (POPs), although this appears to be less of a problem than with COC.

Interactions do not appear to occur with antibiotics or with sodium valproate or clonazepam. Other minor drug interactions are possible.

Metabolic effects

In general, progestogens induce fewer metabolic changes than COC. Effects on lipids (such as total serum cholesterol, high-density lipoprotein- and low-density lipoprotein-cholesterol, triglycerides, free fatty acids or phospholipids) are minimal, even with DMPA and norethisterone enanthate (NET-EN). Minor changes in the insulin response to a glucose load may occur with higher dose methods, but precipitation of a diabetic state must be rare. There is little or no effect on liver, thyroid, pituitary or adrenal function.

Low-dose methods do not appear to influence body weight, although high-dose methods may.

Hypertension

Development of hypertension while using progestogens is uncommon, and is usually not related to use.

Coagulation factors

Adverse effects on all parts of the coagulation and fibrinolytic cascades appear to be minimal, and there does not appear to be any induction of a hypercoagulable state even with higher dose methods. A recent multicentre study (World Health Organization 1998) demonstrated no significant increase in the relative risk of stroke, myocardial infarction or venous thromboembolic disease among women using oral or injectable progestogen-only contraceptives.

Major surgery

Progestogens do not affect blood coagulation and the risk of venous thrombosis, and therefore do not need to be stopped before major surgery.

Overdosage

No harmful effects appear to result from overdosage of any method, even when POP are taken by a child.

DISADVANTAGES

Progestogen-only methods are generally well tolerated and continuation rates are good, but all methods require detailed counselling for optimum long-term usage. Implants require medical intervention for insertion and removal, which may be a disadvantage if appropriately trained medical personnel are not always available. Subjective side effects generally present few problems apart from the almost universal menstrual change, which can sometimes be persistent and distressing. These menstrual effects, as well as other potential side effects, are discussed below in specific detail related to each method.

MODES OF ACTION

Progestogens have a multiplicity of actions within the human reproductive system. The importance of each action probably depends on dosage and type of progestogen. The more important actions are thought to be:

1. Local ovarian effects:
   a. suppression of follicular growth
   b. inhibition of ovulation
   c. suppression of luteal activity.
2. Cervical mucus modification inhibiting sperm penetration.
3. Endometrial modification to prevent implantation.
4. Hypothalamic and pituitary effects to inhibit cyclical release of follicle stimulating hormone and luteinizing hormone, and hence contribute to suppression of follicular development and ovulation.
5. Effects on fallopian tubal function and fertilization are probably relatively unimportant.

Very low-dose progestogen-only methods probably act mainly by interfering with cervical mucus and endometrial structure, with less predictable effects on luteal and follicular function, while higher dose methods usually reliably suppress follicular development and ovulation (Landgren and Diczfalusy 1980, Brache et al 1990). Direct effects also occur on the ovary, and the most sensitive appears to be an effect on luteal function resulting in defective progesterone secretion.

ASSESSMENT FOR USE

History, examination and the woman's preference will determine suitability for a particular progestogen-only method.

History

This should always include details of age, obstetric history, previous contraceptive history, current contraceptive requirements and motivation, and details of medical conditions and drug therapy which might influence choice of progestogen-only method.

Examination

Measurement of blood pressure is the only essential investigation. Weighing of the woman can be valuable as weight gain is a common complaint, especially with DMPA. It is not necessary to examine the breasts or undertake a pelvic examination unless it is indicated by the medical history. A cervical smear should be performed in accordance with local screening policy.

CHOICE OF METHOD

This will usually be determined by the woman's preference for the attributes of a particular method. The most important issues to be considered are the probable duration of required contraception, the extent of user control of the method and previous user experience of other contraceptive methods. Motivation for a specific method is more likely to lead to correct long-term use.

There is little to choose between different POPs and first choice is usually a matter of physician or patient preference based on familiarity rather than actual differences between pills. Changing to another pill is rarely helpful and there is no evidence that one POP is more effective than another, or that one has a different side-effect profile. Nevertheless, some women will occasionally feel better on one particular pill or progestogen.

Choice of one of the very long-acting methods such as Implanon or Mirena generally presupposes that the woman does not plan to try to become pregnant within the next 3 to 5 years. Removal of the device prior to this time may not be cost-effective, although numerous unanticipated reasons may make premature removal appropriate.

INDICATIONS

The general aspects of progestogen-only use are considered in this section and aspects specific to particular methods are discussed in each separate section.

1. As first-choice contraceptives, where the attributes of the method appeal to the woman and no contraindications exist. Local regulations may need to be considered where, for example, DMPA is still only licensed for contraception in women in whom other contraceptives have proved unsuitable. In the UK, DMPA was licensed for general contraceptive marketing in 1995.
2. Where the woman expresses a wish to use hormonal contraception, but:
   a. oestrogens are contraindicated
   b. oestrogens are not well tolerated
   c. the profile of oestrogenic side effects or complications is disliked.
3. For older women and smokers. It is well established that smokers over the age of 35 have an increased risk of cardiovascular incidents and this is exacerbated by use of COC (Ch. 2). This risk does not appear to be enhanced by progestogen-only methods, although long-term data are not so extensive as for COC. Progestogen-only methods can be used up to the menopause, and may even ameliorate the onset of some perimenopausal symptoms.
4. During lactation. Progestogen-only methods are preferable to those containing oestrogen (Ch. 6).
5. For women with:
   a. diabetes mellitus
   b. mild hypertension or where blood pressure is well controlled
   c. homozygous sickle cell disease
   d. migraine, including focal types
   e. as an alternative to COC prior to elective major surgery
   f. for women who are unreliable or unwilling pill-takers (long-acting delivery systems provide excellent contraception for this group)
   g. where there is a need for highly effective, but reversible contraception. The long-acting progestogen-only systems are the most effective, yet easily reversible, methods currently available and are a suitable alternative to sterilization for many women.

CONTRAINDICATIONS

In many countries, regulatory authorities still insist on a lengthy list of contraindications to progestogen-only methods which more accurately reflect the risks with combined oestrogen–progestogen preparations. Many are precautionary and have little epidemiological evidence to support them. However, these warnings need to be carefully considered and, if necessary, discussed with the woman.

Absolute

1. Known or suspected pregnancy, even though there is no convincing evidence of risk to the fetus or mother. Androgenic progestogens in moderate dosage, e.g. NET-EN, may carry a very small risk of masculinization of a female fetus if inadvertently given during the first 4 to 5 months of pregnancy.
2. Menstrual disturbance of uncertain cause, at least until this has been investigated. Most progestogen-only methods will confuse the clinical picture.
3. Any serious side effect which is not clearly oestrogen-related, e.g. hepatic adenoma, and certain other acute or chronic liver conditions such as porphyria.
4. Current history of serious cardiovascular disease, until this has been thoroughly assessed.
5. Injectable methods should preferably not be used in women with bleeding disorders, including long-term anticoagulation, because of the risk of haematoma formation at the injection site.
6. DMPA should not be used in women wishing to conceive soon after the presumed end of the 3-month contraceptive effect.

Relative

1. Those who find irregular bleeding or amenorrhoea unacceptable, especially for cultural or other social reasons.
2. Severe obesity may reduce the efficacy of systemic low-dose methods (not the levonorgestrel untrauterine system), and may sometimes be exacerbated by injectables.
3. Malignant disease of the breast. Some doctors include this as an absolute contraindication, but recent evidence suggests that those women who have had their disease adequately treated are at little or no increased risk of a recurrence with use of progestogens. Specialist consultation is always advisable.
4. After hydatidiform mole until the urine is free of chorionic gonadotrophin.
5. Drugs which may interact.
6. A history of recurrent functional ovarian cysts. Very low-dose methods may exacerbate these, although data are anecdotal.
7. POPs should generally be avoided in teenagers, although subdermal implants may be advantageous in this group.

8. The immediate postpartum period. A tiny amount of progestogen is transferred into breastmilk, and some clinicians advise delaying the start of this contraception until 6 weeks postpartum to avoid possible theoretical effects on the neonatal hypothalamus and liver. Although progestogens usually have no effect on lactation, and may even enhance it, the very occasional woman gives a clear history of interference by progestogens with the milk supply during the early weeks of breast-feeding.
9. Severe hypertension should be well controlled before use of low-dose progestogens, and then carefully monitored.
10. Chronic liver conditions, such as obstetric cholestasis, cirrhosis, which may occasionally be exacerbated.

SIDE EFFECTS

Disturbances of the menstrual pattern

All progestogen-only contraceptive systems alter the menstrual pattern, but there is still limited understanding of the mechanisms underlying these menstrual disturbances. The changes are unpredictable, vary to some extent with method and vary greatly between individual women. In most users, there is an increased incidence of erratic and scanty spotting or break-through bleeding, sometimes with prolonged episodes, and sometimes with oligomenorrhoea or even amenorrhoea (Belsey 1988). Most women experience a decrease in the total volume of blood lost per month. The pattern may change with time, in ways which are specific for each method. Heavy bleeding with progestogen-only contraception is unusual, although it may sometimes occur when it is started in the early postpartum period (within 3 weeks of delivery).

Prolonged or frequent spotting or bleeding

These symptoms are common accompaniments of progestogen therapy, particularly during the first few months of use, and are a major cause of premature discontinuation.

Pathological causes should be kept in mind if abnormal bleeding persists, especially in older women. Pelvic infection (especially chlamydia) and genital tract abnormalities (including cervical or endometrial polyps, submucous fibroids, cervical or endometrial cancer) should be considered. The risk of endometrial cancer is reduced by most, probably all, progestogen methods.

If the risk of intrauterine pathology is felt to be significant, a transvaginal ultrasound scan can identify a thickened 'endometrium' caused by polyps or cancer. A hysteroscopy and endometrial biopsy will give even more precise information about possible intrauterine and endocervical pathology. It must be borne in mind that these causes of abnormal bleeding in progesto-gen-users are very uncommon compared with the breakthrough bleeding and spotting associated with the methods themselves.

Amenorrhoea

This is common with DMPA and NET-EN, but can also occur with all other methods. Pregnancy may need to be excluded, although it is uncommon with the long-acting methods; if in doubt, a pregnancy test should be carried out. Prolonged amenorrhoea with progestogens is not known to be harmful, and many women find it highly acceptable. For those who feel that amenorrhoea is unnatural, a reasonable analogy can be drawn with lacta-tional amenorrhoea.

Pretreatment counselling about the range of possible menstrual changes, including amenorrhoea, is vital with all progestogen-only methods.

Post-treatment menstrual disturbance

Once the effect of the progestogen itself has worn off, menstrual disturbance following any of these methods is uncommon. DMPA-users may find that the depot preparation has an effect for many months after the last injection (see below), but once the progestogen has been cleared from the body the menstrual cycle usually rapidly returns to its previous pattern. Continuing menstrual disturbances should be investigated in the same way as in women who have never used these methods.

Persistent ovarian follicles or follicular cysts

Women using low-dose progestogens sometimes experience temporary breast tenderness and lower abdominal discomfort associated with persist-ing oestradiol-secreting follicles. These follicles often grow slowly up to 5–7 cm diameter, and then undergo slow atresia with fluctuating symptoms over 6 to 8 weeks. Torsion or rupture of these persistent follicles is uncommon. Their presence can be confirmed by the demonstration of a unilateral, unilocular cystic ovarian structure on transvaginal ultrasound. Usually, no active treatment is required and surgery is rarely necessary. In older women, it is essential to ensure that more serious ovarian pathology is not present. The scan can be repeated 1 to 2 months later to confirm spontaneous disappearance.

Other side effects

Headaches, dizziness, nausea, mood changes, abdominal bloating, breast tenderness, loss of libido or a number of vague symptoms may be reported with any progestogen-only method. These usually subside within the first few months. It is unclear how often these reported symptoms are actually caused by the progestogen method since almost all these symptoms are common in daily life. Placebo studies with COC carried out 20 to 30 years ago indicated that there was little difference in the incidence of most of these symptoms between the active pill-taking and placebo groups (even with higher dose pills). Weight gain is rarely caused by low-dose progestogens, but may be a problem for a minority of DMPA and NET-EN users.

Acne

Acne can sometimes be caused or exacerbated by the slightly androgenic progestogens such as levonorgestrel or NET. Good skin care will usually carry the woman through a period of adjustment to the new method, although rarely a user may need to discontinue that particular method.

MANAGEMENT OF CLINICAL PROBLEMS

Treating progestogen-associated breakthrough bleeding can be difficult. Pretreatment counselling about the range of possible menstrual changes, including amenorrhoea and erratic bleeding or spotting, is vital with all progestogen-only methods. There is limited evidence to confirm that a 3-week course of COC or oestrogen alone (ethinyloestradiol 50 µg daily) will stop an episode of prolonged bleeding and perhaps improve the long-term menstrual pattern in Norplant users (Diaz et al 1990). The same effect probably applies with other methods. Oestrogen should not be given to women using very low-dose methods such as POP, because it may counteract the contraceptive effect of the progestogen on cervical mucus. Mefenamic acid (500 mg three times daily) may also help.

Persistent ovarian follicles or cysts will usually settle spontaneously, but if not, or if the pain is severe, transvaginal needle drainage under ultrasound guidance may be curative. Surgery is rarely necessary.

Vague general symptoms will usually subside within a few months. If they do not, POP-users may try a different formulation. No simple guidelines exist for management of these symptoms with long-acting methods, but temporary symptomatic treatment and counselling may be remarkably effective in allowing continuation of a method which is otherwise highly suitable for the woman. If symptoms are persistent and troublesome, the method may need to be terminated. With DMPA and NET-EN, the woman will need to wait until the progestogen is completely out of the system, which may take many weeks, but it is surprsing how infrequently this lack of flexibility causes real problems.

INDIVIDUAL METHODS

Progestogen-only pills

Specific attributes

In a pill-taking society, these have the advantage of familiarity, as well as the flexibility to stop and start whenever the woman wishes. This very flexibility is also the major disadvantage, since the low dosage of POP means that there may be little margin for delay in taking each tablet. In some women, the effect on cervical mucus is already wearing off by 24 hours.

Administration

The pill-taking regimen must be carefully explained. Patient information leaflets are not always clear, and do not replace careful one-to-one instruction. Meticulous attention to timing of daily pill-taking must be emphasized.

Pills are dispensed in bubble packs with the day of the week and direction arrows clearly marked. The number of pills per packet may vary. Currently available preparations in the UK are shown in Table 3.2.

Starting. When the first pill is taken depends on the circumstances.

1. The first pill should be taken:
   a. when starting for the first time: on the first day of the next period
   b. when changing from a combined pill: on the day following the last active pill in the COC packet
   c. after pregnancy: generally 3 to 4 weeks after delivery. Lactation should preferably be well established, since some women notice changes in milk volume in the early weeks. POP may occasionally cause postpartum bleeding disturbances if given before 3 weeks. It is not necessary to await the return of menstruation
   d. after termination of pregnancy: within 24 hours.
2. Further pills are taken every day thereafter without a break.

Pills should ideally be taken at the same time every day. The best time is between 4 and 10 hours before intercourse is likely to take place, when the effect on cervical mucus is maximal. However, timings between 2 and 20

Table 3.2   Progestogen-only pills

Name	Progestogen	Dose	No. of pills per packet
Femulen	Ethynodiol diacetate	500 µg	28
Noriday	Norethisterone	350 µg	28
Micronor	Norethisterone	350 µg	28
Neogest	Levonorgestrel	37.5 µg*	35
Microval	Levonorgestrel	30 µg	35
Norgeston	Levonorgestrel	30 µg	35

* Plus 37.5 µg of inactive isomer.

hours should be reasonably safe. For most women, the optimum time would be a set hour in the late afternoon or early evening, but each woman will need to work out the preferable time for herself and the best time is that when she is most likely to remember to take it. For the 40% of women who continue to ovulate apparently normally while taking POP, these considerations of timing may be very important.

Extra contraceptive precautions. These are recommended for 7 days in the following circumstances:

- if the pill is taken more than 3 hours late.
- if a pill is forgotten – the missed pill should be taken as soon as the mistake is recognized, and the regular pill for the next day at the usual time.
- if vomiting occurs within 3 hours of pill-taking, another tablet should be taken. If this pill is also vomited, additional contraceptive precautions should be taken during the upset and for 7 days after symptoms have subsided.
- if an attack of severe diarrhoea occurs, the pill may not be completely absorbed. Extra contraceptive precautions and normal pill-taking should be continued through the episode and for 7 days afterwards.
- extra precautions may be needed to cover short-term drug interactions.

Emergency contraception. This should be considered if two or more POPs have been missed and intercourse has already taken place. POP use should be resumed the day after emergency contraceptive use, and follow-up planned to exclude pregnancy (see ch. 8).

When transferring from POP to COC. The first new active pill should be taken on the day after stopping POP, and should usually begin during menstruation (unless the woman has lactational or other amenorrhoea).

Effectiveness

Maximum effectiveness depends on meticulous tablet-taking and individual motivation of the woman. Efficacy is clearly related to age with failure rates being of the order of 3 per 100 woman-years (HWY) in a motivated population aged 25–29, but only 0.3 per HWY in women aged 40 years or over (Vessey et al 1985). Higher failure rates occur when tablet-taking is poor, and in some studies have been as high as 10 per HWY.

Preliminary evidence that failure is more common in women who are overweight has not been confirmed.

Efficacy is very high in lactating women.

Some studies have suggested that the rate of ectopic pregnancies might be increased compared with the normal population. This has not been confirmed, but it seems likely that POPs do not decrease the risk of ectopic pregnancies as much as they do intrauterine pregnancies.

Specific indications

a. Use during lactation is the most popular indication for POP in most countries.
b. Where an oral preparation is desired but oestrogen is contraindicated.
c. As an alternative to COC prior to elective major surgery.
d. For women with medical conditions such as diabetes mellitus, migraine or mild hypertension where COC is less desirable.

Specific contraindications

a. Women who are unreliable or unwilling pill-takers.
b. Drugs which may interact.
c. A history of recurrent functional ovarian cysts.
d. POPs should generally be avoided in teenagers whose lifestyle does not lend itself to the strict compliance required.
e. POPs should be avoided in severe obesity because of decreased efficacy.

Specific side effects and complications

a. Menstrual irregularities which typically include unpredictable short or long cycles with variable duration bleeding and/or spotting; amenorrhoea occasionally occurs. Menstrual disturbances with POP tend to be less than with most long-acting, progestogen-only methods.
b. Persistent ovarian follicles and follicular cysts.
c. Rare exacerbation of pre-existing medical diseases such as severe hypertension, obstetric cholestasis, cirrhosis or hydatidiform mole.

Controversies and medicolegal aspects

There are few persisting controversies about POP, which is among the most underused of methods of effective, well-studied and widely available contraception.

Injectables

Specific attributes

The major advantage is simplicity of administration combined with pro-longed duration of action. A 3-monthly injection schedule seems to suit many women well, with shorter intervals being less convenient.

Oestrogen–progestogen once-a-month combined injectables offer the benefit of more regular menstrual bleeding patterns, with the monthly episode of bleeding about 15 days following the injection, but the incon-venience of relatively frequent injections. They are now marketed in an increasing number of countries including the USA, China and several Latin American countries and should be given in the same way as NET-EN (Ch. 18).

Amenorrhoea becomes prominent with prolonged use of DMPA. This is seen as a major advantage by some and unacceptable by others. The effect of DMPA may take many months to wear off after the last injection, resulting in an unpredictable delay in return of fertility. The effects of NET-EN are less pronounced than DMPA. DMPA may have a small effect on rate of loss of bone mineral over many years. This issue remains to be resolved (see below).

Administration

Deep intramuscular injections are given into the gluteal region (or occasionally into the deltoid, especially in the very obese). The injection site should not be massaged since this sometimes dissipates the depot, resulting in higher initial blood levels and shortened duration of action.

The recommended dosage of DMPA is 150 mg and NET-EN is 200 mg.

1. The DMPA vial should be well shaken before loading the syringe; new administration procedures include preloaded syringes in some countries.
2. The NET-EN vial should be warmed close to body temperature.
3. The first injection must be given within the first 5 days of the start of the menstrual cycle.
4. Subsequent injections should be given according to a schedule marked on a calendar for the client; DMPA is usually given every 90 ± 7 days, while the optimal NET-EN schedule is more complicated. For the first 6 months, NET-EN should be given once every 60 ± 5 days, and then at 84 ± 7-day intervals to maximize efficacy and minimize side effects.
5. DMPA has a much greater safety margin for delay in the next injection than NET-EN and can be left with reasonable confidence up to 16 weeks. Longer intervals may still be quite safe, but patients need to be advised about a possible small increased risk of contraceptive failure. For medicolegal reasons, it is wiser to do a pregnancy test if the interval is prolonged beyond 12 weeks.

Effectiveness

Failure rates below 0.5 per HWY for DMPA have been reported in almost all large-scale studies in a wide variety of different communities (Fraser and Weisberg 1981). Failure rates with NET-EN are slightly higher, but are still usually less than 1 per HWY. The incidence of ectopic pregnancies is very low. Once-a-month injectables also have a very low failure rate of less than 0.5 per HWY.

Indications

In the UK, DMPA is now licensed for long-term, general contraceptive use. It may also have particular benefits for contraception for women with certain pre-existing conditions:

a. sickle cell disease (DeCeulaer et al 1982)
b. endometriosis
c. defective ovulation, especially polycystic ovarian disease (in preventing the risk of endometrial carcinoma)
d. certain other medical conditions (see pp **98–101** under special considerations).

NET-EN is licensed in the UK for short-term use (up to two injections) in the following circumstances:

a. in conjunction with rubella immunization
b. for the partners of men undergoing vasectomy, or postpartum women awaiting interval sterilization.

Contraindications

a. Injectable methods should not be used in women with coagulation disorders.
b. DMPA should be avoided in women who may not tolerate amenorrhoea or prolonged erratic spotting.

Specific side effects and complications

Delay in return of fertility. This is only a problem for DMPA-users, who may experience a prolonged interval before normal ovulation returns. The delay is due to persistence of MPA in the circulation, because microcrystals in the injected depot may sometimes dissolve very slowly. The average delay in return of fertility is 7 to 8 months beyond the calculated 3- to 4-month effect of the last injection. This means that some women will take well over a year to conceive.

There is no evidence that DMPA causes permanent sterility. NET-EN causes a very small delay, but the combined injectables are not known to have any lasting effect following the last dose.

Weight gain. This is rarely caused by low-dose progestogens, but may be a problem for a minority of DMPA- and NET-EN-users. A small gain of 1–2 kg often stabilizes during continued use but a very small number of women continue to gain moderate amounts of weight as long as they use the method. The main mechanism appears to be an increase in appetite with laying down of increased fat stores, but a small anabolic effect can occur.

Strict dieting and an exercise programme will help, but many women find this difficult to pursue in the long term. The weight gain is not generally the result of 'fluid retention', and diuretics do not help.

Controversies and medicolegal aspects

DMPA (marketed by Pharmacia Upjohn as Depo-Provera) has been the major focus of a number of concerns arising from different groups in society over the past three decades. Much of the controversy has arisen in the USA where DMPA was first manufactured, but where marketing approval for contraception was only given in 1992 after a lengthy saga where political, media and feminist agendas played a more prominent role than science or clinical medicine. These same influences have resulted in the contraceptive availability of DMPA being restricted in the UK, Australia and some other countries. These controversies are now fading as time passes, and as the main antagonists of this safe, effective and much maligned method have moved on to other issues.

Animal toxicology

There have been a number of real concerns about the possible effects of DMPA on the body, most of which have now been dismissed or put in sensible context. These began with the difficulties of extrapolating from excessive dose animal toxicology, where female beagles on long-term, high-dose DMPA developed increased rates of breast cancer, and rhesus monkeys on lifetime treatment were found to have developed the occasional endometrial cancer. Although these animal cancers have now been demonstrated to have no predictive value for human risk and such toxicology is no longer required by drug regulatory agencies, the stigma caused by repeated negative media publicity has persisted against DMPA.

Cancers

There are now extensive World Health Organization (WHO) epidemiological data on women who have used a variety of hormonal contraceptives. All demonstrated a very similar situation in relation to reproductive cancers (Meirik 1994).

1. DMPA provides a major degree of protection against the development of endometrial adenocarcinoma, and possibly against ovarian cancer (not yet confirmed).
2. In an analysis of the worldwide epidemiological evidence on the relationship between breast cancer risk and use of hormonal contraceptives (Collaborative Group on Hormonal Factors in Breast Cancer 1996), there was some evidence of an increase in the risk among current users of POPs and injectables for use in the previous 5 years. The risk had returned to normal by 10 years after stopping. In contrast to the COC data, the number of users was small.
3. Any increased risks of carcinoma of the cervix with DMPA are very difficult to evaluate because of multiple confounding factors, but all hormonal contraception, including DMPA, may play a very small promoting role.
4. There is no evidence of an increase in risk of liver, pituitary or other tumours.

In utero and neonatal exposure

Concern was expressed at one stage that inadvertent exposure to progestogens of the fetus in utero or of the breast-fed neonate could cause adverse effects on growth and development. This has been extremely difficult to disprove, but adequate long-term data now exist to be reasonably reassuring on both these concerns.

The only uncertain issue is the possible risk of masculinization of a female fetus exposed continuously over the first 4 to 5 months of pregnancy to a weakly androgenic progestogen, such as NET-EN.

Bone loss

The possibility that long-term DMPA use may increase the rate of bone mineral loss (Cundy et al 1991), resulting in a slightly increased risk of osteoporosis in later life, has yet to be completely resolved. There is now an extensive literature of mainly cross-sectional data showing that most women do not show any substantial bone loss while using DMPA, but some do. It is suspected that very low levels of circulating oestradiol in some DMPA-users may be primarily responsible for this bone loss. This issue will require a good prospective longitudinal study before it can be resolved. There is no consensus on the value of undertaking serum oestradiol levels or bone density scans in asymptomatic women receiving DMPA but it would seem sensible to pay particular attention to women with other risk factors for osteoporosis, e.g. heavy smoking or steroid use.

Feminist and consumer concerns

As the first of the successful long-acting methods, DMPA has drawn the attention of a number of feminist and consumer groups spanning a wide spectrum of philosophies. These groups still express real worries about the potential for misuse or even abuse of some methods, and they emphasize the difference between 'informed consent' and 'informed choice' of method.

There is a need for women to feel that they have control over their decisions, particularly in relation to technology which they do not understand. This requires the provision of simple but full information about the advantages and disadvantages of new methods, and this may include brief discussion of controversies. Willingness for dialogue on the part of feminist, consumer and media groups may be important for successful introduction of new technologies where consumer choice is involved.

Subdermal implants

Specific attributes

These systems are all made with a non-biodegradable polymer, such as polydimethyl siloxane or polyethylene vinyl acetate, with the active progestogen contained in the core of a capsule or evenly dispersed through a polymer rod. They have very prolonged duration of action (1 to 5 years) and very high contraceptive efficacy which requires no action on the part of the user. They require small operations under local anaesthesia for insertion and removal, and are usually inserted just under the skin of the forearm where they can be palpated for easy removal but are not obvious on inspection. They provide very constant and low blood levels of contraceptive steroid, by steady diffusion from the rod or capsule, which decline very slowly over the lifespan of the device. They can be removed when required with very rapid return of fertility.

In common with all progestogen-only methods, menstrual bleeding patterns tend to be erratic and unpredictable in the first few months following insertion, but gradually become more regular with time as serum levels decline. Implanon appears to produce a higher incidence of amenorrhoea than Norplant or Jadelle.

Norplant is a six-capsule system manufactured by Leiras, Finland and now marketed worldwide jointly by Schering & Wyeth. It contains levonorgestrel in the core of each capsule.

Norplant has now been withdrawn voluntarily from the market in the UK because the manufacturers perceived that it was no longer a good commercial proposition following medicolegal and media activity, even though the legal class action against it had collapsed (p. 97).

Two new subdermal contraceptive implants have recently become available on the market in Europe. Jadelle and Implanon are both highly effective, safe and acceptable contraceptives and have similar attributes. They are already marketed in several countries in Europe and North America. Uniplant is also effective and safe but has a much shorter duration of action. It is marketed in several Latin American countries.

Implanon is a single-rod system which releases etonogestrel (previously known as 3-keto-desogestrel), 60–70 µg/day in week 5–6, decreasing to 35–45 µg/day at the end of 1 year and to 25–30 µg/day at the end of 3 years. It is easy to insert and remove and has an excellent pharmacological and clinical profile. This new method has been reviewed in detail in several publications (Archer et al 1998, Edwards and Moore 1999).

Jadelle is a two-rod system which releases levonorgestrel (around 35 µg/day by 18 months) and has a pharmacological and clinical profile which is almost identical to Norplant. Its major advantage compared with Norplant is the relative ease of insertion (with a well-designed preloaded inserter) and removal.

Uniplant is also a single-rod system marketed in several Latin American countries and utilizes nomogestrol acetate as the progestogen. It is effective for 1 year.

Administration

Health professionals need to be carefully trained in the techniques of insertion and removal of subdermal implants, and users need to be given thorough counselling and written information prior to insertion.

Many countries have developed formal training programmes with certification of competence to ensure that subdermal implants are used optimally. It is strongly recommended that all doctors using new implants should be appropriately trained in their use prior to prescribing them, to avoid potential medicolegal pitfalls.

Norplant insertion is carried out using standard sterile precautions and local anaesthesia through a 3–5 mm incision in the skin of the inner aspect of the upper arm. Insertion usually takes 10 to 15 minutes.

Although Norplant is no longer marketed in the UK, there are a number of Norplant-users who will need to have the implants removed in due course. Removal is also carried out with sterile precautions and local anaesthesia through a 3–5 mm incision at the site of original insertion. Removal is usually very straightforward if the capsules have been inserted correctly in the first place. Each capsule is palpated and manipulated in turn so that the lower end protrudes at the incision. The tip is grasped with forceps, the thin overlying fibrous sheath is split with a second pair of forceps and the Norplant capsule withdrawn.

Implanon is a single-implant system and therefore particularly easy to insert, and the inserter is well designed and simple to use (Fig. 3.1). Removal is also straightforward and is carried out using standard techniques, as above. On average, 30 minutes of counselling and 3 minutes are required for insertion.

Jadelle is easy to insert using a specially designed preloaded inserter which allows placement of each rod in a slightly different position under the skin of the forearm. A simple, narrow fan shape is usually utilized. Removal is carried out using the same techniques as Norplant, but is much easier because of the small number of implants.

Effectiveness

Norplant. Excellent long-term efficacy data demonstrate that this is one of the most effective reversible contraceptives currently marketed. Most studies have demonstrated pregnancy rates of less than 0.5 per HWY even after 5 years of use (Sivin 1988). Early data indicating somewhat lower efficacy in women over 70 kg after 3 years of use (owing to reduced blood levels) appear to have been corrected by modifications to the device. Very obese women may still face an increased failure rate, but data are limited. Ectopic pregnancies are rare.

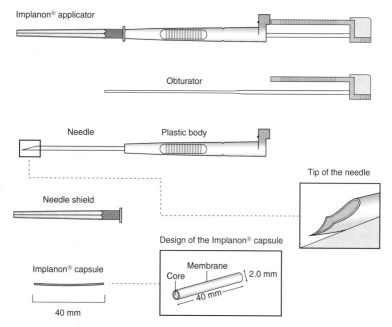

Figure 3.1 Implanon – a single capsule with a disposable inserter.

Jadelle. This has virtually identical contraceptive effectiveness to Norplant, and is marketed as a 5-year method.

Implanon. This newly marketed method has extremely high contraceptive efficacy with no pregnancies at all being recorded in the phase III trial. It is marketed for 3-year use.

Specific indications

a. All are first-choice methods for those who wish them.
b. Requirement for long-acting contraception for 1 to 5 years or more.
c. Unreliable or unwilling pill-takers.
d. Women who like the convenience of prolonged action.

Specific contraindications

a. Intolerance of amenorrhoea or unpredictable menstrual disturbance.
b. Uncertainty about intentions for another child in the near future.

Specific side effects and complications

a. The major problem is menstrual disturbance (see above).
b. WHO, the Population Council and Family Health International have undertaken a major 5-year postmarketing surveillance study involving Norplant, IUDs and female sterilization. This is due to appear in a series of publications in late 2000, and shows that Norplant is remarkably free of side effects and serious complications.

Controversies and medicolegal aspects

Norplant has engendered a great deal of medicolegal activity in the USA, and a smaller amount in the UK. Initially doctors were sued for difficult removals, resulting in unsightly scarring of the arm. This was extended to include legal action for a multitude of recognized side effects on the basis of the doctor having 'failed to warn' adequately of the severity of these effects. The class action in the UK collapsed because the Legal Aid Board withdrew support, but then Norplant was voluntarily withdrawn because it had become commercially 'non-viable'. In the USA, most suits (including some class actions) which have been concluded have been settled in favour of the distributing pharmaceutical company. However, the cost of successfully defending such cases has become unreasonably expensive, and the pharmaceutical company has made an offer to pay all remaining plaintiffs a limited sum in settlement, without admission of liability, in order to conclude the outstanding cases.

It is anticipated that the medicolegal problems faced by Norplant will not affect other implants provided that doctors using the products will be willing to participate in approved training programmes.

Intrauterine systems (IUS)

The uterus appears to be a particularly suitable route for administration of low-dose, long-acting contraceptive progestogen, with delivery of a sufficiently high local dose to provide highly effective contraception as well as greatly reducing the volume of the menstrual periods and providing other health benefits (Ch. 4).

SPECIAL CONSIDERATIONS

Adolescents

While the compliance necessary for POP use probably precludes this method for many teenagers, some find long-acting methods such as the subdermal implants and DMPA to be highly acceptable (Ch. 9). Double protection with condoms may be appropriate for those at some risk of exposure to sexually transmitted infections.

Older women and the perimenopause

Progestogen-only methods of all types may be very suitable for older women (Ch. 17).

Women with pre-existing medical disorders

Progestogen-only methods may be the best choice for many such women, although patient information leaflets often still provide a counsel of excessive caution against their use. It is also essential to weigh up the risks of unplanned pregnancy in women with these conditions, while balancing the small uncertainties about long-term progestogen use.

Women with pre-existing medical conditions must be given reasonable information about the advantages and disadvantages of the relevant contraceptive choices in the light of their own particular condition, bearing in mind that there will always be a small degree of uncertainty about how a method will affect any individual.

Cardiovascular system

1. A history of superficial or deep venous thromboembolism does not appear to be a contraindication to use of any progestogen-only method. Pregnancy may be a significant risk for these women.
2. Myocardial infarction or stroke is not thought to be a contraindication to progestogen use, although extensive data do not exist. Low-dose methods are probably preferable because they allow secretion of endogenous ovarian oestradiol which is important for normal vascular endothelial cell function and protection against further cardiovascular episodes. Norplant, Jadelle, Implanon and Mirena are satisfactory choices because of their very high contraceptive efficacy.
3. Hypertension:
   a. Mild hypertension or where blood pressure is well controlled. Progestogen-only methods are generally suitable, and the low-dose methods are preferable. Blood pressure control should be kept under regular review
   b. Moderate or severe hypertension. Low-dose progestogens may be prescribed with careful supervision. It may be sensible to begin with a method which can be easily stopped if the woman experiences a significant rise in blood pressure attributable to the method. This risk appears to be small.

It is uncertain whether long-term progestogen use interacts adversely with severe hypertension or the risk of cardiovascular disease.

Breasts

1. Benign breast disease may improve with progestogens, although the response is variable.
2. Women with breast cancer should probably avoid use of progestogen-only methods, unless alternatives are unsuitable. It is possible that a small proportion of breast cancers in young women may be stimulated by progestogen exposure, although others may even be inhibited. Data on these effects are limited. Progestogens are a reasonable choice for women in whom breast cancer has been adequately treated.

Genital tract

1. Women with pre-existing endometriosis, adenomyosis or uterine fibroids may benefit from progestogen-only contraception in contrast to COC. Endometriosis is most likely to benefit from higher dose treatment. Adenomyosis often continues to cause symptoms of erratic and painful bleeding, but in some patients will improve.

Fibroids may continue to grow, but some will stabilize in size and symptoms reduce.
2. Malignant diseases of the genital tract are not contraindications to progestogen use. It is usually recommended that hormonal contraceptives are avoided in women with hydatidiform mole until β-human chorionic gonadotrophin levels have returned to zero, and in women with choriocarcinoma until cure is confirmed. High-dose progestogens like DMPA and NET-EN may be contraceptives of choice in women with a history of endometrial hyperplasia or adenocarcinoma.

Liver

1. Women with a previous history of hepatic adenoma should not use steroid contraception of any kind, although the risk of recurrence with low-dose progestogens must be very small.
2. Severe active hepatitis could be exacerbated by progestogens, as may poor hepatic function in chronic cirrhosis. If progestogens are to be used in women with any degree of liver failure, low-dose preparations should be used, and liver function monitored.
3. Previous hepatitis with normal liver function is not a contraindication.
4. Porphyria is usually felt to be a contraindication to use of any hormonal contraceptive, although it is more prominently related to oestrogen exposure than progestogens.
5. There is no evidence that gallstones are exacerbated or precipitated by progestogen-only methods, but data are limited.
6. Obstetric cholestasis is less likely to recur with low-dose progestogens than with COC.

Autoimmune disease

Exacerbations of autoimmune diseases, such as systemic lupus erythematosus, are not usually increased during progestogen-only contraceptive use, although progress of the condition should be monitored carefully during the first few months of use of any new medication.

Nervous system

1. Focal migraine (with unilateral neurological signs) is another phenomenon which is often exacerbated by oestrogen, but rarely by progestogen. Therefore, low-dose progestogens may be suitable contraceptives for these women.

2. Epilepsy is rarely exacerbated by progestogens, but higher dose progestogens should generally be used because of occasional drug interactions which may reduce the contraceptive efficacy of the lower dose preparations (see above).

Skin

Chloasma is an oestrogen-stimulated phenomenon and will usually fade steadily during progestogen use. These women should be advised to wear hats and use 'block-out' sunscreens when exposed to direct sunlight for any length of time.

Diabetes mellitus

Low-dose progestogen-only methods do not appear to make the management of diabetes more difficult or increase the risk of complications. Injectables may alter the dosage requirements for diabetic control, but there is no evidence of increase in complications.

Sickle cell disease

There is good evidence that DMPA will improve the haematological picture and reduce the incidence of painful sickling crises, and this may be the contraceptive of choice for them (DeCeulaer et al 1982). Other progestogens may provide acceptable alternatives, but oestrogen should be avoided.

There are no data on other haemoglobinopathies or other progestogens in sickle cell disease.

Drug interactions

These are less of a problem for progestogen-users than COC-users, although women using low-dose methods such as POP, implants or vaginal rings may run some risk with certain drugs. Higher dose methods, such as DMPA or NET-EN, are preferable in women using rifampicin or most anti-epileptic drugs.

If doctors are suspicious that an interaction is occurring between progestogen contraceptives and any other drug, they should notify the Committee on Safety of Medicines on the appropriate yellow card.

Future fertility and pregnancy

There is no evidence to suggest that any progestogen method causes infertility following the end of expected contraceptive effect. It needs to be remembered that 10–15% of all couples will consult a doctor at some time about difficulty in conceiving, and several studies have indicated that this rate does not appear to be increased after hormonal contraception.

Before starting DMPA, potential users must be warned that there may be a substantial temporary delay in return of fertility beyond the normal duration of effective action of the drug.

There is no evidence that women who become pregnant immediately after stopping a progestogen method are at increased risk of fetal abnormality, and there is no justification for advising any delay before attempting to conceive.

Occasionally, a woman may inadvertently continue with use of her hormonal contraceptive after conceiving. There is no evidence of a significant increase in risk of birth defects in these women.

Interpretation of laboratory tests

Progestogen-only methods have little or no effect on common biochemical tests.

Indications for stopping progestogen-only contraception

There are few medical indications for stopping progestogen-only methods. These include:

1. Confirmed pregnancy when the woman does not wish to consider termination.
2. Acute liver disease.
3. Significant and maintained increase in blood pressure which requires treatment.
4. Side effects which are unacceptable to the patient.
5. When another pregnancy is desired.
6. When contraception is no longer required. With very long-acting methods, such as implants or the IUS, the woman may wish to leave her system in place in case of future requirement for contraception.
7. When menopause is reached (Ch. 17).

CONCLUSION

In many countries, progestogen-only methods have not yet gained the popularity that might have been expected. This particularly applies to POP which has not been widely promoted by manufacturers, but deserves more widespread use, especially in older women. The resolution of several controversies, the introduction of new delivery systems and increasing public awareness will undoubtedly lead to an increase in the use of progestogen-only methods. With increased use will come many more questions about side effects, especially about the management of menstrual bleeding irregularities. The provision of clear and simple information at the time of starting the method, with reinforcement at follow-up, has been shown to lead to high rates of satisfaction and excellent continuation rates of use with all these methods.

REFERENCES

Archer D, Kovacs L, Landgren BM (eds) 1998 Implanon, a new single-rod contraceptive implant; presentation of clinical data. Contraception 58: 75S–115S

Belsey E, Task Force on Long-Acting Systemic Agents for Fertility Regulation 1988 Vaginal bleeding patterns among women using one natural and eight hormonal methods of contraception. Contraception 38: 181–206

Brache V, Alvarez-Sanchez F, Faundes A, Tejada AS, Cochon L 1990 Ovarian endocrine function through five years of continuous treatment with Norplant subdermal implants. Contraception 41: 169–177

Collaborative Group on Hormonal Factors in Breast Cancer 1996 Breast cancer and hormonal contraceptives: Collaborative reanalysis of individual data on 53,297 women with breast cancer and 100,293 women without breast cancer from 54 epidemiological studies. Lancet 1996; 347: 1713–1727

Cundy T, Evans M, Roberts H, Wattie D, Ames R, Reid IR 1991 Bone density in women receiving depot medroxyprogesterone acetate for contraception. British Medical Journal 303: 13–16

DeCeulaer K, Gruber C, Hayes R, Serjeant GR 1982 Medroxyprogesterone acetate and homozygous sickle cell disease. Lancet i: 229–231

Diaz S, Croxatto HB, Pavez M, Belhadj H, Stern J, Sivin I 1990 Clinical assessment of treatments for prolonged bleeding in users of Norplant implants. Contraception 42: 97–109

Edwards JE, Moore A 1999 Implanon: a review of clinical studies. British Journal of Family Planning 24: 3–16

Fraser IS, Weisberg E 1981 A comprehensive review of injectable contraception with special emphasis on depot medroxyprogesterone acetate. Medical Journal of Australia 1 (Suppl 1): 1–19

Landgren BM, Diczfalusy E 1980 Hormonal effects of the 300 µg norethisterone (NET) minipill. 1. Daily steroid levels in 43 subjects during a pretreatment cycle and during the second month of NET administration. Contraception 21: 87–113

Meirik O 1994 Updating DMPA safety – Preface to an issue on DMPA and cancer. Contraception 49: 185–188

Sivin I 1988 International experience with Norplant and Norplant-II contraceptives. Studies in Family Planning 19: 81–94

Vessey MP, Lawless M, Yeates D, McPherson K 1985 Progestogen-only oral contraception. Findings in a large prospective study with special reference to effectiveness. British Journal of Family Planning 10: 117–121

World Health Organization 1998 Cardiovascular disease and use of oral and injectable progestogen-only contraceptives and combined injectable contraceptives. Results of an international multicentre, case-control study. Contraception 57: 315–324

4

Intrauterine contraceptive devices

Meera Kishen

Types of intrauterine
  device   106
  Inert (non-medicated)
    devices   106
  Copper-bearing devices   107
  Hormone-releasing devices   108
Mode of action   108
Effectiveness   109
Advantages   109
  Compliance and
    continuation   109
  Cost   110
  Gynaecological benefit   110
  Reversibility   111
  Malignancy   111
Disadvantages   112
  Menstrual bleeding
    pattern   112
  Infection   112
  Expulsion   113
  Perforation   113

Indications   113
Contraindications   113
  Absolute contraindications   113
  Relative contraindications   114
Clinical management   115
  History   115
  Examination   115
  Choice of device   115
  Insertion   115
  Client instructions   119
  Follow-up   119
  Removal   119
  Removal technique   119
Complications and their
  management   120
  Bleeding and pain   120
  Vaginal discharge   121
  Pelvic infection   122
  Pregnancy   123
  Lost threads   124
  Lost devices   125

Intrauterine contraceptive devices (IUDs) are an effective, safe and convenient contraceptive option for many women. They are the most commonly used reversible method of contraception worldwide with about 100 million current users, most of them in China. The current generation of IUDs is more than 99% effective in preventing pregnancy over 1 year of use.

Like most methods of contraception, the IUD has been the subject of adverse publicity. In the past, there has been concern about an association between IUD use and increased risk of pelvic inflammatory disease (PID) and subsequent infertility. Recent research has clarified some of these concerns showing that the IUD by itself does not cause PID or infertility. There is virtually no increased risk of infertility in a woman using a copper IUD who is in a mutually monogamous sexual relationship. The commonest side effect – heavy and painful periods – that often results in discontinuation of IUD use can now be overcome by use of a hormone-releasing intrauterine system (IUS). Using an IUD is many times safer than undertaking a normal pregnancy.

TYPES OF INTRAUTERINE DEVICE

Presently available IUDs belong to three main groups: inert, copper-bearing and hormone-releasing. IUDs come in many shapes and sizes (Fig. 4.1). All currently available devices have one or two nylon filaments attached to the lower end to facilitate removal.

Inert (non-medicated) devices

The World Health Organization (WHO) does not recommend insertion of inert IUDs, because copper-bearing and hormone-releasing devices are

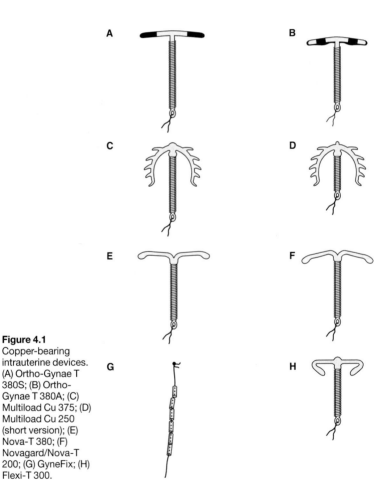

Figure 4.1
Copper-bearing intrauterine devices. (A) Ortho-Gynae T 380S; (B) Ortho-Gynae T 380A; (C) Multiload Cu 375; (D) Multiload Cu 250 (short version); (E) Nova-T 380; (F) Novagard/Nova-T 200; (G) GyneFix; (H) Flexi-T 300.

much more effective. They are no longer manufactured although some older women may still have them in situ.

Copper-bearing devices

Copper-bearing IUDs are generally licensed for use over 5 to 10 years with some variations from country to country. The Nova-T 380 is licensed for 5 years and the Copper T 380 is licensed for up to 10 years continuous use in western Europe. They all consist of a plastic frame with copper wire round the stem and some have copper sleeves on the arms. The surface area of the copper determines the effectiveness and active life of the device. The lifespan of many devices actually exceeds the manufacturer's specifications.

Frameless devices

A frameless copper intrauterine implant, GyneFix (Fig. 4.2) has been developed in an attempt to reduce the common side effects associated with framed copper IUDs (Wildermeersch et al 1999). GyneFix consists of a non-biodegradable, monofilament, polypropylene thread and six copper beads providing a total surface area of 330 mm^2. The upper and lower beads are crimped onto the thread to keep the others in place. A knot at the upper end of the filament serves as an anchor which is implanted into the fundal myometrium. A version of the device with a slightly bigger anchoring knot

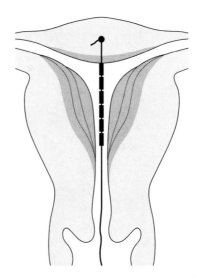

Figure 4.2
GyneFix at insertion. The line drawings represent different cavity shapes.

has also been developed for immediate insertion after childbirth or abortion. The device is licensed in Europe for 5 years' use.

Hormone-releasing devices

The levonorgestrel-releasing intrauterine system (LNG-IUS) (Fig. 4.3) was developed by the Population Council. Approved for use in Finland and Sweden since 1990, it was licensed in the UK in 1995 under the tradename of 'Mirena' ('Levonova' in other European countries). It consists of a Nova-T frame with a column of LNG within a rate-limiting membrane around its vertical stem. It contains 52 mg LNG released at a rate of 20 µg/day. It is licensed in Europe for 5 years' use but trials have shown no loss of efficacy after 7 years' use.

MODE OF ACTION

All IUDs cause a foreign-body reaction in the endometrium, with increased prostaglandin production and leucocyte infiltration. This reaction is enhanced by copper, which affects endometrial enzymes, glycogen metabolism and oestrogen uptake and also inhibits sperm transport. The number of spermatozoa reaching the upper genital tract is reduced in copper-bearing IUD-users. Alteration of uterine and tubal fluid impairs the viability of the gametes and both sperms and ova retrieved from copper-bearing IUD-users show marked degeneration (WHO 1997). Early hormone surveillance shows

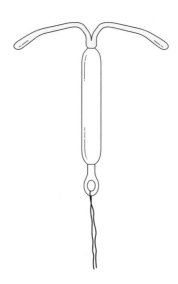

Figure 4.3
Mirena – levonorgestrel-
releasing intrauterine system.

Table 4.1   Mechanisms of action of intrauterine devices

Mechanism of action	Copper-bearing IUD	Hormone-releasing IUS
1. Interferes with ability of sperm to pass through uterine cavity	Yes	Yes
2. Interferes with fertilization process in the fallopian tube before ovum reaches the uterine cavity	Yes	Yes
3. Inhibits implantation if a fertilized egg enters the uterus by causing local inflammatory response in the endometrium	Yes	Yes
4. Interferes with sperm movement by thickening cervical mucus	No	Yes
5. May interfere with implantation through hormonally-induced endometrial changes	No	Yes

no evidence of pregnancy in users of modern copper-bearing IUDs. Prevention of implantation is therefore not the most important mechanism of action except when a copper-bearing IUD is used for postcoital contraception.

The LNG-IUS induces endometrial atrophy and the development of hostile cervical mucus, further enhancing its effectiveness (Table 4.1).

EFFECTIVENESS

IUDs are more effective in practice than oral contraceptives. Efficacy has improved, from pregnancy rates at 1 year of 2–3% with early inert and copper-bearing devices to less than 0.5% with newer devices which contain over 300 mm^2 of copper (Fig 4.4). Failure rates are even lower in older women whose natural fertility is declining. Ectopic pregnancy rates with IUD use have likewise declined (Fig. 4.5). Pregnancy rates for GyneFix are less than 1% per year (Van Kets et al 1995).

The LNG-IUS has an annual pregnancy rate of around 0.2 per 100 woman years of use with no observed increase in the rate of ectopic pregnancy.

For all devices, the rates of pregnancy, spontaneous expulsion and removal for bleeding tend to fall with continuing use.

ADVANTAGES
Compliance and continuation

IUDs require very little compliance for successful use. Apart from the initial visits for counselling and insertion, there is little demand on time or effort on the woman's part to achieve contraceptive efficacy. It is a method of

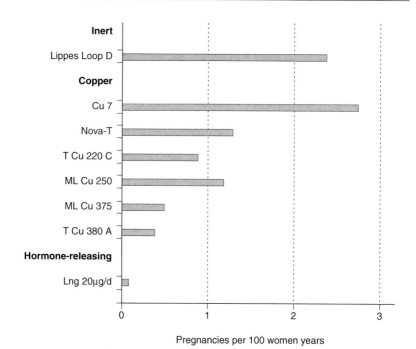

Figure 4.4   Rate of intrauterine pregnancies with intrauterine devices. (Adapted with permission from Farley TMM 1997 Evolution of IUD performance. IPPF Medical Bulletin 1(4) August.)

contraception that is totally unrelated to coitus, which makes it attractive to many users. Any copper-bearing IUD inserted in a woman over 40 years of age can be left in situ until the menopause without concern regarding its continued effectiveness.

Cost

Modern IUDs are effective and long acting and copper-bearing devices are extremely inexpensive. They provide contraception for up to 10 years and are therefore highly cost-effective. However, the LNG-IUS is expensive, just under £80 in the UK compared with under £10 for framed copper-bearing devices and around £20 for the frameless GyneFix.

Gynaecological benefit

The LNG-IUS has additional benefits beyond contraception and is increasingly being used for the management of gynaecological problems (Sturridge

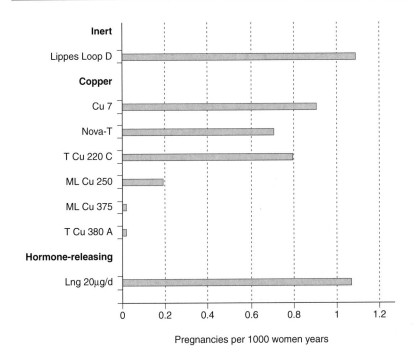

Figure 4.5   Rate of ectopic pregnancies with intrauterine devices. (Adapted with permission from Farley TMM 1997 Evolution of IUD performance. IPPF Medical Bulletin 1(4) August.)

and Guillebaud 1997). It markedly reduces menstrual flow and dysmenorrhoea and can be useful in the treatment of menorrhagia (Anderson and Rybo 1990). Frequent spotting, however, often precedes the development of oligoamenorrhoea, especially during the first 3 months of use.

Reversibility

IUDs are generally removed very easily and return of fertility is rapid (conception rates of 78–88% after 12 months and 92–97% at 3 years after removal). Fertility returns immediately after removal of an LNG-IUS.

Malignancy

In contrast to hormonal methods, there are no concerns about increased risks of malignant disease.

DISADVANTAGES

Menstrual bleeding pattern

Heavier and more prolonged menstrual periods are a common side effect of copper-bearing IUDs. Over 10% of IUD-users report menstrual problems. Removals for medical reasons, primarily for increased menstrual bleeding, pain and intermenstrual spotting, are around 4% per annum. Though periods do still get heavier with GyneFix, removal rates for pain and bleeding are generally low.

Infection

The overall PID rate in IUD-users is around 1.4 to 1.6 cases per 1000 woman years of use which is double the risk compared to women using no method of contraception. The risk is increased during the first 20 days following insertion (9.7 per 1000). This is related to the introduction of infective organisms into the uterine cavity at the time of insertion, especially if the woman has an undetected infection or if the provider fails to use proper aseptic techniques. Although the IUD itself does not cause pelvic infection, the sexual behaviour of the woman and her partner may increase the risk of acquiring sexually transmitted infections (STIs) and consequently pelvic infection (Farley et al 1992). Tubal damage and subsequent infertility are serious consequences of pelvic infection in women.

Expulsion

IUDs can become spontaneously displaced or expelled from the uterine cavity. Spontaneous expulsion rates of modern IUDs (including LNG-IUS) range from around 3 to 10% in the first year of use, depending on the age and parity of users, timing of insertion and type of IUD, as well as the expertise of the person inserting the device (Fig. 4.6). Expulsion rates in the second and subsequent years for framed devices remain very low. Postplacental IUD insertion is associated with much higher expulsion rates. Early indications are that GyneFix is associated with a low expulsion rate of less than 1% per year.

Perforation

Perforation of the uterus is a rare event (less than 1 in 1000 insertions) and is related to the type of IUD, insertion technique, and the skill of the provider. There is some evidence to suggest that the risk of fundal perforation is greater early in the postpartum period before the uterus is fully involuted. Special care is required during postpartum insertion whether or not the woman is lactating.

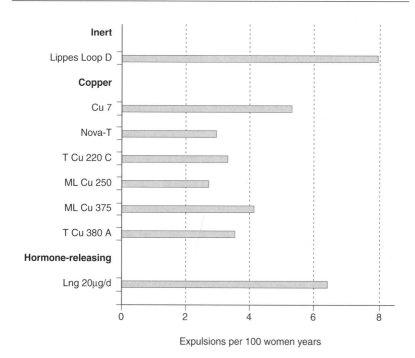

Figure 4.6   Rate of expulsions with intrauterine devices. (Adapted with permission from Farley TMM 1997 Evolution of IUD performance. IPPF Medical Bulletin 1(4) August.)

INDICATIONS

The IUD can be considered as a first choice contraceptive method for a woman in a mutually monogamous couple, even if she is nulliparous. It is particularly appropriate for women who have difficulties in using a contraceptive method which demands compliance. Immediately reversible, the IUD is well suited to women who are spacing pregnancies. It also offers long-term effective contraception to those who may have completed their families but wish to avoid or defer sterilization. Copper-bearing, but not hormone-releasing, devices are highly effective as emergency contraception (Ch. 8).

The LNG-IUS may be particularly indicated for women with menorrhagia as it combines effective contraception with reduction in menstrual loss.

CONTRAINDICATIONS
Absolute contraindications

1. Known or suspected pregnancy.
2. Undiagnosed abnormal vaginal bleeding. However, once uterine or cervical pathology has been excluded, an IUD can be fitted.

3. Suspected malignancy of the genital tract. An IUD can be fitted after local therapy for early lesions of the cervix.
4. Active or recent (in the past 3 months) STI or PID.
5. Severely distorted uterine cavity that prevents proper insertion/placement, e.g. large fibroids.
6. Copper allergy or Wilson's disease (rare) – for copper-bearing devices only.

Relative contraindications

1. Menorrhagia and anaemia. This is a relative contraindication to copper-bearing IUDs but an indication for the LNG-IUS.
2. Multiple sexual partners. If the woman is in a new or unstable relationship, the risks of PID and infertility have to be weighed against her inability or unwillingness to use another method and the risk of an unplanned pregnancy
3. Recent history of treated pelvic infection. Past history of a single episode of confirmed PID adequately treated is not a contraindication to IUD use provided there are no continuing, predisposing risk factors. However, recurrent episodes of PID must be viewed as a strong relative contraindication to IUD use.
4. Age and nulliparity. Age and nulliparity by themselves do not constitute a contraindication to IUD use. In general, however, younger women are at higher risk of acquiring STIs because of higher levels of sexual activity and possibly more sexual partners. In view of the potential damage to future fertility, adequate counselling of young, nulliparous women wishing to use an IUD is essential.
5. Valvular heart disease. There is a risk of sub-acute bacterial endocarditis, especially at the time of IUD insertion. Appropriate antibiotic cover at the time of insertion should be given to women with a prosthetic heart valve.
6. Systemic corticosteroid treatment, immunosuppressive therapy and HIV infection or AIDS. These conditions affect the immune system, thereby increasing the risk of infection. An IUD may not be the ideal contraceptive for these women. All alternative options must be considered first.
7. Recent benign trophoblastic disease. Bleeding irregularities associated with IUD use may cause difficulties in the follow-up and management of the condition.
8. Current anticoagulant therapy. Use of a copper-bearing IUD may lead to particularly heavy periods in women on heparin or taking warfarin. The LNG-IUS is more appropriate for these women as it is likely to reduce menstrual flow.

CLINICAL MANAGEMENT

Successful IUD use depends on more than a well-designed and tested IUD. Providers must ensure a woman's suitability for an IUD based on good history-taking, including assessment of risk of STIs; correct insertion technique; informative and empathetic counselling to enable informed choice and satisfaction.

The assessment of a woman prior to IUD-fitting should include a detailed history and a pelvic examination, including investigations to exclude reproductive tract infection if indicated.

History

History should include details of age, past contraceptive use, menstrual history, past obstetric and gynaecological history, past history of STIs/pelvic infection, and nature and duration of current relationship to enable assessment of risk of STIs in future. Exploring the woman's reason for choosing an IUD, her knowledge of other contraceptive options and a detailed discussion of the risk/benefit profile of the IUD for her will allow fully informed choice.

Examination

1. Examine the vagina and cervix with a speculum to exclude abnormality and infection.
2. Take swabs (vaginal and endocervical) to exclude infections if indicated.
3. Pelvic examination to determine the size, shape and position of the uterus and to confirm that the appendages are normal.

Choice of device

Currently, the Copper T 380 is the gold standard among copper-bearing IUDs in terms of efficacy and duration of action. A woman's previous experience with IUDs may sometimes determine the device chosen, e.g. unexplained expulsion of a device or pain related to past IUD use uncomplicated by infection may lead to consideration of GyneFix. Problems with a current IUD may dictate a change, e.g. menorrhagia may require consideration of LNG-IUS.

Insertion

If the insertion procedure has been explained and the woman's questions and concerns have been addressed, she is likely to be more relaxed during the procedure thus facilitating insertion and minimizing discomfort. The correct insertion technique substantially reduces the risks of pregnancy and complications – expulsion, bleeding and pain, perforation and infection.

Equipment required for insertion

Light source.
Bivalve speculum.
Bacteriological swabs (when appropriate).
Cotton wool swabs.
Antiseptic solution.
Clean gloves.
Disposal bags for used instruments and clinical waste.
Sterile kidney dish/tray (receptacle for insertion instruments).
Sterile 10-inch sponge-holding forceps.
Sterile malleable uterine sound graduated in centimetres.
Sterile 12-inch tissue forceps or single-toothed tenaculum with blunted tips.
Pair of scissors which are long enough to allow the threads to be cut.

Timing of insertion

An IUD may be inserted at any time during the menstrual cycle provided pregnancy has been excluded. It may be inserted immediately after suction termination of pregnancy or evacuation of spontaneous abortion, and 6 weeks after childbirth whether by vaginal or caesarean delivery. Post-placental insertion (within 48 hours after delivery) is safe and convenient, particularly in settings where subsequent contact with healthcare providers may be difficult, but is associated with high expulsion rates.

Insertion during a menstrual period has conventionally been recommended for the following reasons: pregnancy is unlikely; the cervix is softer and the internal os slightly open, possibly making insertion easier; post-insertion bleeding is disguised by menses. However, there are disadvantages – expulsion rates are slightly higher as uterine contractility is increased and some women prefer not to be examined during menstruation.

For IUD insertion as an emergency method of contraception, see Chapter 8.

Insertion technique

As the method of insertion is different for each device, insertion is safest if the manufacturer's instructions are followed meticulously.
1. Throughout the whole procedure, a 'no-touch' technique should be employed. The part of the sound and the loaded introducer which enter the uterus must not be touched, even by a gloved hand, at any time. Hence, use of clean gloves (non-sterile) is sufficient.

2. Following bimanual examination of the pelvis, the cervix is exposed with a speculum while the woman lies in a modified lithotomy or lateral position.
3. The cervix is cleansed with antiseptic and grasped with 12-inch atraumatic forceps (long Allis's forceps are often used). Gentle traction to straighten the uterocervical canal helps achieve fundal placement.
4. A uterine sound is passed gently to determine the depth and direction of the uterine cavity and the direction and patency of the cervical canal. If cervical spasm/stenosis is encountered, local anaesthetic administration and dilatation of the cervical os may need to be considered.
5. The device is loaded into the introducer in such a way that it will lie flat in the transverse plane of the uterine cavity when it is released.
6. The device should not remain in the introducer tube for more than a few minutes as it will lose its 'memory' and become distorted in shape.
7. The introducer tube is carefully inserted through the cervical canal, the IUD released according to the specific instructions for each device, and the introducer withdrawn.
8. Following insertion, further sounding of the canal to exclude low placement of the device is recommended. Fundal placement is essential to achieve a low incidence of expulsion and pregnancy.
9. The IUD threads should be trimmed with long scissors to about 3 cm from the external os.

Note. IUDs must be inserted and removed by trained personnel. Studies show no difference in complication rates between insertions performed by doctors and by other trained providers.

The technique of GyneFix insertion is simple but different from that of conventional IUDs. Special training in the insertion technique is recommended to ensure proper implantation into the fundus.

Problems at insertion

Syncope and bradycardia. Severe pain associated with vasovagal syncope – 'cervical shock' – is rare, but may be caused by dilatation of the internal cervical os with the sound or introducer. Adequate preparation of the client by counselling and appropriate selection for local analgesia (surface analgesia by gel/spray, intra- or para-cervical block) can reduce the incidence of cervical shock.

The vasovagal episode is usually transient and self-limiting and the insertion procedure can be completed safely. If severe, insertion may have to be abandoned and the woman resuscitated. If the woman fails to recover quickly with basic resuscitation manoeuvres, the IUD may have to be removed to facilitate recovery.

If a woman develops a bradycardia during the insertion procedure:

1. The procedure must be stopped and the foot end of the bed elevated and oxygen administered if available through a face mask.
2. A clear airway must be maintained – by supporting the chin or use of an airway. Any tight clothing, especially around the neck, should be loosened.
3. Pulse, blood pressure and breathing should be monitored.

If the bradycardia is persistent:
4. The IUD should be removed.
5. Atropine 0.5 mg should be administered intravenously.

If the woman becomes unconscious:
6. Call for help/emergency ambulance to transfer the woman to a nearby hospital.
7. Check and maintain airway, breathing and circulation.

Epileptic attacks. These are sometimes precipitated by IUD insertion, especially in women with a past history of epilepsy.

Resuscitation

1. IUD insertion must always be carried out in the presence of a nurse/trained assistant who should monitor the condition of the woman during IUD insertion.
2. The necessary equipment and drugs to deal with cervical shock/convulsions/cardiac arrest should always be available in IUD clinics (Box 4.1).
3. All professionals fitting IUDs must be trained and updated in basic resuscitation skills.

Perforation. This is rare and occurs in no more than 1.3 per 1000 inser-tions. Careful insertion technique can prevent most perforations. Perforation may be partial, with just part of the IUD piercing the uterine or cervical wall, or complete, with the IUD passing through the uterine wall into the peritoneal cavity. Most perforations occur at the time of insertion and may go unnoticed unless the clinician is vigilant. Perforations occur most often at the uterine fundus and heal quickly without any treatment. If perforation occurs at the time of sounding, the procedure should be stopped

---

Box 4.1   Contents of a resuscitation box

1. Airway
2. Face mask
3. Atropine (0.5 mg/mL ampoules)
4. Rectal diazepam (10 mg in 2.5 mL suppositories)
5. Adrenaline (1 in 1000 solution – 1 mg in 1 mL ampoules)

and the client observed for signs of internal bleeding. If the perforation is recognized only after the device has been inserted, the woman should be referred for removal of the device by laparoscopy/laparotomy. Copper-bearing devices cause an intense inflammatory reaction within the peritoneal cavity leading to adhesions.

Failure to insert. This may be due to client anxiety, poor operator technique or anatomical abnormality of the cervix or uterus. If unusual difficulty is encountered, the fitting should be abandoned and the woman asked to return at a later date to see a more experienced clinician in IUD fittings. Care should be taken to provide interim contraception for the woman.

If a difficult IUD insertion is anticipated, vaginal administration of misoprostol 400 μg the night before will soften and dilate the cervix to allow easier insertion, particularly in older women.

Client instructions

Most women do not experience any problems following IUD insertion. Some report mild-to-moderate, lower abdominal pain, nausea and rarely, syncope. Women are generally advised to rest for 10 to 15 minutes following IUD insertion. Simple analgesics often relieve pain/discomfort.

Before the woman leaves the clinic, she should be given a written record of the date and type of IUD inserted. She should be instructed to check the IUD threads regularly. She should check for the threads often in the first few weeks of use and thereafter on a monthly basis at the end of her period.

Follow-up

The woman should be seen at least once around 6 to 12 weeks after IUD insertion to ensure that she is not experiencing any problems. Her ability and confidence in checking the threads should be confirmed. A vaginal examination is advisable to check that the IUD is in position. Women are usually advised to attend for review annually thereafter. Such regular contact with healthcare providers affords an opportunity to assess any other reproductive health needs.

Removal

IUD removal is usually straightforward. It can be done at anytime in the menstrual cycle. If the woman does not wish to become pregnant in that cycle, she should avoid intercourse in the 7 days prior to removal or the IUD should be removed during menstruation and alternative contraception started immediately. If, for any reason, the IUD must be removed without application of the '7-day rule', emergency contraception must be offered. Removal of GyneFix is simple and is by the same technique.

Removal may be difficult if IUD threads are not visible or if the IUD has become partially embedded in the uterus. If the IUD cannot be removed easily, the woman should be referred to an experienced clinician.

Removal technique

Threads visible

1. Expose the cervix with a speculum and clearly visualize the IUD threads.
2. Grasp the thread(s) firmly near the external os with a pair of straight artery forceps.
3. Apply gentle downward traction. Usually the IUD will be withdrawn without difficulty and with minimal pain. If resistance to removal is encountered, or if the patient experiences pain, stop traction and:
4. Check the size and position of the uterus by bimanual examination.
5. Grasp the cervix with tissue forceps and apply gentle traction to straighten out the uterocervical canal.
6. Continue traction on the threads and remove in the usual way.
7. Sometimes it may be necessary to administer local anaesthesia to reduce discomfort to the woman during removal.

If threads break

During removal, the cervical canal should be explored gently with the straight artery forceps to check if the lower end of the device has descended into the canal. If felt, the vertical stem of the device can be grasped and removed. If the device remains totally within the uterine cavity, exploration of the cavity with a long, thin, curved forceps or a 'hook' may be carried out to locate and remove the device. Cervical dilatation may be achieved by prior preparation with a single dose of misoprostol 400 µg vaginally prior to uterine exploration. Only doctors experienced in intrauterine techniques should attempt to carry out such procedures.

Intrauterine device changes

IUDs should not be replaced before the recommended intervals as removal and re-insertion increase the risk of failure, expulsion and infection. In a woman aged 40 or over, copper-bearing IUDs may be left unchanged until 12 months after the final menstrual period.

COMPLICATIONS AND THEIR MANAGEMENT
Bleeding and pain

Increased menstrual bleeding, often with pain, is the commonest problem associated with IUD use. Some 15% of women request removal of the device within a year of insertion because of problems related to bleeding. Pre-insertion counselling, that gives women realistic expectations of the method, and adequate follow-up both influence continuation rates.

Menstrual irregularities

For the first few months intermenstrual bleeding or spotting may occur, but decreases with time. Pre-and post-menstrual spotting lasting 2 to 3 days is also common.

Increased menstrual loss

Despite great individual variability, all copper-bearing devices increase the amount and/or duration of bleeding. Hormone-releasing devices reduce the amount of menstrual loss to less than pre-insertion levels, though it must be emphasized to the user that it may take between 3 and 6 months for this to happen.

All medical management of IUD-related menorrhagia is empirical. Non-steroidal anti-inflammatory drugs (NSAIDs) and even the combined oral contraceptive pill have been used with varying success. If the main concern is development of/aggravation of anaemia, oral iron supplementation must be considered. If intolerable menorrhagia persists despite treatment, or recurs after a time-limited period of treatment, the IUD should be removed.

Pain

Pain may persist for a few days following insertion and usually responds to rest and analgesics. IUD use may cause or exacerbate dysmenorrhoea which may be alleviated by NSAIDs. It has been postulated that irritation of the uterine wall by the transverse arms of framed devices may exacerbate dysmenorrhoea, hence the development of the frameless device, Gynefix. Pelvic pain other than dysmenorrhoea must be investigated to exclude other possibilities such as incorrect placement of the device or infection.

Vaginal discharge

Watery or mucoid discharge is common in IUD-users. It may cause concern to the woman as discharge is usually perceived to be associated with infection. It is important to explain the basis of such 'non-infective' discharge at pre-insertion counselling.

In the presence of a low-grade, anaerobic infection, the discharge may become offensive. If profuse or persistent, vaginal and endocervical swabs should be taken to exclude infection. Bacterial vaginosis is commoner among IUD-users than among women not using an IUD. It usually responds to a short course of oral metronidazole but often recurs. Women must be given information on the nature of the infection and reassured that it is not sexually transmitted. In the event of persistent or recurrent symptomatic vaginal infection, the IUD may have to be removed.

Pelvic infection

The diagnosis of PID associated with IUD use is notoriously inaccurate as it is usually based on clinical criteria. Patients with vaginal discharge and/or uterine pain are commonly labelled as suffering from PID – particularly if they have an IUD in place – yet these symptoms do not by themselves signify infection.

A woman is most likely to develop PID just after IUD insertion. Analysis of 13 WHO clinical trials found that women were 6.3 times more likely to develop PID in the 20 days following IUD insertion than at any later time. This risk can be minimized by proper screening of clients and by meticulous attention to preventing infection during the insertion procedure. There is no rationale for routine antibiotic cover for all women undergoing IUD insertion; it will have no effect on the future risk of IUD-users acquiring STIs which remains the main cause of PID related to IUD use. Providers should describe the symptoms of PID (Ch. 13) and encourage women to seek medical help promptly if symptoms appear, especially in the first month post-insertion.

The type of IUD may influence the risk of PID. The Dalkon Shield with multifilament threads was five times more likely to be linked to PID than other IUDs. Moreover, the increased risk persisted in long-term users of the Dalkon Shield unlike other devices. There is little evidence, however, to suggest that cutting the threads off a standard copper IUD to provide a tailless device reduces the incidence of PID. A European multicentre study reported significantly lower rates of PID associated with the LNG-IUS than with Nova-T, a copper-bearing device. However, further studies have not confirmed that the LNG-IUS actually protects against PID.

The uterine cavity is free of bacteria 3 to 4 weeks after IUD insertion. Pelvic infection developing more than 4 months after IUD insertion is due to other factors such as acquisition of an STI.

For diagnosis and management of PID, see Chapter 13.

Actinomycosis

Actinomycosis of the genital tract is very rare. The presence of actinomyces-like organisms (ALOs) in the cervical smears of IUD-users has in the past created concern as clinicians have associated this with a potential risk of pelvic actinomycosis. In the absence of any symptoms, smears revert to normal within 3 months of removing or replacing the IUD. The presence of ALOs on cervical smears is not considered clinically significant in an asymptomatic IUD-user although current opinion is however divided as to whether IUD removal is necessary (Cayley 1997). Once the situation has been explained, an asymptomatic woman who is happy to be monitored may retain the IUD. The smear should be repeated after 6 months.

Pregnancy

Intrauterine pregnancy

In the rare event of a woman becoming pregnant with an IUD in situ, she has a higher risk of spontaneous early or mid-trimester pregnancy loss (which may be associated with sepsis), premature labor and increased perinatal mortality if the device is left in situ. If pregnancy is confirmed in an IUD-user up to 12 weeks gestation, the device should be removed if the threads are accessible. If the threads are not seen or felt at the cervical os, the presence or absence of the IUD within the uterus should be confirmed by ultrasound scan. If the woman wishes to continue with the pregnancy, she can be reassured that there is no evidence for an increased risk of congenital malformation.

After 12 weeks gestation, the threads have usually been drawn up into the enlarged uterine cavity. Even if they are visible, there is a greater likelihood of the device being firmly wedged alongside the conceptus. The device should be left in place.

At delivery, the IUD is usually expelled with the placenta and membranes. If not, an ultrasound examination and/or abdominal X-ray should be carried out early in the puerperium to locate it.

Ectopic pregnancy

If a woman using an IUD is suspected of being pregnant, the possibility of ectopic pregnancy should always be considered. Modern IUDs are highly effective and reduce the risk of all types of pregnancy including ectopic pregnancy, particularly when compared with women not using contraception. However, when pregnancy occurs with an IUD in utero, the risk of it being an ectopic pregnancy is increased as IUDs provide more protection against intrauterine than extrauterine pregnancy.

The symptoms of ectopic pregnancy – pain and menstrual irregularity – may be mistakenly attributed to PID or even to the IUD itself. Classical symptoms of pregnancy such as amenorrhoea may be absent. The diagnosis should be suspected if there is any unexplained pelvic pain, lower abdominal cramps, any irregular bleeding and especially if a period is scanty, late or missed (Ch. 15). Sensitive β-hCG tests that are currently available for clinic-based urinary testing are likely to confirm a pregnancy even at low levels of hCG. If the clinical picture is suspicious of an ectopic pregnancy, even if the pregnancy test is negative, the woman must be referred for urgent gynaecological assessment.

Lost threads

Short IUD threads can create difficulties for both the woman and the clinician in locating the threads at routine checks to confirm the presence of the IUD in utero.

Threads not visible

If threads are not visible at the time of examination, the following possibilities should be considered:

1. Threads drawn into the uterine cavity – alongside the device in a normal or an enlarged uterus (exclude pregnancy).
2. Expulsion of the device.
3. Delayed perforation/transmigration of the device.

To locate missing threads

1. Carefully expose the cervix, in a good light, as this will allow short threads in the cervical canal to be seen.
2. If no threads are seen, clean the cervix and explore the endocervical canal (up to the level of the internal os) with Allis forceps, opening and closing the instrument within the canal. In about one-third of cases, the threads will be brought down.
3. Gently sound the uterine cavity, applying tissue forceps to the cervix to straighten out the canal. An IUD in the canal or uterus will usually be felt with the sound.
4. A thread retriever (Emmett or Retrievette) should be passed into the uterine cavity and gently rotated before being withdrawn. This will retrieve the threads in about 50% of cases (Bounds et al 1992). If IUD removal is desired, one or more of a variety of IUD retrievers, such as an IUD hook or Patterson alligator forceps, may be used to retrieve the device itself.
5. If these procedures fail to locate the IUD or retrieve the threads, ultrasonography should be performed to locate the position of the missing IUD. The woman should be advised that she should use another reliable contraceptive until the intrauterine position of the device has been confirmed. Only 4% of women with lost threads will ultimately require uterine exploration under general anaesthesia (Bounds et al 1992).

Lost devices

Expulsion

Most spontaneous expulsions occur in the first year of use, especially in the first 3 months after insertion, and often during a menstrual period. Although expulsion is uncommon, women should be advised to examine towels and tampons, especially in the first 3 months, to check this. They should also report unexplained pelvic pain or intermenstrual bleeding as these may signify expulsion.

Complete expulsion of the device may be diagnosed if the threads are not seen on examination and if ultrasound examination of the pelvis and/or X-ray of the abdomen fail to reveal the presence of the IUD in the uterus or the abdominal cavity. If the woman wishes, another IUD may be inserted. Second insertions, even of the same type of IUD, are associated with lower expulsion rates than first insertions.

Partial expulsion is much more common than complete expulsion. Part of the device, usually the end of the vertical stem, is found protruding from the cervical canal. The woman may feel the hard tip of the device during routine self-examination or she may present with pain or intermenstrual bleeding and the clinician may detect the tip at IUD check. If the device is found partially expelled, it should be removed, and if the woman wishes, another inserted immediately. If for any reason it is not possible to re-insert the device at that visit, coital history should be obtained to ensure that emergency contraception may be provided if appropriate.

Perforation/transmigration

Perforation of the uterus is rare and almost always occurs during insertion. In large clinical trials, perforation rates of 1.3 per 1000 insertions have been reported. Transmigration of IUDs is usually the consequence of unrecognized partial perforation at insertion. The management involves:

1. If perforation is recognized prior to insertion, usually no treatment is required as fundal perforations heal quickly without further complications.
2. If perforation is recognized during or just after insertion of the device, the procedure should be stopped and the device removed immediately.
3. If the perforation is recognized within a few days or weeks after insertion, copper-bearing and hormone-releasing IUDs should be removed by laparoscopy or laparotomy.
4. If the perforation is not recognized at insertion and is diagnosed only when the woman presents some time after insertion with missing threads, the decision to remove the device surgically will depend on a number of factors, including the type of device, symptoms if any, risks of

surgical exploration and the woman's personal views. Lost inert devices have remained in the peritoneal cavity for years without producing problems. However, they do tend to migrate and may be found anywhere in the abdomen. Open or linear devices theoretically cause few problems but closed devices could cause intestinal obstruction. Copper-bearing devices cause a sterile inflammatory reaction and rapidly become adherent to the omentum or bowel. The woman may often be asymptomatic or present with abdominal pain. If complete or partial perforation is suspected or confirmed, the woman must be referred to a gynaecologist for evaluation and further management.

Displacement of intrauterine device within the uterine cavity

Occasionally, rotation of the IUD within the uterine cavity can occur. This will cause pain and bleeding and will necessitate removal of the device. Very rarely, downward displacement of the IUD may lead to cervical perforation. In both cases, referral to a gynaecologist for removal is advised.

REFERENCES

Anderson K, Rybo G. 1990 Levonorgestrel-releasing intrauterine device in the treatment of menorrhagia. British Journal of Obstetrics and Gynaecology 44: 473–480
Bounds W, Hutt S, Kubba A, Cooper K, Guillebaud J, Newman GB 1992. Randomized comparative study in 217 women of three disposable plastic IUCD thread retrievers. British Journal of Obstetrics and Gynaecology 99: 915–919
Cayley J 1997 Actinomyces-like organisms and intrauterine devices. British Journal of Family Planning 23:73.
Farley TMM 1997 Evolution of IUD performance. IPPF Medical Bulletin (4) August
Farley TMM, Rosenberg MJ, Rowe PJ, Chen JH, Meirik O 1992 Intrauterine devices and pelvic inflammatory disease: an international perspective. Lancet 339: 785–788
Sturridge S, Guillebaud J 1997, Gynaecological aspects of the levonorgestrel-releasing intrauterine system. British Journal of Obstetrics and Gynaecology 104: 285–289
Van Kets H, Wildermeersch D, Van der Pas H, et al 1995 The frameless GyneFix intrauterine implant; a major improvement in efficacy, expulsion and tolerance. Advances in Contraception 11: 137–142
Wildermeersch D, Batar D, Webb A, Gbolade B A, et al 1999 GyneFix. The frameless intrauterine implant – an update. For interval, emergency and postabortal contraception. British Journal of Family Planning 24: 149–159
World Health Organization (WHO) 1997 Intrauterine devices. Technical and managerial guidelines for services. WHO, Geneva

5

Barrier methods

Ailsa Gebbie

Occlusive pessaries (caps)   127
  Diaphragm   128
  Cervical cap   138
  Vault cap   142
  Vimule   143
  New types of occlusive
    pessaries   144
  Damage to occlusive
    pessaries   145
Female condom   145
Home-made barriers   147
Condoms   147
Spermicides   151

Creams and gels   151
Vaginal pessaries   151
Foaming tablets   151
Aerosol foam   151
Spermicidal film   153
The vaginal contraceptive sponge   154
Alternative spermicidal agents and
  delivery systems   157
**Adaptations of coital
  technique   158**
  Coitus interruptus   158
  Coitus outwith the vagina   159
Risks/benefits   159

A barrier method of contraception interrupts the process of human reproduction by blocking the progress of sperm from the male partner to the female and thereby preventing fertilization. From earliest times, an extensive array of barrier methods has been used by couples attempting to control their fertility. Nowadays, barrier methods still offer considerable advantages in terms of safety and reversibility. Their efficacy depends critically on quality of use. The failure rates of barrier methods are reduced significantly when they are used consistently and correctly by well-motivated individuals.

A marked decline in the use of barrier methods occurred following the widespread availability of oral contraception in the 1960s and 1970s. The spread of HIV infection into the heterosexual population has focused attention on barrier methods. The 'Safe Sex' campaign in the UK, promoting use of condoms to combat spread of the virus, has attempted to break down many traditional taboos concerning the openness with which sexuality and contraception may be discussed and dealt with.

OCCLUSIVE PESSARIES (CAPS)

For hundreds of years women have attempted to avoid pregnancy by preventing the access of sperm to the cervix. Various materials such as sponges and pads of cotton were used, but occlusive pessaries did not appear until the 19th century. The German gynaecologist Hasse (using the pseudonym

Mensinga) is credited with introducing the diapragm in 1882. Wilde described the use of a rubber pessary made to a wax model of the patient's cervix almost 50 years earlier. Since the 1950s, the diapragm or 'Dutch cap' has been by far the most commonly used type of occlusive pessary in the UK. Overall, female barrier methods are an unpopular method of contraception and a recent UK survey showed they are used by less than 1% of sexually active women aged 16 to 44 years (Schering Healthcare, unpublished data).

Types. Four main occlusive pessaries are in current use – the diaphragm, cervical cap, vault cap and the vimule.

Diaphragm

A diaphragm consists of a thin, latex rubber hemisphere, the rim of which is reinforced by a flexible flat or coiled metal spring. Sizes of the external diameter range from 55 to 95 mm, in 5 mm increments, but in practice most women use the 70–85 mm sizes (Fig. 5.1).

Variations

1. The flat-spring diaphragm has a firm watch-spring (Fig. 5.2A), remains in the horizontal plane on compression and is easily fitted. It is suitable for the normal vagina and is usually tried first.
2. The coil-spring diaphragm has a spiral coiled spring (Fig. 5.2B), is considerably softer than the flat-spring, and is particularly suitable for a woman who has tight vaginal musculature and is sensitive to the pressure of the flat-spring type. With the largest sizes, handling and insertion may be slightly less easy because of a tendency to twist on compression.

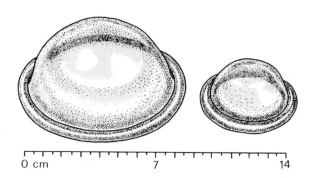

Figure 5.1
Large and small
diaphragms.

| 0 cm | 7 | 14 |

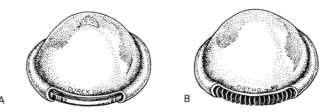

Figure 5.2 (A) Flat-spring Durex diaphragm to show rim in cross-section;
(B) Coil-spring Ortho diaphragm to show rim in cross-section.

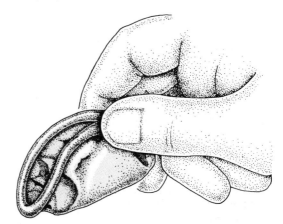

Figure 5.3
Arcing diaphragm.

3. The arcing diaphragm combines features of both the above and exerts strong pressure on the vaginal walls (Fig. 5.3). It is particularly useful when the vaginal walls appear lax or the length and position of the cervix make reliable fitting of the more common types of diaphragm difficult.
4. Variations in colour, texture and packaging have been introduced in an attempt to improve acceptability.

Mode of action

The diaphragm acts as a physical barrier during sexual intercourse to prevent sperm reaching the cervical mucus and thereby gaining access to the upper genital tract. It should lie diagonally across the cervix (see Fig. 5.7, p. **133**), reaching from the posterior vaginal fornix to behind the pubic symphysis. The largest comfortable size should be used as the vagina expands during sexual arousal.

Effectiveness

When a diaphragm is used correctly in conjunction with spermicide, the failure rate is 4–8 per 100 woman years (HWY). With less careful use, the failure rate may reach 10–18 per HWY (Bounds 1994). Higher efficacy is found when diaphragms are used by experienced users who have completed their families rather than by women who are spacing their pregnancies.

Because a sperm-tight seal between the rim of the diaphragm and the vaginal walls is impossible to achieve, the use of a spermicide in conjunction with all caps is recommended in order to provide maximum effectiveness. As spermicides add greatly to the 'messiness' of the method, a few women may decide to depend on the barrier function of the diaphragm alone. This cannot be recommended and one small study has demonstrated increased efficacy of the diaphragm when used with spermicide (Smith et al 1995).

Causes of failure, apart from poor motivation, are incorrect insertion or fitting, displacement during intercourse, and unnoticed defects in the diaphragm.

Indications

1. When a couple wish the woman to use a barrier method of contraception and find other contraceptive methods unacceptable.
2. When there are medical reasons that exclude the woman from taking hormonal contraception.
3. When a couple need intermittent, or infrequent, yet reliable contraception.

Contraindications

1. Poor vaginal muscular support or prolapse, although this may be overcome by careful assessment of the size and type of diaphragm fitted. Fitting should be delayed until at least 6 weeks postpartum to allow muscle tone to return.
2. Psychological aversion, or inability to touch the genital area.
3. Inability to learn insertion technique.
4. Lack of hygiene or privacy for insertion, removal and care of the diaphragm.

Advantages

1. No systemic side effects.
2. Effective when fitted and used correctly.
3. Does not interfere with lactation.

4. Spermicide provides extra lubrication if vaginal dryness is a problem.
5. Significant reduction in the risk of pelvic inflammatory disease relative to that of women using no method of contraception. Estimation of the degree of protection from the diaphragm alone is difficult as additional spermicide is almost always used and this may be the protective factor.
6. Reduction in the risk of pre-malignant disease and carcinoma of the cervix. Again, the use of spermicidal agents may be the actual protective factor.

Disadvantages

1. Requires premeditation, and thereby there is loss of spontaneity with intercourse.
2. Spermicide makes the method rather 'messy'.
3. May cause:
   a. Discomfort to the wearer or her partner during intercourse
   b. Loss of cervical and some vaginal sensation.
4. Has to be fitted and checked regularly by a trained doctor or nurse.
5. Does not provide protection against the transmission of HIV and other viral infections.
6. Sensitization to rubber or spermicide may develop.
7. Significantly more frequent candidal infections although the incidence of bacterial vaginosis is not increased.
8. Increased incidence of symptomatic urinary infection. This is thought to be the result of altered bladder neck angle and increased vaginal colonization with coliforms in diaphragm users. Women with recurrent urinary infections should be advised to use an alternative method of contraception.
9. Toxic shock syndrome following prolonged retention of a diaphragm has been reported in a very small number of cases.
10. Efficacy depends on correct use and sustained motivation.

Fitting a diaphragm requires time and patience on the part of trained personnel. Models and diagrams of the female anatomy will often improve understanding. An initial examination should be performed to assess the following:

1. Position and condition of the uterus and cervix.
2. Length of vagina and muscle tone.
3. Measurement of the distance between the posterior fornix and the posterior aspect of the pubic symphysis.

Screening procedures (e.g. cervical smear) should be carried out according to routine practice.

Selection and fitting

1. A diaphragm, corresponding roughly in size to the distance between the posterior fornix and the symphysis pubis, is chosen (Figs 5.4 and 5.5).
2. With the woman supine, the labia are separated, the diaphragm is compressed and inserted into the vagina, downwards and backwards into the posterior fornix, before being released (Fig. 5.6).
3. The anterior rim is tucked behind the pubic symphysis and the position of the cervix checked (Fig. 5.7).

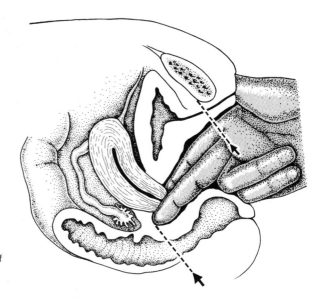

Figure 5.4
Estimating the size of diaphragm to be fitted.

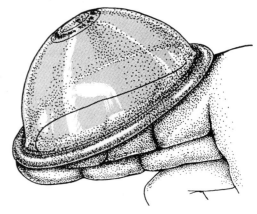

Figure 5.5
Size of diaphragm on hand.

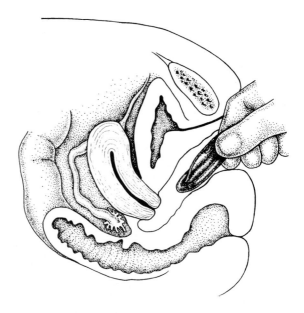

Figure 5.6
Diaphragm being
inserted.

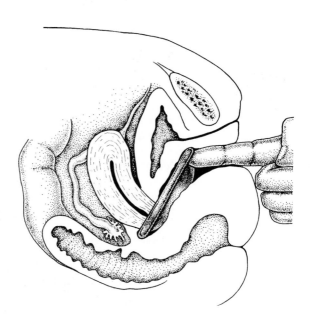

Figure 5.7
Checking the position
of the diaphragm.

4. Secure fitting is checked. When the woman strains down, the anterior rim of the diaphragm should not project or slip.
5. Too large a diaphragm may project anteriorly, be immediately uncomfortable, or become uncomfortable or distorted after being worn (Fig. 5.8A).
6. If the diaphragm is too small, a gap will be felt between the anterior rim and the posterior surface of the symphysis pubis, or it may even be inserted in front of the cervix (Fig. 5.8B).
7. Persistent anterior protrusion of the diaphragm may be due to a mild cystocele, and may be discovered only after the woman strains or stands up. In this case, a cap other than a diaphragm is required.
8. The flat-spring diaphragm is usually used dome-upwards and, if reversed (to increase retention behind the pubic symphysis), is slightly more difficult to remove. The coil-spring type is normally recommended for use dome-downwards. However, the decision which way up the diaphragm is fitted is crucial in only a few women.
9. The diaphragm is removed by hooking the index finger under the anterior rim and pulling gently downwards.

Teaching the woman

1. The woman squatting, or with one foot on a chair, or occasionally lying on her back, according to her preference, is first taught to feel the cervix (Fig. 5.9).
2. The instructor then inserts the diaphragm for the woman, allowing her to feel the cervix covered with the thin rubber. This is extremely important since correct placement of the diaphragm over the cervix is vital to its success.
3. The woman then removes the diaphragm by hooking her finger under the anterior rim and pulling downwards (Fig. 5.10).
4. She is then taught to insert the diaphragm herself, the instructions being precisely those given for fitting by the doctor or nurse. Emphasis is placed on the downward and backward direction in which the compressed diaphragm is inserted into the vagina. After releasing the diaphragm, the correct covering of the cervix must always be rechecked (Fig. 5.11), as should the snug fit of the anterior rim behind the pubic symphysis.
5. Variation in the order of teaching these techniques may be required for some women, depending on their aptitude.
6. If the woman repeatedly inserts the diaphragm into the anterior fornix, this can often be overcome by:
   a. The use of a larger diaphragm
   b. The use of an introducer (Fig. 5.12), or an arcing diaphragm where the difficulty is due to the length of the cervix

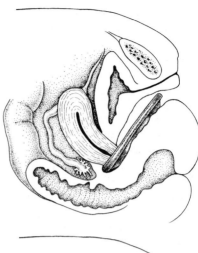

Figure 5.8A
Diaphragm too large.

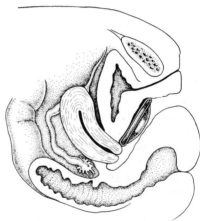

Figure 5.8B
Diaphragm too small.

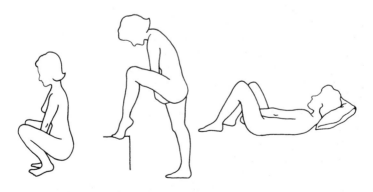

Figure 5.9   Positions for inserting a diaphragm.

   c. The partner being willing and able to learn the technique of insertion on the woman's behalf

   d. Allowing the woman to teach herself in privacy with the aid of a hand cassette instructor.

Instructions for use

1. The diaphragm may be inserted at any convenient time prior to intercourse to minimize the loss of spontaneity.
2. Insertion of the diaphragm can be incorporated as part of the woman's regular nightly routine, whether or not intercourse is planned.
3. To ensure maximum effectiveness, the diaphragm should always be used with spermicidal cream or gel.
4. A ribbon of cream or gel approximately 5 cm long is placed on the upper side of the diaphragm prior to insertion.
5. If the diaphragm has been in place for more than 2 hours prior to intercourse, additional spermicide should be inserted into the vagina.
6. The diaphragm should be left in position for at least 6 hours after the last act of intercourse.
7. Care of the diaphragm is essential, and after removal it should be washed in warm, soapy water and dried carefully. It should be restored to its normal rounded shape and stored in its container in a cool place. It should never be boiled. Perfumed soap, disinfectants or detergents should never be used to clean it, nor talcum powder to dry it.

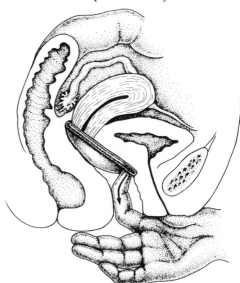

Figure 5.10
Removing the diaphragm
(standing position).

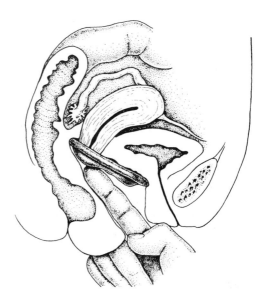

Figure 5.11
Checking the diaphragm
covering the cervix (standing
position).

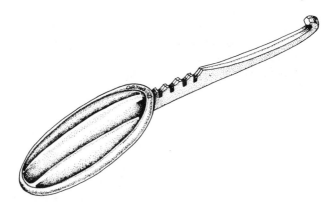

Figure 5.12
Introducer.

Follow-up

It is customary, but not mandatory, to provide a woman with a practice diaphragm for 1 week. This allows her to gain confidence in the technique of insertion, removal and care of the diaphragm and to assess whether it is comfortable. Practice caps were formerly sterilized and re-used but this is no longer recommended, and practice caps should be for single-patient use only and then discarded. The diaphragm should not be used for contraceptive purposes during this practice week.

The second visit allows rechecking of the size and fitting. The woman should be reviewed after 3 months, and yearly thereafter.

A diaphragm should be replaced annually, or immediately if any defect develops. The size and fitting should be reviewed if the woman loses or gains 4 kg in weight, and after pregnancy or vaginal surgery.

Cervical cap

This cap is shaped like a thimble and is designed to fit closely over the cervix. It is held in place by precise fitting onto the cervix and by suction, not by spring tension as in the diaphragm.

Variations

The Prentif cavity-rim cap, made of firm pink rubber with an integral thickened rim incorporating a small groove, is the most commonly used. This groove is intended to increase suction to the sides of the cervix. Sizes, measured from the internal diameter of the rim, range from 21 to 31 mm (Fig. 5.13). Other one-size rubber or silicone caps are now available (see below).

Mode of action

By covering the cervix, the cap acts as a physical barrier to the entrance of sperm into the cervical canal.

Effectiveness

Recent studies found pregnancy rates varying from 8 to 20 per HWY. Approximately half the pregnancies were due to user failure, and the other major cause was accidental dislodgement of the cap during intercourse.

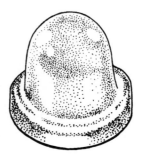

Figure 5.13
Cervical cap.

Indications

When there is a request for an occlusive pessary by a woman who is unsuitable for a diaphragm, provided the cervix is normal and healthy, pointing down the axis of the vagina and not acutely backwards.

Contraindications

1. Short or damaged cervix.
2. Purulent cervical discharge suggesting infection.
3. Inability to reach the cervix with the fingers.

Advantages

1. Suitable for women with poor muscle tone and some cases of uterovaginal prolapse.
2. Not felt by the male partner.
3. No reduction in vaginal sensation.
4. Fitting unaffected by changes in the size of the vagina, either during intercourse or as a result of changes in body weight.
5. Unlike a diaphragm, a cervical cap may be kept in place for several days. Some have proposed leaving it in situ for as long as the intervals between menses, although this is not recommended. In the UK, the standard practice is to advise patients not to wear it for longer than 24 hours at a time.
6. Unlikely to produce urinary symptoms.

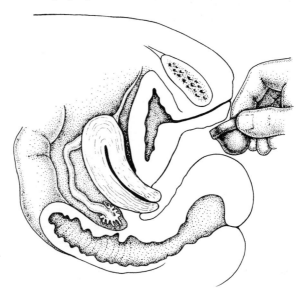

Figure 5.14
Cervical cap being inserted.

Disadvantages

1. Requires accurate selection of cap size and fitting to avoid displacement during intercourse.
2. Self-insertion and removal of a cervical cap are more difficult than with a diaphragm.
3. An unpleasant odour may develop if the cap is left in place for more than a day or two.

Selection and fitting

1. The correct size is that which allows the rim to touch the vaginal fornices easily without a gap, comfortably accommodates the cervix, and is not displaced when the woman bears down.
2. With the woman in the supine position, the labia are separated, the rim of the cap is compressed and then guided along the posterior vaginal wall until the posterior rim is just behind the cervix. The thumb and first two fingers are used as illustrated in Figure 5.14.
3. The cap is allowed to open by removing the thumb and then it is pushed upwards onto the cervix with the fingertips (Fig. 5.15). A final check is made to ensure that the cervix is palpable through the bowl and that no gap is left above the rim.
4. The cervical cap is removed by inserting a fingertip between the rim of the cap and the cervix, easing the cap downwards and withdrawing it with the index and middle fingers.

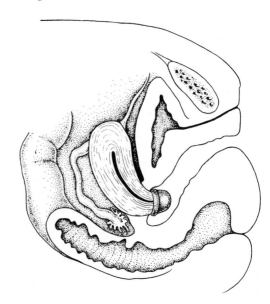

Figure 5.15
Cervical cap in situ.

Teaching the woman

The woman is taught to feel her cervix, and to insert and remove the cap, according to the instructions given above for fitting. In time, an experienced user will often develop her own technique for inserting and removing a cervical cap and, provided it is effective, this is quite acceptable.

Instructions for use and follow-up

The instructions for use of the diaphragm also apply to the cervical cap:

1. Spermicidal cream or gel is strongly advised and should be used to fill one-third of the bowl of the cap.
2. Further spermicide should be inserted into the vagina immediately prior to intercourse.
3. The position of the cervical cap should always be rechecked prior to each act of coitus to ensure that accidental dislodgement has not occurred.
4. The schedule of follow-up visits is the same as for the diaphragm.

Vault cap

This cap, made of rubber, is an almost hemispherical bowl with a thinner dome through which the cervix can be palpated (Fig. 5.16).

It is designed to fit into the vaginal vault, stays in place by suction, and covers, but does not fit closely to, the cervix. Five sizes are available ranging from 55 to 75 mm, in 5 mm steps.

Indications

1. Wish to use an occlusive cap.
2. Unsuitability for, or inability to use, a diaphragm.
3. Unsuitability of the cervix because of its shape or position for a well-fitting cervical cap.

Selection, fitting and teaching

These instructions are precisely the same as for the cervical cap, with modifications only in the siting of the upper rim. The correct size should cover

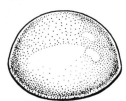

Figure 5.16
Vault cap (Dumas).

the cervix without exerting pressure on it, and fit snugly into the vaginal vault (Fig. 5.17).

Instructions for use and follow-up

These are identical to those of the cervical cap, with a spermicidal agent being used to fill one-third of the bowl of the vault cap prior to insertion.

Vimule

This is a variation of the vault cap with a thimble-shaped prolongation of the dome (Fig. 5.18). There are three sizes – small (45 mm), medium (48 mm) and large (51 mm). The vimule has fallen into some disrepute because of its association with the development of vaginal abrasions, possibly because of the relatively sharp-edged rim.

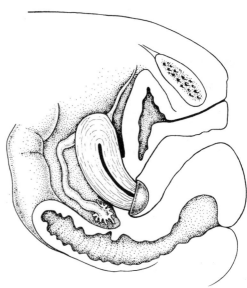

Figure 5.17
Vault cap in situ.

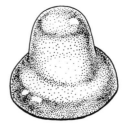

Figure 5.18
Vimule.

Indications

It is used specifically for the woman requiring a vault cap to accommodate a cervix which is so long that it prevents suction being exerted by a cervical cap on the vaginal vault.

Selection, fitting and teaching

Again, this is identical to that of the cervical cap apart from the exact siting of the upper rim (Fig. 5.19). A vimule may often provide the solution for a woman who proves difficult to fit with an occlusive pessary. A string attached to the vimule facilitates removal while learning, but should be removed once the user is confident.

Instructions for use and follow-up

These are identical to those for the cervical cap, using a spermicide in the same manner.

New types of occlusive pessaries

Lea's shield

This is a silicone, re-usable, one-size female barrier that can be purchased over the counter in North America and several European countries. When used in conjunction with spermicide, it can be left in situ for 48 hours and has a valvular device which allows the escape of cervical secretions and

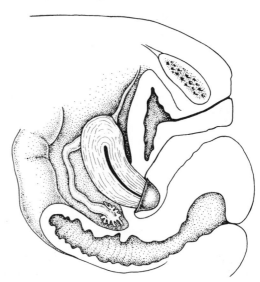

Figure 5.19
Vimule in situ.

trapped air. Preliminary data suggest it is as effective as other female barrier methods and no fitting or medical supervision is required (Mauck et al 1996). Some women and their partners have described discomfort during intercourse with Lea's shield but it appears very acceptable to a small select group of women.

Oves cervical cap

This is a thin, flexible silicone cervical cap that is disposable and designed to remain in situ for up to 3 days. A small amount of spermicide is placed in the cap prior to insertion and there is no requirement to re-apply spermicide thereafter. It has been developed in France and and is designed to be purchased over the counter. Three sizes of 26, 28 and 30 mm are available but there is very little data on efficacy of the Oves cap.

Damage to occlusive pessaries

Some oil-based vaginal or rectal suppositories, pessaries, ointments, creams and gels can damage latex rubber barriers. Women should be warned routinely against using diaphragms during treatment with such preparations and advised about alternative methods. Occlusive pessaries manufactured in plastic are not affected in this way.

FEMALE CONDOM

The female condom is a polyurethane sheath, 15 cm long by 7 cm in diameter, its open end attached to a flexible polyurethane ring (Fig. 5.20). A

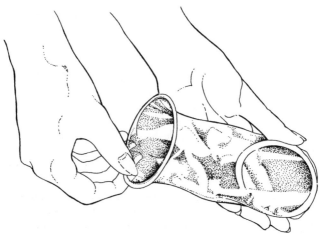

Figure 5.20 Female condom.

removable polyurethane ring inside the condom serves as an introducer and anchors the device in the vagina.

The condom comes in a single size, has a silicone-based, non-spermicidal lubricant and is for single use only. It is available over the counter under the trade name Femidom (Reality in North America and Femy in Spain). Initial adverse responses to female condoms undoubtedly become less when couples become familiar with their use.

Mode of action

In common with all barrier methods, female condoms prevent spermatozoa gaining access to the female upper genital tract.

Effectiveness

Studies on the efficacy of the female condom suggest that it is as effective as the diaphragm with failure rates ranging from 5 to 21 per HWY. Motivated women who use female condoms correctly and consistently would be expected to have low failure rates.

Indications

1. When a couple wish the woman to use a reversible, barrier method of contraception.
2. For maximum protection against sexually transmitted infections (STIs).

Contraindications

Some couples find female condoms psychologically unacceptable.

Advantages

1. An effective method of contraception that is controlled by the woman.
2. Available over the counter for purchase in most pharmacies and free from some family planning clinics.
3. Affords very high protection against STIs by protecting the vulva and urethra. In vitro studies show no leakage of HIV or cytomegalovirus through the female condom (Hicks 1996).
4. Stronger than latex male condoms with less risk of splitting and not weakened by oil-based vaginal preparations.
5. Less diminution of sensation for the man than with latex condoms.
6. Can be inserted a long time (i.e. hours) in advance of intercourse and also left in some time after ejaculation thereby allowing less disruption of the sexual act.

Disadvantages

1. Unattractive appearance.
2. Altered sensation and a 'rustling' noise during intercourse.
3. Some initial difficulty with insertion may be experienced but this improves quickly with repeated use.
4. Can occasionally be pushed completely into the vagina or penetration can take place outside it.
5. Expensive. Research is underway to establish if female condoms can be washed and re-used.

Instructions for use

1. Insert the female condom squatting, with one foot on a chair, or lying down.
2. Squeeze the sheath-covered inner ring between thumb and other fingers and slide the condom into the vagina similar to inserting a tampon.
3. Once the condom is in the vagina, push the inner ring as high as possible so that it will remain there during intercourse.
4. The outer ring should lie closely against the vulva.
5. Immediately after intercourse, hold the outer ring together and gently pull the condom out.
6. Discard in a bin and not down the toilet.

HOME-MADE BARRIERS

These cannot be advocated in any way, but their use is widespread, particularly in developing countries. For centuries, women have used pads or sponges as barriers to conception, and when soaked in household substances such as vinegar, lemon juice, butter, cooking oil, Coca-Cola or even fluoride toothpaste there will be a mild spermicidal effect. Detergents or caustic substances must never be used as they will damage the vaginal mucosa.

Postcoital douching should be discouraged.

CONDOMS

The condoms first described historically were used for decoration, and thereafter for protection against disease. Fallopio, the Italian anatomist, described the use of a linen sheath in 1544 to protect the wearer from syphilis. With the development of vulcanized rubber and then liquid latex, condoms could be inexpensively mass-produced resulting in worldwide availability and an effective, reversible male method of contraception.

The condom is recognized by such familiar names as French letter, Johnny, sheath, rubber and protective. They may be purchased from pharmacies, supermarkets and vending machines, by mail order and around 10% of those used in the UK are provided free by family planning clinics. General practitioners are currently unable to prescribe condoms free on prescription but may have access to providing them free through an HIV-prevention budget. Condoms have been extensively promoted in the 'Safe Sex' campaign as an effective barrier against the spread of HIV. Prominent advertising has attempted to increase the public's awareness of the risks of unprotected intercourse and to encourage condom use. New trends in marketing and packaging condoms aim to increase consumer appeal and to escape from their association with clandestine sex.

Types. A large range of types is now available:

1. Most condoms are made of fine latex rubber and consist of a circular cylinder (approximately 3.0–3.5 cm diameter, 15–20 cm long, 0.03–0.08 mm thick) with one closed, plain or teat-shaped end and an integral rim at the open end. They are packaged individually, rolled to the rim and hermetically sealed in impermeable foil. If the packaging is cracked or torn, deterioration of the condom inside is rapid (Free et al 1996).
2. For many years, only one size was available but the need for both larger and smaller sizes has been recognized and these are now available.
3. Lubricated, spermicide-incorporating, coloured, flavoured, scented and textured variations have been introduced in an effort to improve acceptability.
4. Allergy condoms, made of low-residue latex rubber and which are not pre-lubricated, are available for individuals who develop hypersensitivity.
5. Condoms which are thicker and exceed the British Standards are marketed primarily for anal intercourse in homosexual men to offer extra protection against infection with HIV.
6. Condoms manufactured from polyurethane are widely available now (sold under the trade name of Avanti in the UK). They are roughly the same thickness as latex condoms but are less constricting and are not harmed by oil-based lubricants. In studies comparing plastic condoms to latex condoms, most male users preferred the sensitivity provided by polyurethane condoms although they had a clinical breakage rate significantly higher than that of the latex condom (Frezieres et al 1998). They are particularly suitable for use by individuals with allergy to latex rubber but are significantly more expensive than latex condoms.
7. Condoms made from sheep's intestine (Fourex) are available. Despite their unaesthetic appearance, they have improved sensitivity compared with latex condoms but their efficacy against STIs is unknown.

Mode of action

Like all barrier methods, condoms prevent spermatozoa from reaching the female upper genital tract.

Effectiveness

The published efficacy of condoms ranges from 3 to 23 per HWY. Failure rates are consistently low when condoms are used perfectly by well-motivated individuals. In order to ensure high quality, three major agencies worldwide have established condom manufacturing standards for size, resistance to breaking, freedom from holes, packaging and labelling.

Users become technically more competent with experience and have fewer accidents. Tightness of condoms may be a factor in their failure and larger condoms may be needed by some individuals. If the condom is not used at the beginning of intercourse or is applied only just before ejaculation, pre-ejaculatory secretions may contain sufficient sperm to cause pregnancy. Poor practices such as snagging the condom with fingernails or rings, tearing the condoms while opening the pack, unrolling the condom prior to putting it on and re-using condoms obviously cause higher failure rates.

Indications

1. When a couple wish the man to use a reversible method of contraception.
2. During the period of instruction in the use of a cap.
3. Following childbirth or therapeutic abortion, before another method is adopted.
4. Condoms may be used for personal protection against STIs, even when contraception is not required or a hormonal method is used to prevent pregnancy.
5. When other methods are unacceptable or additional contraception is required (e.g. when oral contraceptive pills are forgotten).

Contraindications

1. When they are psychologically unacceptable.
2. Any malformation of the penis.
3. When either partner is allergic to latex rubber.

Advantages

1. Effective when used correctly and consistently.
2. Widely available, inexpensive and often provided free. No requirement to consult healthcare professionals.

3. Simple to use with no local or systemic side effects.
4. A very high level of protection against STIs, including HIV infection.
   Intact latex condoms are impermeable to sexually transmissible
   organisms including viruses when tested in vitro (Feldblum 1998).
5. Protection against carcinoma and pre-malignant disease of the
   cervix.
6. Improvement of performance in some patients with premature
   ejaculation.

Disadvantages

1. Unattractive appearance.
2. Diminution of pleasurable sensation during intercourse, particularly
   transmission of body heat.
3. Requires application prior to coitus and prompt removal thereafter,
   which couples may find an unacceptable interruption to sexual
   activity.
4. Erectile difficulty may be increased, though some men in later years find
   the use of a condom helps to maintain an erection.

Instructions for use

1. If the condom is not pre-lubricated with a spermicide, the woman
   should insert a spermicidal cream, jelly or pessary into the vagina
   before intercourse. Some condoms come packaged with spermicidal
   pessaries.
2. The condom is unrolled onto the erect penis before any contact with the
   vulva is made, leaving the tip of the condom empty to accommodate the
   ejaculate.
3. During withdrawal, the condom should be held firmly at the base of the
   penis so that it remains in place until after the penis has been
   withdrawn.
4. The penis should be washed before any further contact with the woman
   occurs.
5. Disposable condoms should not be re-used.
6. Condoms should not be used after the expiry date marked on the packet.
   The older the condom, the more likely it is to break during use.
7. Oil-based lubricants such as Vaseline, baby oil and petroleum jelly
   drastically reduce the tensile strength of condoms. Other vaginal
   creams and pessaries such as antifungal and oestrogen preparations can
   be oil-based and could theoretically affect the strength of latex
   condoms.
8. Condom-users should always be informed about the availability of
   emergency contraception should the condom burst or slip off.

SPERMICIDES

These contraceptive agents comprise a chemical capable of destroying sperm, incorporated into an inert base. The commonly used spermicides contain non-ionic surfactants that alter sperm surface membrane permeability, causing osmotic changes which result in sperm death. Nonoxynol-9 was the original agent to be developed and is still the active constituent of most products.

It is emphasized that the use of spermicides as a contraceptive measure alone is not recommended and their main role is to improve the contraceptive effect of other barrier methods. A recent small study showed that women using spermicidal film only had a pregnancy rate similar to women using no method of contraception (Steiner et al 1998).

Spermicides may be purchased from pharmacies and by mail order. They are available free from family planning clinics and free on prescription from general practitioners. Spermicidal products are available in a variety of different forms; most are suitable for all purposes (Table 5.1).

Creams and gels

The chemical is incorporated in a stearate soap base in a cream, or in a water-soluble base in a gel. Both liquefy at body temperature and disperse rapidly throughout the vagina.

Vaginal pessaries

The base consists of gelatin, glycerine or wax. They are foil-packed and easy to handle. Since they spread less easily throughout the vagina, weight for weight they are probably less effective than creams and gels but women often find them more convenient.

Foaming tablets

These are hard white discs which effervesce on contact with moisture, releasing the spermicide and forming CO_2 foam.

Aerosol foams

The spermicide is incorporated in an emulsion of oil and water and is stored under gas pressure in a rigid container. It is released into an applicator as required, by pressure on a valve on top of the container.

Spermicidal film

This consists of squares of water-soluble, semi-transparent film which dissolve rapidly in the vagina to release nonoxynol-9.

Mode of action of spermicides

The action of spermicides is two-fold:

1. The base material of the preparation physically blocks sperm progression.
2. An active chemical kills sperm without damaging other body tissues.

Effectiveness

Nonoxynol-9 and its derivatives are unable to diffuse into cervical mucus. Sperm, which enter the cervical mucus before being immobilized by spermicide within the vagina, can survive and ascend the genital tract. Therefore, when used in isolation, spermicides are ineffective contraceptives. Failure rates have been reported to range from 3 to 28 per HWY.

Indications

1. Spermicides are used in conjunction with diaphragms, condoms and coitus interruptus to increase the effectiveness of these methods.
2. To give some measure of protection against STIs. Nonoxynol-9 has been shown to reduce the risk of gonococcal and chlamydial infections in women and also appears to inactivate HIV rapidly in vitro. To date, no data exist to show unequivocally that spermicides prevent HIV infection. Human papilloma virus does not appear to be affected by nonoxynol-9.

Contraindications

1. Allergy in either partner.
2. Aerosol foam should not be used with the diaphragm because, if pressure builds up in the vagina, the cap could possibly be displaced.

Advantages

1. Provide extra lubrication if dryness is a problem.
2. Readily available without a prescription.

Table 5.1 Commonly used spermicides

Product	Manufacturer	pH	Chemical constituent	Storage	Shelf-life	Re-application if intercourse delayed
Gels						
Duragel	LRC Products Ltd	6.0–7.0	Nonoxynol-11 2%	30 °C	3 years	3 hours
Gynol II	Ortho	4.5–4.7	Nonoxynol-9 2%	Cool place	2 years	Any subsequent coitus or delay of a few hours
Creams						
Duracreme	LRC Products Ltd	6.0–7.0	Nonoxynol-11 2%	30 °C	3 years	3 hours
Orthocreme		6.0	Nonoxynol-9 2%	Room temp.	3 years	Any subsequent coitus or delay of a few hours
Pessaries						
Ortho-forms	Ortho	4.5–5.0	Nonoxynol-9 5%	Cool place	3 years	1 hour
Double check	FP Sales Ltd	5.0	Nonoxynol-9 6%	Cool place	2 years	1 hour
Foams						
Delfen	Ortho	4.5–5.0	Nonoxynol-9 12.5%	Room temp	3 years	1 hour
Sponge	FP Sales Ltd	4.7	Nonoxynol-9 1 g	Room temp.	3 years	Effective for 24 hours

3. No evidence of topical vaginal toxicity and very limited, if any, systemic absorption.
4. Probable protection against carcinoma of the cervix (p. **131**).

Disadvantages

1. Unacceptably high failure rate when used alone.
2. Require premeditation prior to intercourse.
3. Varying degrees of 'messiness' according to the preparation.
4. Pessaries are unsuitable for use in tropical countries, as they melt. However, melted pessaries will solidify if cooled in the pack, and still retain their activity.
5. Aerosol preparations may be difficult to use if the container is not shaken properly. They are also expensive and environmentally unfriendly.
6. Occasional complaints of an unpleasant odour, stinging or discomfort in the vagina. A few individuals are allergic to nonoxynol-9 and its derivatives.
7. Usage of spermicides in excess of normal dosages can cause irritation and ulceration in the vaginal mucosa and the effect appears to be dose related. The damaged vaginal epithelium may potentially enhance the entry of sexually transmissible organisms such as HIV.
8. There is no apparent increase in spontaneous abortion or fetal abnormality associated with using spermicides in the periconceptional phase despite concerns in the past over this issue.

Instructions to users

1. Creams and gels may be inserted into the vagina with an applicator 2 to 3 minutes before intercourse, or on an occlusive pessary (pp **132–144**). A dose of 2 g is adequate.
2. Foaming tablets are slightly moistened and inserted high into the vagina 3 to 10 minutes before intercourse.
3. Pessaries are inserted about 15 minutes before intercourse.
4. One applicatorful of foam should be inserted into the vagina just before intercourse (Fig. 5.21). The aerosol can is shaken well to ensure adequate mixture of the spermicide and the foam.
4. If spermicide is inserted more than 2 hours before intercourse takes place, a second application of spermicide should be used.

The vaginal contraceptive sponge

The Today sponge is an 'over-the-counter' method which has not achieved popularity in the UK compared to North America. At the present time, it has been withdrawn by its manufacturers because of marketing reasons but is scheduled to be reintroduced. It consists of a soft, white circular sponge 5.5 cm in diameter, made of polyurethane foam and impregnated with 1 g nonoxynol-9. A polyester loop is attached to facilitate removal (Fig. 5.22). It should be inserted high into the vagina, with the indented surface positioned over the cervix. The spermicide is activated when the sponge is moistened prior to insertion.

Mode of action

The Today sponge prevents pregnancy in three ways: as a barrier, as a mechanism for absorbing semen and as a carrier for spermicide.

Effectiveness

UK studies comparing the sponge and diaphragm found the sponge to be much less reliable. However, women have found it a very acceptable addition to the range of barrier methods of contraception.

Indications

1. Women who want to use a vaginal method of contraception but do not wish to seek medical advice or fitting.
2. Women of lower fertility, such as lactating mothers or perimenopausal women, and those spacing pregnancies.

Advantages

1. One size is suitable for most women, although it has been suggested that a larger size of sponge may reduce the risk of pregnancy in parous women. It can be purchased across the counter without the need for fitting or prescription.
2. Women find it convenient and simple to use, and particularly like the absence of messiness.
3. There is no need for additional spermicide before each act of intercourse.

Disadvantages

1. The relatively high failure rate.
2. Small numbers of cases of toxic shock syndrome have been reported, but the overall risk appears to be in the region of 1 case per 2 million sponges used, which is reassuring. Traumatic manipulation, lengthy periods of

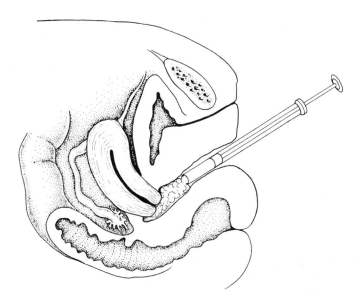

Figure 5.21   Foam insertion.

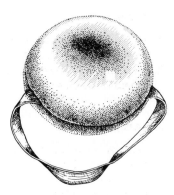

Figure 5.22
Today vaginal contraceptive sponge.

insertion and use during menstruation or in the immediate postpartum period increase the risk of toxic shock syndrome.
3. A very small number of women or their partners may be sensitive to the spermicide.
4. Expensive.

Instructions for use

1. The sponge must be moistened thoroughly and inserted high into the vagina (Fig. 5.23).

2. It may be left in situ for up to 24 hours.
3. Intercourse may be repeated as often as desired during this time.
4. The sponge should be kept in place for at least 6 hours after the last intercourse, removed and then thrown away.
5. Use during menstruation should be avoided.
6. It may be kept in place whilst swimming or bathing.

Alternative spermicidal agents and delivery systems

There is widespread global interest and investment currently in developing new agents which combine virucidal and spermicidal activities to combat the spread of STIs including HIV and AIDS.

Chlorhexidine. This broad-spectrum antiseptic has spermicidal action comparable to nonoxynol-9. However, in contrast to nonoxynol-9, it can permeate cervical mucus and exert undiminished spermicidal action within the mucus. It also appears active against STIs including HIV.

Benzalkonium chloride. This agent has spermicidal and antiseptic properties. It is available in some countries in a cream, pessary and impregnated tampon (Pharmatex). It is a useful alternative for women who are allergic to nonoxynol-9. It is however inactivated by soaps which must be avoided after intercourse for several hours.

Cholic acid. This exerts strong spermicidal and antiviral activity. It is being evaluated in combination with low concentrations of nonoxynol-9 and benzalkonium chloride in the new Protectaid sponge. This sponge can be obtained over the counter and may offer contraception with particularly effective anti-HIV action.

Gramicidin. This polypeptide has antimicrobial properities and appears to exert marked HIV inactivation in vitro. It completely impairs sperm motion and is therefore a potential spermicide with antiviral activity.

Propranolol. Currently being evaluated as a vaginal contraceptive, this appears to be as effective as conventional spermicides and acts by inhibition of sperm motility. It is unlikely to offer protection against STIs but may be effective in combination with nonoxynol-9.

ADAPTATIONS OF COITAL TECHNIQUE
Coitus interruptus

This is the oldest method of birth control, widely used in Christian and Muslim communities but less so in Oriental countries. It was first described in the Bible (Genesis 38, verse 9), when Onan spilled his seed on the ground to prevent conception when forced to have sexual intercourse with his brother's wife. St Augustine based his condemnation of contraception on this, leading eventually to the doctrine set out in the Papal encyclical *Humanae Vitae* which still today condemns the practice of coitus interruptus.

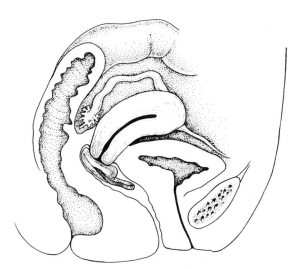

Figure 5.23
Today sponge in
situ.

Description

Coitus interruptus is the withdrawal of the erect penis from the vagina
before ejaculation. It is described by users as 'being careful', 'withdrawal'
and by local euphemisms implying stopping before the effective 'end of the
line'. When questioned, users often claim not to use contraception, and
unless asked specifically about coitus interruptus a false history of infertility
may be assumed. The method requires discipline on the part of the male
and is practised most successfully by men able to recognize the imminence
of orgasm and to withdraw quickly prior to ejaculation. Unfortunately,
it is often the method practised unsuccessfully by young inexperi-
enced men.

It has been estimated that around 4% of the sexually active population in
the UK rely on coitus interruptus as their method of contraception.

Mode of action

Since ejaculation occurs outside the vagina, semen is not deposited within
the vagina and therefore pregnancy should not follow. However, pre-
ejaculatory secretions containing thousands of sperm may escape from
the urethra during penetration, resulting in pregnancy.

Effectiveness

Failure rates vary with the age and experience of the couple and estimates
range from 5 to 20 per HWY.

Advantages

1. No supplies, preparation or medical supervision required.
2. Costs nothing.
3. No serious side effects.
4. Allows total privacy about the couple's sexual relationship.

Disadvantages

1. High failure rate.
2. No protection from STIs.
3. Limits full enjoyment of sexual intercourse.

Coitus outwith the vagina

Oral and anal sex are now widespread sexual practices. Individuals may request specific advice on them, especially in relation to STIs (Ch. 13).

RISKS/BENEFITS

Selection of a barrier method of contraception is frequently a matter of compromise between the advantages and disadvantages. Any method of contraception is always better than none, and the most effective method is the one the couple chooses to use. Sexual health advisers can help individuals to use barrier methods effectively. Failures with these methods do occur and a woman may be at risk of pregnancy following a burst condom or dislodgement of a diaphragm. Individuals using barrier methods must be informed of when to use emergency contraception and where to obtain it (Ch. 8).

REFERENCES

Bounds W 1994 Contraceptive efficacy of the diaphragm and cervical caps used in conjunction with a spermicide – a fresh look at the evidence. British Journal of Family Planning 20: 84–87
Feldblum PJ 1998 Pregnancy and STD prevention. In: McNeill ET, Gilmore CE, Finger WR, Lewis JH, Schellstede WP (eds) The latex condom: recent advances, future directions. Family Health International, Research Triangle Park, North Carolina, p 5–11
Free MJ, Srisamang V, Vail J, Mercer D, Kotz R, Marlowe DE 1996 Latex rubber condoms: predicting and extending shelf life. Contraception 53: 221–229
Frezieres RG, Walsh TL, Nelson AL, Clark VA, Coulson AH 1998 Breakage and acceptability of a polyurethane condom: a randomized, controlled study. Family Planning Perspectives 30: 73–78
Hicks D 1996 The risks and benefits of contraceptive method regarding sexually transmitted infection. British Journal of Family Planning 22: 34–36
Mauck C, Glover LH, Miller E et al 1996 A study of the safety and efficacy of a new vaginal barrier contraceptive used with and without spermicide. Contraception 53: 329–335

Smith C, Farr G, Feldblum PJ, Spence A 1995 Effectiveness of the non-spermicidal fit-free diaphragm. Contraception 51: 289–291

Steiner MK, Herz-Picciotto I, Schulz KF, Sangi-Haghpeykar H, Earle BB, Trussell J 1998 Measuring contraceptive efficacy. A randomised approach – condom versus spermicide versus no method. Contraception 58: 375–378

6

Natural family planning

Lora Green

The biological basis of natural family
  planning 163
  The menstrual cycle 163
Natural family planning methods 164
  Calender method 164
  Temperature method 164
  Ovulation (mucus or Billings)
    method 166
  Cervical palpation method 167
  Symptothermal method 168
  Multiple index method (double
    check method) 168
  Personal fertility monitor 168
Effectiveness 169
Indications 170
Advantages 170
Disadvantages 171

Teaching natural family planning 171
Breast-feeding as a contraceptive
  method 171
  The effect of breast-feeding on
    fertility 172
  Lactational amenorrhoea
    method 172
Postpartum contraception 174
  Timing 174
  Barrier methods and
    spermicides 174
  Intrauterine devices 175
  Combined hormonal
    contraception 175
  Progestogen-only methods 175
  Emergency contraception 176
  Sterilization 176

It has long been recognized that there are only a few days during the menstrual cycle when conception can occur. A variety of symptoms and signs can be used to detect the so-called 'fertile period'. These indicators, together with knowledge of the average duration of a woman's cycle, the normal timing of ovulation and the lifespan of the ovum and sperm can be used to determine when a couple should abstain from intercourse if they wish to avoid pregnancy.

In the presence of an increasing number of extremely effective artificial methods of contraception, professionals are sometimes surprised and even intimidated by a request to discuss natural family planning (NFP) in a routine family planning consultation. Yet NFP is an attractive option for some, facilitating a woman's interpretation and subsequent control of her fertility. If the rules are correctly applied, NFP is an effective method that requires commitment, abstinence from penetrative sex during the fertile period and a caring, understanding relationship. Motivation and commitment to the method are essential if the method is to be used successfully.

THE BIOLOGICAL BASIS OF NATURAL FAMILY PLANNING

A thorough understanding of the menstrual cycle is essential for couples who use NFP and for healthcare and other professionals who teach the method. The hormonal changes which take place during the cycle, together with the indicators of fertility are shown in Figure 6.1.

The menstrual cycle

The average menstrual cycle lasts for 28 days with a normal range from 21 to 35 days. The first day of the cycle, day 1 of the period, is the start of the shedding of the endometrium. In the first half of the cycle (follicular phase), follicle stimulating hormone (FSH) from the pituitary gland acts directly on the ovary to stimulate the development of up to 30 Graafian follicles, only one of which will mature sufficiently to release the ovum. The developing follicle produces oestrogen allowing proliferation of the endometrium in preparation for implantation of a fertilized ovum. Rising oestrogen concentrations reach a peak approximately 24 hours before ovulation, stimulating the mid-cycle surge of luteinizing hormone (LH) from the pituitary. LH acts on the ovary to stimulate release of the ovum (ovulation). In the second half of the cycle (luteal phase), the cells of the ruptured ovarian follicle change their characteristics to form the corpus luteum which secretes progesterone. Concentrations of progesterone reach a peak approximately 7 days after ovulation (mid-luteal phase). Progesterone acts on the uterus to stimulate the development of secretory phase endometrium, an effect which is essential for successful implantation.

If the ovum has not been fertilized, concentrations of both oestrogen and progesterone decline, the endometrium can no longer be maintained and menstruation begins again.

The length of the follicular phase varies between individuals and between cycles within any one individual. The duration of the normal luteal phase is much more constant and is, on average, 14 days. Around the time of ovulation some women experience mild abdominal pain (mittelschmerz) and slight vaginal spotting. During the follicular phase, rising concentrations of oestrogen facilitate the production of stretchy fertile mucus from the cervical glands which allows sperm transport into the uterus. After ovulation, the effect of progesterone on the cervical glands results in the production of scanty, sticky infertile mucus which prevents transport and survival of sperm.

The physiological changes associated with alterations in the steroid environment, regardless of cycle length, allow a woman to identify the fertile time of her cycle and thereby to time intercourse either to prevent or achieve a pregnancy. The rules for all methods of NFP must take into

HORMONES OF THE MENSTRUAL CYCLE

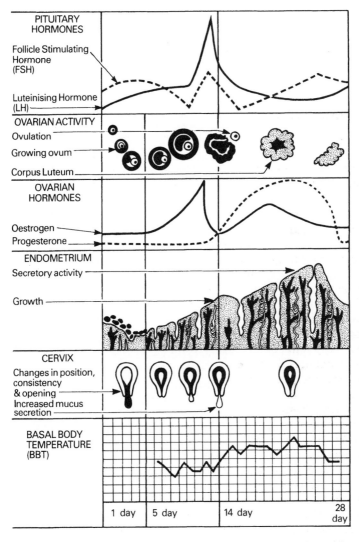

Figure 6.1 Changes in pituitary and ovarian hormones, folllicle growth, endometrial development, position and characteristics of the cervix and mucus and changes in basal body temperature during the ovarian cycle.

account the lifespan of the egg and sperm which last a maximum of 24 hours and 6 days respectively.

NATURAL FAMILY PLANNING METHODS
Calender method

This method of NFP is also known as the 'rhythm method' or 'Russian roulette' (the latter referring to the high failure rate). The method is based on an algorithm derived from information collected over a number of consecutive menstrual cycles. The duration of at least six and preferably 12 cycles is documented, 20 days are subtracted from the shortest cycle to identify the first fertile day and 11 days from the longest cycle to identify the last fertile day. Thus, if a woman's cycles vary in length from 28 to 35 days, then the fertile phase starts on day 8 and ends on the 24th day. The variability and length of the cycles dictate the number of days of abstinence required, in this case 17 days. Women with very regular cycles therefore get away with a shorter period of abstinence. To ensure maximum effect-iveness, the calender method should be used in combination with other fertility indicators.

Temperature method

At ovulation, the rise in progesterone produces a rise in the basal body temperature (BBT) of approximately 0.2°C–0.4°C, which is maintained until the onset of menstruation. The rise in temperature is an indication that ovulation has occurred. For 3 days afterwards – allowing some leeway in the survival time of the egg – abstinence from sexual intercourse is necessary. Thus the temperature method identifies the end of the fertile period but not the beginning. Intercourse must also be avoided before ovulation (i.e. throughout the follicular phase) if the method is to be effective. For this reason, the temperature method is usually used in conjunction with other fertility indicators.

Using the temperature method

A new temperature chart, obtainable from fertility organizations, is started at the beginning of menses and maintained throughout the cycle (Fig. 6.2). The temperature can be taken orally (for 5 minutes), vaginally or rectally (for 3 minutes) but the chosen route must be maintained throughout the cycle. Commercially available ovulation thermometers with wider markings are easier to read than a normal thermometer. Battery-operated digital thermometers which contain no mercury and can be read within 45 seconds are also available.

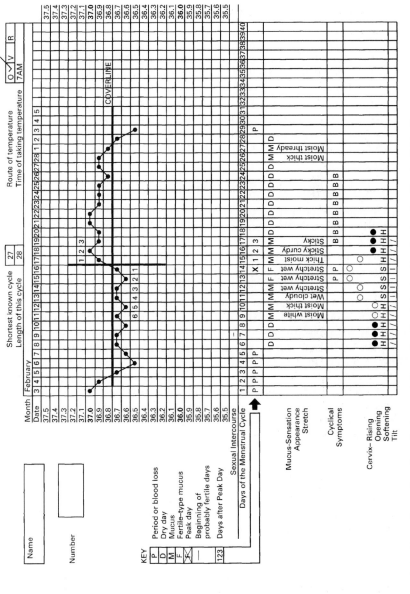

Figure 6.2 Chart of recordings from the to symptothermal method of natural family planning. P, pain; B, bloating.

The temperature must be taken at the same time each day, before getting up and before drinking or eating, and can be affected by a number of factors including late nights, alcohol the evening before, viral or bacterial illness and stress.

To be indicative of ovulation, the rise in temperature must be maintained for 3 days and must increase by at least 0.2°C on at least one day. A vertical line is drawn on the temperature chart on the first-rise day of the rise in temperature and a horizontal line drawn through the preceding 6 days (the '3 over 6 rule'). The junction where the two lines meet is called the coverline and is regarded as the day of ovulation.

The temperature chart can sometimes be difficult to interpret, particularly if there is an unexpected rise in temperature which is not maintained. If charts are persistently difficult to understand, a good teacher will be required to help with interpretation.

Ovulation (mucus or Billings) method

This method, too, can be used on its own or in combination with other fertility indicators. The woman is taught to recognize the characteristics of cervical mucus as described earlier (Fig. 6.3). Fertile mucus has the classic appearance of raw egg white which, if stretched for several centimetres between the finger and thumb, does not break (spinnbarkheit). It appears some days before ovulation (stimulated by the growing follicles) and the final day of fertile mucus is considered the day when ovulation is most likely to occur (so-called 'peak day'). Abstinence must be maintained from the day when fertile mucus is first identified until 3 days after the peak day. The end of the fertile period is characterized by the appearance of infertile mucus which is scanty and viscous.

Some women are already aware of mucus changes in their cycle before learning the method. They know that there are times in their cycle where they appear to be wetter at the vagina in the absence of sexual excitement. 93% of women are able to identify fertile mucus within the first month of

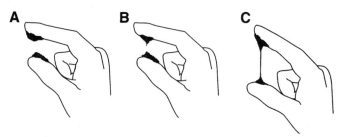

Figure 6.3   Changes in cervical mucus characteristics. A, infertile mucus – cloudy, white and sticky; B, intermediate mucus – less cloudy but not sticky; c, fertile mucus – clear, slippery and stretchy.

charting (WHO 1981a). However, it takes time to learn to interpret the chart and apply the rules.

Using the mucus method

1. First-time users of the method are advised to abstain from sexual intercourse during the entire first cycle of using the method.
2. Couples should abstain from intercourse during menses in case fertile mucus is present but undetectable.
3. Starting on the first day of her cycle, cervical mucus characteristics are recorded on a dedicated chart. Before every micturition, the vulva is wiped with coloured toilet tissue and examined for mucus. The peak day of mucus is likely to be preceded by the slippery wet mucus but sticky mucus prior to the peak day can also prove to be fertile mucus. Hence, teachers of the method emphasize that any change of mucus, whether sticky or stretchy, may herald ovulation. The average number of dry days prior to a change to fertile mucus is $3\frac{1}{2}$ and mucus is identifiable for an average of 6 days before the peak day (WHO 1983).
4. Using sticky labels or coloured pens, menstrual bleeding, dry days and mucus days are recorded (Fig. 6.4). Dry or infertile mucus days are marked in a different colour or symbol from fertile mucus days. The mucus pattern may change during the day and it is the most fertile mucus which should be recorded on the chart.
5. At the first sign of mucus, intercourse should be avoided until the 4th night after the peak day. Thereafter, couples can have sex until the end of the cycle. Since the presence of seminal fluid in the vagina may make the characteristics of cervical mucus more difficult to interpret, couples are advised to have intercourse only on alternate days.

Cervical palpation method

The cervix itself is also sensitive to changes in the steroid environment and certain characteristics alter during the cycle. It can be palpated on a daily

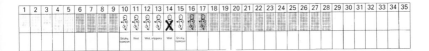

Figure 6.4   Charting the mucus method. On or around the 10th day, the mucus is sticky and opaque, the 11th day it is wet, the 12th and 13th days it is wet and slippery and the 14th (peak) day it is wet again, with the mucus becoming sticky and opaque on the 15th day. The couple must abstain from intercourse from the first sign of mucus to the fourth night after peak mucus.

basis as another fertility indicator, particularly if cervical mucus changes are difficult to interpret, e.g. during irregular cycles or the perimenopause. During the infertile period, the cervix feels lower in the vagina and is firm and dry. As ovulation approaches, the cervix rises up, by about 1–2 cm towards the body of the uterus and feels wet and soft to the touch. The cervical os opens slightly.

Symptothermal method

This method combines the temperature and mucus methods and incorporates other minor indicators of hormone changes such as pain, spotting or bleeding, breast tenderness, mood swings and bloatedness. Women may not previously have been aware of the relevance of such symptoms but may begin to see a pattern which assists further interpretation of the cycle.

Multiple index method (double check method)

Recording and interpreting the indicators of fertility requires considerable commitment, particularly if all the indicators are used as in the multiple index method. In this approach, the calendar and cervical mucus methods are used to identify the beginning of the fertile phase while the temperature and mucus methods define its end.

Personal fertility monitor

It is widely recognized that fertility indicators are not always easy to identify and that the number of days of abstinence required makes natural methods of fertility regulation quite demanding to use. Attempts have been made to harness scientific and technical developments to identify the fertile period with more accuracy. A personal hormone monitoring system (Persona, Unipath UK, Fig. 6.5) is available for women to use as a substitute for (or addition to) physiological fertility indicators (Bonnar et al 1999).

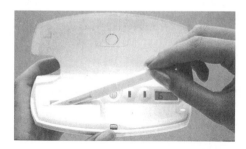

Figure 6.5
Persona (Unipath, UK).

Some choose to use the monitor in combination with abstinence, while others use condoms during the fertile period.

The device consists of a hand-held monitor and a set of disposable dipsticks which measure oestrone-3-glucuronide (E3G) and LH concentrations in urine. The monitor is switched on on the first day of menses. It displays a light which when green indicates that it is safe to have intercourse and when red that there is a risk of conception. For about 8 days each cycle, a yellow light appears indicating that a dipstick should be used to test an early morning urine sample. The monitor takes about 5 minutes to read the test and then displays either a red or a green light depending on the concentrations of LH, E3G and the ratio between them. The computer within the monitor stores information from the users last six cycles thus personalizing the algorithm with increasing accuracy as time passes. Persona is designed to detect concentrations of E3G at a level typical of that reached 5 to 6 days before ovulation, and concentrations of LH that define the ovulatory LH peak. Thus it is able to define both the start and end of the fertile period. The days of abstinence shown by the red light take into account the lifespan of both sperm and egg and the algorithm is such that the median number of days warning of the LH surge is 6. In the UK, the Persona fertility monitor can be bought from pharmacies at a cost of £64.95. A packet of dipsticks costs £9.95, making it an expensive method of contraception which is not available on the NHS.

Inevitably, Persona has had its share of bad publicity and a number of newspaper articles have appeared with detailed stories of pregnancies occurring despite apparently perfect use of the monitor. The method does in fact demand quite a lot of the user. Urine must be tested within 3 hours before or after the time when the machine is first switched on at the start of the cycle (the testing window). Thus, if the monitor is started at 8 a.m. on the first day of the user's cycle, urine must be tested by no later than 11 a.m. each day. If the test is delayed until 11.05, it will not be read. If a test is not done on a day when it is requested, then the accuracy of the monitor is significantly reduced as the biochemical information required for the algorithm is missing. A smart card can be inserted into the machine to obtain a record of testing and the hormone concentrations recorded. It appears that many of the 'failures' result from inadequate testing or from disobeying the rules and having intercourse on a red light day.

EFFECTIVENESS

1. The calendar method has a failure rate of up to 20 per hundred women years (HWY). In some studies, rates as high as 40 per HWY have been reported.
2. The temperature method used by itself has a method-related failure rate of 1.2 per HWY and a user failure of 6.6 per HWY. Used in

combination with the calendar method, it has a method-related failure of 5.0 per HWY, presumably because intercourse is allowed during the first half of the cycle and so the risk of pregnancy is significantly increased.

3. A large multicentre study involving women in three developing and two developed countries (WHO 1981 b) tested the efficacy of the mucus method. Among 725 women, after a 3-month teaching period, the failure rate of the method was 2.8 pregnancies per HWY. For couples who knowingly broke the rules, the failure rate was 15.4 per HWY. The overall failure rate (user plus method failures) was 22.3 per HWY. An average of 15.4 days of abstinence was required per cycle.

4. In the European Multi-centre Study of Natural Family Planning (Freundl 1993), the typical failure rate for the symptothermal method was 17.7 per HWY although if condoms were used during the fertile period, the failure rate fell to 3.6 per HWY.

5. In the same study, perfect use of the double check method was associated with a pregnancy rate of 2.6 per HWY, decreasing to 2.3 per HWY if condoms were used during the fertile period.

6. Persona, used correctly and avoiding intercourse on days when a red light shows, is said to be associated with a method failure rate of 6.2 per HWY, i.e. the efficacy of the method is 93.8%.

INDICATIONS

In the UK, an estimated 2% of the population use NFP. In some developing countries, social, cultural and economic reasons dictate a higher usage. A woman or a couple may wish to use NFP for the following reasons:

1. Their religion or culture is opposed to artificial methods of birth control.
2. Individual preference prevents use of hormonal or other methods of contraception which are regarded as 'unnatural' or invasive.
3. Couples find that natural methods which demand shared responsibility for contraception enhance their relationship.

ADVANTAGES

1. An effective method of contraception when all the rules are followed.
2. Promotes a couple's understanding of each other within their physical and emotional relationship.
3. Enhances the woman's familiarity with her body and control of her fertility.
4. A non-hormonal, non-invasive method of fertility regulation.
5. Can be taught and used in developing countries (where the cost of artificial methods is high), regardless of the individual's level of education.
6. May be used to either achieve or prevent a pregnancy.

DISADVANTAGES

1. Requires long periods of abstinence from intercourse – an average of 15 to 17 days of the cycle.
2. There is a long learning period of 3 months, requiring a good teacher.
3. Symptoms must be recorded every day.
4. The rules of the method are often found to be too demanding so people break them.
5. Not a suitable method for those not in a stable relationship.
6. Much more difficult to use if menstrual cycles are irregular and for this reason is not ideal for use during the perimenopause or postpartum period unless the user is already familiar with the method.
7. It is also not a suitable method for women who have reservations about exploring their bodies.
8. It has been suggested that if NFP fails and conception occurs with an ageing ovum or ageing sperm, there may be an increased risk of spontaneous abortion or fetal abnormality. There is no evidence for this. Nor is there any evidence to substantiate the claim that intercourse on a particular day in relation to ovulation affects the sex of the offspring
9. NFP does not protect against sexually transmitted infections.

TEACHING NATURAL FAMILY PLANNING

While doctors and nurses who offer contraceptive advice should have an overview of the advantages and disadvantages of natural methods of family planning and how they are used, it is essential that those who teach NFP should be properly taught themselves. If there is no-one in the clinic or practice who is qualified to teach NFP, information about the nearest recognized teacher can be sought from Fertility UK (Clitherow House, 1 Blythe Mews, London W14 0NW)

BREAST-FEEDING AS A CONTRACEPTIVE METHOD

Breast-feeding is associated with a delay in the resumption of fertility after childbirth and can be used as a natural method of contraception. Patterns of breast-feeding which reliably confer infertility are associated with amenorrhoea and it is the suppression of ovulation (associated with the lack of menstrual bleeding) and not the breast-feeding per se which is the contraceptive.

The effect of breast-feeding on fertility

After childbirth, high circulating concentrations of oestrogen, progesterone and prolactin (PRL) associated with pregnancy fall precipitously. In the absence of breast-feeding, gonadotrophin levels increase rapidly, PRL concentrations return to normal within about 4 weeks and by the 8th week postpartum, most bottle-feeding women show evidence of follicular development and will ovulate soon after. In contrast, among breast-feeding women, PRL concentrations remain elevated as long as frequent suckling occurs and acute episodes of PRL secretion occur with each breast-feed. Although FSH concentrations return to normal within a few weeks postpartum, circulating concentrations of LH remain suppressed throughout the period of lactation. Importantly, the normal pulsatile pattern of release of LH is disturbed and it is this which is thought to be the underlying cause of the suppression of normal ovarian function. LH pulsatility is a reflection of the pulsatile release of gonadotrophin releasing hormone (GnRH) from the hypothalamus and, although the mechanism of lactational infertility is not completely understood, it is thought that nipple stimulation by the baby acts, through some neuroendocrine mechanism, on the hypothalamus to alter pulsatile GnRH secretion. Whether PRL is involved directly in the suppression of ovarian activity is not known and it may simply be a reflection of the intensity of the suckling stimulus.

As the frequency and duration of breast-feeding episodes decline with time, and particularly with the introduction of food other than breastmilk, the effect on the hypothalamo–pituitary–ovarian axis weakens and ovarian activity resumes. Patterns of infant feeding and time postpartum therefore influence the duration of lactational infertility. The resumption of menstruation may be preceded by ovulation or by follicular development with sufficient oestrogen production to stimulate endometrial growth (and shedding when oestrogen levels fall). Thus the onset of menses is a sign of impending fertility.

In 1988 at a Consensus Conference held in Bellagio Italy, scientists pooled clinical and endocrine data obtained from 13 prospective studies of the effects of lactation on fertility. They agreed that a woman who is fully or nearly fully breast-feeding her child and who remains amenorrhoeic has less than a 2% chance of pregnancy during the first 6 months after childbirth (Kennedy et al 1989).

Lactational amenorrhoea method

The Bellagio guidelines were formalized into a method of family planning known as the lactational amenorrhoea method or LAM (Labbok et al 1994). LAM is essentially an algorithm (Fig. 6.6) which enables a woman to determine whether or not her pattern of infant feeding, combined with her pattern of menstruation, confers effective contraception.

A number of studies undertaken in developing countries studies have tested LAM prospectively. Perez et al (1992) demonstrated a cumulative 6-month pregnancy rate of 0.45%. Among women who remained amenor-

Ask the mother, or advise her to ask herself, these three questions:

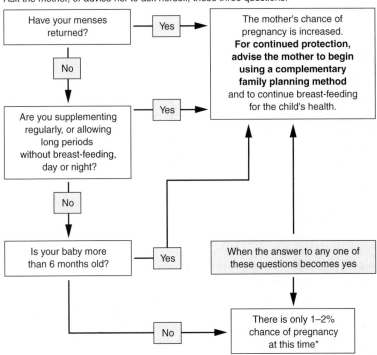

* However the mother may choose to use a complementary method *at any time*

Figure 6.6   The lactational amenorrhoea method (LAM) (after Labbok et al 1994).

rhoeic for 1 year (regardless of whether fully or nearly fully breast-feeding or not), the pregnancy rate was 1.12% (Kazi et al 1995). It is likely that in societies where prolonged breast-feeding is the norm, the rules of LAM can be extended beyond 6 months postpartum since ovarian activity is suppressed for much longer.

There is little doubt that LAM is effective but in developed countries the average duration of breast-feeding is short. In the UK, despite efforts to encourage breast-feeding, in 1990 65% of mothers in England and 50% in Scotland breast-fed their babies and 39% of them were giving supplementary bottle-feeds by 6 weeks (Office of Population Censuses and Surveys 1992). Few women are fully or nearly fully breast-feeding their babies beyond 4 months postpartum. With these sorts of infant-feeding patterns, LAM could not be used beyond 4 months postpartum and many women could not use it at all. In developing countries – particularly in rural areas – women breast-feed for much longer and the potential to use LAM is much greater. In countries where few contraceptive methods are available, where they are expensive or where services for contraceptive delivery are poor, LAM is likely to have an important role in birth spacing.

POSTPARTUM CONTRACEPTION

The choice of a method of contraception after childbirth will depend on a multitude of factors (Ch. 1) but clearly the method of infant feeding is important. The combined oral contraceptive pill (and combined injectable methods where they are available) is contraindicated during breast-feeding as oestrogen inhibits the production of breastmilk. Progestogen-only methods do not interfere with breastmilk production and do not have any effect on infant growth or health.

Timing

Since first ovulation in non-breast-feeding women has been observed, on average, at 45 days postpartum, women who bottle-feed their babies are advised to start using contraception from 4 weeks after delivery. In the UK, the routine postnatal check done by the general practitioner is classically undertaken at 6 weeks postpartum. Not all hospitals provide contraceptive supplies to women being discharged home after childbirth but fortunately sexual activity is often minimal or non-existent in the early weeks of the puerperium so that very early conceptions are a rarity. As discussed above, breast-feeding delays the return of fertility and in theory the use of contraception can be postponed for longer. In practice, however, breast-feeding women are also usually advised to start contraception at 4 weeks. Although this advice displays ignorance of reproductive physiology, it is probably pragmatic since many women in developed countries breast-feed for only a very short time and tend to introduce supplementary feeds early. For women relying on lactational amenorrhoea for contraception, the rules of LAM should be followed.

Barrier methods and spermicides

Barrier methods are often particularly acceptable to women in the postpartum period because of limited sexual activity. Additional lubrication is recommended for breast-feeding women who are relatively hypo-oestrogenic but may also be of benefit to women who have had an episiotomy and who are therefore more likely to find intercourse uncomfortable. Spermicides have no effect on breastmilk or on infant health. Diaphragms and caps should not be fitted until 6 weeks postpartum when involution of the uterus is complete.

Intrauterine devices

Immediate insertion of an intrauterine device (IUD) after delivery of the placenta (postplacental insertion) is often the norm in developing countries where accessibility to contraceptive services is limited. Post-placental insertion is associated with a higher rate of expulsion but not with an increased rate of infection or perforation. It may become more common in the UK with availability of the postpartum Gynefix IUD (Ch.4). Interval IUD insertion should not be carried out until 6 weeks postpartum by which time the risks of expulsion and perforation are no different from those associated with insertion at any other time. Women delivered by caesarean section can have an IUD inserted at 6 weeks postpartum. Since there is no evidence for any adverse effect of progestogens on infant growth or health, and since the dose of levonorgestrel is so small, there is no reason why the Levonorgestrel-releasing intrauterine system (LNG-IUS) (Ch. 4) should be contraindicated for breast-feeding women.

Combined hormonal contraception

The combined oral contraceptive pill is contraindicated for breast-feeding women as the oestrogen component of the pill inhibits the production of breastmilk. Combined methods are suitable for women who do not breast-feed but their initiation should be delayed until 4 weeks postpartum because of the increased risk of venous thromboembolism (VTE) during the puerperium.

Progestogen-only methods

Progestogen-only methods do not increase the risk of VTE and, as discussed, are not contraindicated during breast-feeding. The World Health Organization recommends delaying initiation until 6 weeks after childbirth because of theoretical risks of exposure of the neonate to steroids. This advice is widely ignored particularly in developing countries where childbirth may be the only opportunity when contraception can be initiated. Implanon is not licensed for use by breast-feeding women. It is unlikely however in Europe that any new method will be licensed for use during lactation since the expense and difficulty involved in undertaking the research required for regulatory approval is probably not warranted by the size of the potential market.

Emergency contraception

Requests for emergency contraception by breast-feeding women are surprisingly common. Although the theoretical risks of pregnancy may be small, particularly if the baby is being nursed frequently and during the night, most women are highly motivated to avoid short interbirth intervals and emergency contraception should not be withheld. The Yuzpe regimen may theoretically reduce breastmilk production for a couple of days and levonorgestrel is probably the method of choice.

Sterilization

Female sterilization can be done within the first 3 days postpartum via mini-laparotomy or at the time of caesarean section. Immediate postpartum sterilization, however, is associated with higher failure rates, perhaps because the fallopian tubes are very vascular and somewhat oedematous at this time so that the clips, rings or ties become looser when the tubes shrink to their pre-pregnancy size. It is also associated with a higher incidence of regret and unless women have been carefully counselled during the antenatal period, particularly if elective caesarean section is planned, is usually avoided in favour of laparoscopic interval sterilization. Vasectomy is often delayed until after the baby is born because of fears of mishap such as stillbirth or neonatal death and subsequent regret about sterilization.

REFERENCES

Bonnar J, Flynn A, Freundl G, Kirkman R, Royston R, Snowden R. 1999 Personal hormone monitoring for contraception. British Journal of Family Planning 24: 128–134

Freundl G 1993 The European Natural Family Planning Study Groups. Prospective European multi-centre study of natural family planning (1989–1992). Advances in Contraception 9: 269–283

Labbok MH, Perez A, Valdez V et al 1994 The lactational amenorrhoea method (LAM): a postpartum introductory family planning method with policy and program implications. Advances in Contraception 10: 93–109

Kazi A, Kennedy K, Visness CM, Khan T 1995 Effectiveness of the lactational amenorrhoea method in Pakistan. Fertility and Sterility 64: 717–723

Kennedy KI, Rivera R, McNeilly AS 1989 Consensus statement on the use of breastfeeding as a family planning method. Contraception 35: 477–496

Office of Population, Census and Surveys 1992. Infant Feeding 1990. HMSO: London, p. 127

Prerez A, Labbok MH, Queenan TJ 1992 Clinical Study of the lactational amenorrhea method of family planning. Lancet 339: 968–970

World Health Organization 1981a A prospective multicentre trial of the ovulation method of natural family planning. I. The teaching phase. Fertility and Sterility 36: 152–158

World Health Organization 1981b A prospective multicentre trial of the ovulation method of natural family planning. II. The effectiveness phase. Fertility and Sterility 36: 591–598

World Health Organization 1983 A prospective much centre trial of the ovulation method of natural family planning. III. Characteristics of the menstrual cycle and the fertile phase. Fertility and Sterility 40: 773–778

7

Sterilization

Anna Glasier

Female sterilization 177	Contraindications 190
Laparoscopy 177	Advantages 190
Mini-laparotomy 178	Disadvantages 190
Techniques 179	Counselling 191
Clinical management 182	Effectiveness 192
Complications 183	Reversibility 192
Vasectomy 184	Risks/benefits 193
Techniques 184	**Appendices 195**
Clinical management 186	Sterilization of the female by
Complications 188	laparoscopy 195
Indications 189	Male sterilization 197

It has been estimated that worldwide more than 150 million women have chosen sterilization as their method of contraception. Vasectomy is becoming increasingly acceptable and is used by over 50 million couples throughout the world, the majority of whom live in developing countries.

In Britain, almost 30% of all couples, and almost 50% of those over 40, are using either female or male sterilization as their method of contraception.

FEMALE STERILIZATION

Female sterilization usually involves blocking both fallopian tubes which can be reached either by laparotomy or mini-laparotomy or, more commonly, laparoscopy. In their recent evidence-based guidelines, the Royal College of Obstetricians and Gynaecologists (RCOG 1999) in the UK has recommended laparoscopy, wherever possible as a day case, as the procedure of choice.

Sterilization may also be achieved by the removal of both tubes (salpingectomy) or by hysterectomy, if either procedure is indicated by the presence of gynaecological disease such as hydrosalpinx or fibroids.

Laparoscopy

General anaesthesia (GA) is normally used, although spinal or local anaesthesia (LA) is more common in the USA and in developing countries where skilled anaesthetists may not be available. A pneumoperitoneum is created by the insufflation of nitrous oxide or carbon dioxide into the peritoneal cavity. Through a small subumbilical incision, a trochar and cannula are introduced into the gas-filled abdomen and the trochar replaced by the laparoscope (Fig. 7.1). With a fibre-optic light source connected, the pelvic organs are inspected. Operating forceps are introduced through a second cannula inserted either suprapubically or in the iliac fossa. Sterilization is performed either by diathermy or the application of clips or rings to both tubes (see below). After the release of gas from the peritoneal cavity, the instruments are withdrawn and the skin incisions closed with sutures (absorbable or non-absorbable), clips or staples.

Mini-laparotomy

Laparotomy using a small (3–5 cm) suprapubic incision avoids the need for sophisticated equipment and can be done almost as quickly as laparoscopic sterilization. The uterus is manipulated vaginally to bring the fallopian tubes to the level of the incision. The tubes are delivered through the incision and rings or clips applied. Alternatively, the tubes may be ligated using a variety of methods, most of which involve excision of a small portion of tube.

In the UK, mini-laparotomy is most commonly used when sterilization is performed immediately postpartum as at that time the uterus is large, the pelvis very vascular, and the risks of laparoscopy are increased.

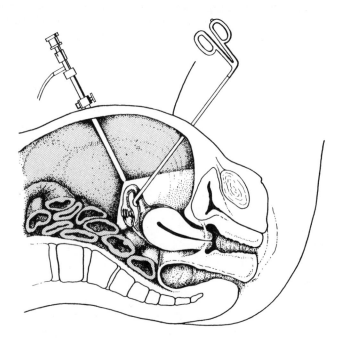

Figure 7.1
Laparoscopy.

Mini-laparotomy may be performed as a day-case procedure but many surgeons prefer the patient to stay in hospital overnight.

Techniques

Whatever the approach, the fallopian tubes may be blocked or divided in a number of ways.

Clips

A variety of clips have been designed for tubal occlusion. The clips destroy a much smaller length of tube (Fig. 7.2) and thus allow easier reversal, but special care must be taken to ensure that the whole width of the tube is occluded – some surgeons routinely apply two clips to each tube. Those most commonly used in the UK are probably the Hulka–Clemens clip (Fig. 7.3A) made of stainless steel and a polycarbonate, and the smaller Filshie clip (Fig. 7.3B) made of titanium lined with silicone rubber.

Falope ring

The ring is made of silicone rubber and, using a specially designed applicator, is placed over a loop of tube (Fig. 7.4). It destroys 2–3 cm of tube and may be difficult to apply if the tube is thick or fibrotic. Ischaemia of the loop causes significant postoperative pain. The application of local anaesthetic to the tube at the time of the procedure (in addition to traditional postoperative pain relief) has been shown to be of benefit.

Diathermy

One or more areas of the tube are cauterized by diathermy (Fig. 7.5). Unipolar diathermy has been replaced by the potentially safer technique of bipolar diathermy which allows only the tissue held between the jaws of the forceps to be cauterized. Local burns may still occur as the temperature of the cauterized tube may reach 300°C–400°C and thus can cause thermal injury if allowed to touch adjacent structures. Failure to cauterize all the layers of the tube results in a relatively high failure rate and cautery near the cornual portion of the tube is thought to increase the risk of ectopic pregnancy. The RCOG guidelines recommend diathermy only if for some reason mechanical methods of occlusion are difficult to apply.

Laser

Recent advances in laser technology have led to attempts at division of the tubes by laser vaporization. The carbon dioxide laser divides the tube very cleanly, which ironically may allow a high incidence of spontaneous tubal

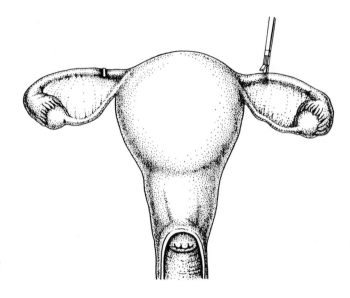

Figure 7.2
Application of
clips.

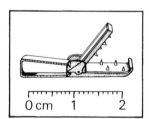

Figure 7.3
(A) Hulka–Clemens clip.

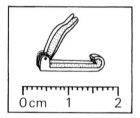

Figure. 7.3
(B) Filshie clip.

recanalization, and therefore failure. The Nd:Yag laser, although probably more effective, is extremely expensive.

Non-surgical methods

A number of chemical agents have been tested for their ability to occlude the fallopian tube when instilled into the tube either directly or via the

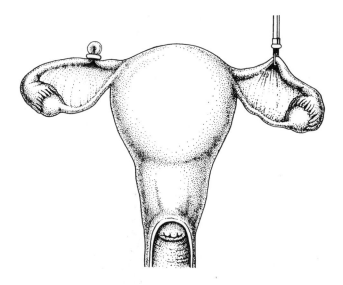

Figure 7.4
Application of
falope rings.

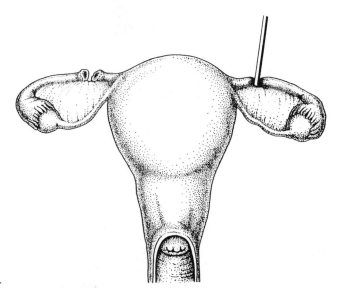

Figure. 7.5
Diathermy
coagulation of
fallopian tubes.

uterus. The best known is quinacrine. Quinacrine pellets are inserted into
the uterine cavity through the cervical canal via a modified intrauterine
device (IUD) inserter. Two insertions are made 1 month apart causing
inflammation, fibrosis and occlusion of the intramural segment of the tube.
Efficacy can be increased by adding adjuvants such as antiprostaglandins or
by increasing the number of quinacrine insertions. The method is cheaper

than surgical sterilization, and can be performed by non-medical personnel. A trial of the method in Vietnam reported a failure rate of 2.6% after 1 year (Hieu et al 1993). However, the Indian Medical Research Council in 1998 abandoned their trial because of very high failure rates and the use of quinacrine for female sterilization has now been banned in India. Interest in non-surgical methods was revived in the latter half of 1999 and studies of the toxicology of quinacrine are underway.

Clinical management

Examination

1. General physical examination should identify any risks for anaesthesia and any factors which might contraindicate or complicate the operation, such as previous abdominal operations or gross obesity.
2. Pelvic examination, to exclude existing pathology such as ovarian cyst or fibroids, is mandatory and a cervical smear should be taken if indicated.

Timing of operation and preoperative advice

1. Sterilization can be performed at any time in the menstrual cycle. A pregnancy test must be performed preoperatively if a woman has a late period or thinks she might be pregnant.
2. Routine curettage at the time of the procedure in order to prevent luteal phase pregnancy is not recommended and would risk contravening the Abortion Act.
3. Reversible contraception should be continued until the operation. It is not necessary to stop the combined pill before sterilization as the risk of thromboembolic complications is negligible. If an IUD is in situ, it should be removed, unless the operation is being done at mid-cycle and intercourse has taken place within the previous few days.
4. Immediate postpartum or post-abortion sterilization is more likely to be regretted and, as discussed earlier, carries more risks.
5. It is not necessary to shave the pubic area or abdomen before laparoscopy or mini-laparotomy.

Postoperative advice

1. Skin incisions closed with absorbable sutures require no further treatment. If clips or non-absorbable sutures are used they will be removed before leaving hospital, or arrangements made to have this done at home. The wounds will usually heal within 10 days.
2. Slight bruising and discomfort may sometimes be experienced around the wounds for a few days.

3. Gas remaining in the peritoneal cavity often causes abdominal discomfort or shoulder pain for 24 to 48 hours.
4. Most women return to work within 48 hours of sterilization.
5. A mini-laparotomy wound takes a few days longer to heal and heavy lifting should be avoided for about 3 weeks.
6. Female sterilization is effective immediately and sexual activity may be resumed when the couple feel like it.

It is helpful to provide a leaflet containing a summary of this information (Appendix 7.1).

Follow-up

The resumption of menses may be delayed in women who have stopped using the combined pill. However, if the patient is amenorrhoeic, pregnancy should always be excluded as she may have already been pregnant at the time of sterilization. If she was previously using an IUD, check that it has been removed; occasionally it gets forgotten!

Complications

Immediate complications

1. The operation carries a small operative mortality – < 8 per 100 000 operations.
2. Vascular damage or damage to bowel or other internal organs may occur during the procedure and is usually recognized at the time of operation. Women should therefore be made aware of the rare need for a laparotomy and consequent longer stay in hospital. Unrecognized bowel damage should be suspected in any patient with unexplained pain, pyrexia and abdominal rigidity occurring within the first 2 weeks of sterilization. Such cases should be referred to hospital urgently.
3. Thromboembolic disease is rare, but is more likely if the procedure is done immediately postpartum.
4. Infection or oozing from the wound does occasionally occur and can be managed symptomatically.

Late complications

1. *Menstrual bleeding patterns*. Female sterilization does not alter ovarian activity or menstruation (Gentile et al 1998). Women who stop using the combined pill, however, will almost certainly notice that their periods become heavier, perhaps more painful and less predictable, and should be warned of this. In contrast, women whose previous method of

contraception was an IUD will notice an improvement in their bleeding patterns. Despite this there have been a number of studies which have demonstrated an increased incidence of hysterectomy among women who have been sterilized (Hillis et al 1998). Bearing in mind the inevitable changes in menstrual bleeding patterns associated with advancing age and with stopping the combined pill (the most commonly used method of reversible contraception), it may be that women who have been sterilized are more likely to seek hysterectomy, or more willing to accept it, if they are already incapable of further childbearing.

2. The term *post-tubal sterilization syndrome* was coined to describe a variety of symptoms that have been reported after sterilization and which women may attribute to the procedure. These symptoms include abdominal pain, dyspareunia, exacerbation of premenstrual syndrome or dysmenorrhoea and emotional and psychosexual problems. Laparoscopy fails to demonstrate any pathology. A recent review of the literature (Gentile et al 1998) concluded that sterilization is not associated with an increased risk of these problems except among women sterilized before the age of 30 in whom the symptoms may sometimes be a manifestation of regret.

3. *Bowel obstruction* from adhesions is a very rare complication.

4. *Ectopic pregnancy* has been reported in up to 50% of failures following cautery and in 4% following mechanical occlusive methods. A large collaborative study undertaken in the USA and involving over 10 000 women was reported in 1996 (Peterson et al 1996). The 10-year cumulative probability of ectopic pregnancy was 7.3 per 1000 procedures.

Women should be advised that **if they miss a period and have symptoms of pregnancy they should seek medical advice urgently**.

5. Several studies have suggested that tubal sterilization may reduce the risk of ovarian cancer. In one large American study, the hazard ratio was 0.64 (Miracle-McMahill et al 1997). The reason for this association is not at all clear.

VASECTOMY

Techniques

Vasectomy involves the division or occlusion of the vas deferens to prevent the passage of sperm. It can be performed under LA or GA. A variety of techniques for vas occlusion is available but the principle is the same in all of them.

Division and ligation

The vas is palpated through the skin of the upper scrotum and fixed either instrumentally or between the fingers and thumb. The vas within its fascial sheath is exposed through a small skin incision, the fascia is opened longitudinally and the vas ligated and divided (Figs 7.6 and 7.7) or occluded with clips or by diathermy. Interposing the fascial sheath between the cut ends of the vas is thought to increase the effectiveness of the procedure. The sheath and scrotal skin are closed separately. The vas may be approached either by a single midline incision or by two incisions, one on each side. Variations in technique include:

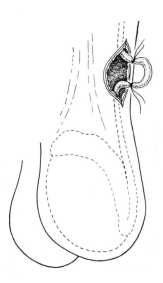

Figure 7.6
Vas ligated.

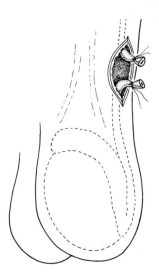

Figure 7.7
Vas divided.

1. *Excising a small portion of vas.* It is unlikely that this increases effectiveness unless at least 4 cm of vas is excised and excision makes reversal more difficult. It does however allow the portion of vas to be examined histologically which may help in subsequent cases of litigation but also increases the expense of the procedure.

2. *Looping* each cut end of vas back on itself.

3. *Occlusion using a small silver clip.*

4. *Occlusion using unipolar diathermy* with a specifically designed probe which is passed 1 cm proximally and distally down the divided vas, coagulating the tissue for 3 to 4 seconds until the muscle becomes opaque.

5. *The 'no-scalpel vasectomy' (NSV),* developed in China in 1974 and now quite widely used, makes use of specially designed instruments for isolating and delivering the vas through the scrotal skin and substitutes a small puncture for the skin incision. Any of the standard methods of occlusion may be used. NSV is quick and is associated with a lower incidence of infection and haematoma. A comparison between NSV and conventional vasectomy in Thailand reported a complication rate of 0.4% compared with 3.1% (Nirapathpongporn et al 1990). Training in the technique can be arranged through the Association for Voluntary Surgical Contraception in New York.

6. *Open-ended vasectomy* – the vas can simply be divided and the cut ends left open. This technique is seldom used as it almost certainly increases failure rates but it does facilitate reversal.

7. *Non-surgical techniques* – percutaneous injection of sclerosing agents such as polyurethane elastomers or occlusive substances such as silicone is being used in China. The technique avoids any skin incision and furthermore the silicone plug is said to be easily removed and pregnancy rates of 100% up to 5 years after vasectomy reversal have been claimed.

No large randomized controlled studies have been done to determine whether one method is any more effective than the other and efficacy probably depends most on the experience of the surgeon.

Clinical management

Assessment

In addition to the points covered in counselling (pp **191–192**), a history should be taken to exclude any factors which may complicate the operation and which may determine whether LA or GA should be used. These should include:

1. A history of previous genital or inguinal surgery, e.g. orchidopexy.
2. A history of reaction to LA or contraindications to GA (including fear or extreme anxiety).

Examination

In some family planning clinics, where vasectomy is done under LA, the man is counselled by a nurse or doctor and not seen by the surgeon until the time of operation. In this case it is good practice to examine the man prior to recommending him for vasectomy. It is annoying for the patient and a waste of operating time if a problem which precludes vasectomy under LA is not discovered until the patient is being prepared for surgery.

Timing of operation

Some surgeons refuse to perform a vasectomy on men whose wives are pregnant and insist that the operation is delayed until after the safe delivery of a healthy baby. While this would seem sensible to most clinicians, some couples see pregnancy as an extremely convenient time during which the vasectomy can become effective. Each couple should be considered individually in respect of timing of the operation.

Preoperative and postoperative advice: follow-up

1. The patient is usually asked to shave the upper scrotum himself before he presents for operation – this saves both time and embarrassment.

2. He is advised to wear underpants which give good scrotal support for a few days after the procedure.

3. Most men return to work the following day but the risk of haematoma formation is probably reduced if strenuous physical exercise is avoided for 3 or 4 days.

4. It **must** be made clear that it takes some time for remaining sperm to disappear from the distal portion of the vas and that an alternative method of contraception **must** be used until there is azoospermia. The rate at which azoospermia is achieved depends on the frequency of ejaculation. In developing countries where laboratory facilities for examining seminal fluid do not exist, couples are advised to use other contraception until after 20 ejaculations. In the UK, seminal fluid is examined after 12 and 16 weeks and, if sperm are still present, usually monthly thereafter. Not until two consecutive negative samples have been confirmed can the vasectomy be considered to be complete. Instructions for the collection of specimens and their delivery to the laboratory should be given to the patient who should be informed once the vasectomy is complete.

5. Men who experience complications or in whom vasectomy fails seem to be particularly ready to sue. In order to avoid successful litigation, it is imperative that counselling for vasectomy is clear and detailed and covers every eventuality. We have a checklist which counsellors tick as they cover all the points in the discussion with the couple. In Edinburgh, a detailed

information leaflet (Appendix 7.2) is sent out with the first appointment informing the couple about complications and the failure rate before they attend for counselling. They are asked to sign a form stating that they have read and understood the information sheet in addition to the standard form consenting to operation.

Complications

Immediate

1. *Bruising and haematoma*. Almost everyone will experience scrotal bruising but in 1–2% of men postoperative bleeding will be sufficient to cause a haematoma. Local support and analgesia are usually adequate treatment but a small number of men will require admission to hospital for drainage of the haematoma.
2. *Wound infection* occurs in up to 5% of men and may need treatment with antibiotics.
3. *Failure* – up to 2% of men fail to achieve azoospermia. If sperm continue to appear in the ejaculate for months, the vasectomy can be re-done. The timing of a 're-do' or exploration is a matter for discussion between the patient and surgeon. The continued presence of sperm may be due to infrequent ejaculation but if this does not appear to be the case and if many sperm are present, it seems a little hard to ask the patient to provide specimens month after month before admitting defeat.

Late

1. *Sperm granulomas* – small lumps may form at the cut ends of the vas as a result of a local inflammatory response to leaked sperm. These may be painful and palpable and pain can persist for years. Excision usually solves the problem. Sperm granulomas may also physically unite the cut ends of the vas and increase the chance of failure.
2. *Chronic intrascrotal pain and discomfort* (post-vasectomy syndrome) – some men complain of a dull ache in the scrotum which may be exacerbated by sexual excitement and ejaculation. The symptoms are probably due to distension and granuloma formation in the epididymis and vas deferens. Pain may also result from scar tissue forming around small nerves. Chronic pain associated with progressive induration, tubular distension and granuloma formation in the epididymis may require excision of the epididymis and obstructed vas deferens.
3. *Late recanalization* – failure can occur up to 10 years after vasectomy despite two negative samples of seminal fluid following the procedure. It is rare (1 in 1000) but pregnancy as a result of late recanalization is always a sensitive issue. It is not tactful to cast any doubt on the paternity of the pregnancy. Seminal analysis can be offered but if no sperm are seen in the ejacu-

late this may cause major domestic problems for the couple concerned. Every case must be handled individually but it is sometimes best simply to offer a re-do without semen analysis.

4. *Antisperm antibodies* – after vasectomy, most men develop detectable concentrations of autoantibodies presumably in response to leakage of sperm. Their presence may compromise fertility if reversal is sought.

5. *Cardiovascular, endocrine and autoimmune disease* – concerns about a possible link between vasectomy and cardiovascular disease were raised in the 1970s following the observation that vasectomy increased athero-sclerosis in rhesus monkeys. It was suggested that this may be attributable to increased levels of auto-antibodies which might alter the risk of autoimmune disease in general, including joint disease and multiple sclerosis. Several large studies, including a cohort study in the USA of over 10 000 vasectomized men, have failed to substantiate increased rates of 98 diseases and in fact suggested that vasectomy was associated with a lower death rate (Massey et al 1984). See McDonald (1997) for a useful review of the long-term effects of vasectomy on health.

6. *Cancer* – two epidemiological studies from the USA and Scotland (Strader et al 1988, Cale et al 1990) suggested an increased risk of testicular cancer following vasectomy. This observation has not been substantiated by later research. A large study of over 73 000 Danish men (Moller et al 1994) concluded that testicular cancer is no more common in men who have been vasectomized than in other men. A number of large epidemiological studies from the USA have also suggested an increased risk of prostate cancer following vasectomy (McDonald 1997). At a meeting in 1991, the World Health Organization (WHO) reviewed biological and epidemiological evidence and concluded that there was no known biological mechanism to account for any association and that any causal relationship between vasectomy and prostate cancer was unlikely. The National Institute of Health in the USA in 1993 endorsed the WHO conclusions and recommended that there was insufficient basis to change policies regarding vasectomy. A review of the literature in 1998 by Peterson and Howards concluded that vasectomy is unlikely to be a major risk factor for prostate cancer.

Indications

1. Couples who are absolutely certain that their family is complete.
2. Individuals or couples who choose to have no children.
3. When one partner:
   a. carries a significant risk of transmitting an inherited disorder
   b. suffers from chronic ill-health which would (in the case of the woman) contraindicate pregnancy or affect the couple's ability to bring up children.

In the last two instances, it is sensible to sterilize the affected partner.

Contraindications

Unless couples are absolutely certain that, for whatever reason, they want no, or no more, children, sterilization should not be performed. It is not unusual, however, for a woman to request sterilization because no other method of contraception suits her, or because she believes that the procedure will enhance her libido or improve her pattern of menstruation. Rarely, the referring doctor implies the same misconception.

Up to 10% of couples regret the decision to undergo sterilization and 1% will seek reversal (Chi and Jones 1994). Factors which are known to increase the risk of regret include:

1. Marital/relationship problems.
2. Young age.
3. Timing of sterilization – women who are sterilized immediately postpartum or post-abortion are more likely to seek reversal.
4. Psychiatric illness in either partner.

Advantages

Both *male and female sterilization* provides highly effective long-term contraception without the need for continued motivation or compliance.

The advantages of *male as opposed to female sterilization* are:

1. It is a simpler procedure.
2. It can be performed under local anaesthetic as an outpatient procedure.
3. It requires no sophisticated equipment and is much cheaper to perform.
4. Mortality and significant operative morbidity are virtually non-existent.
5. Its efficacy can be checked. Perhaps for this reason failure rates are lower.

The advantages of *female as opposed to male sterilization* are:

1. It is immediately effective.
2. A woman's reproductive life is finite; a man retains his fertility for many years and has potentially more opportunity to regret the decision to be sterilized.

Disadvantages

1. Female sterilization carries a risk of operative mortality and morbidity (pp **183–184**).
2. Sterilization cannot always be reversed (pp **192–193**).

3. Sterilization is more complicated than alternative methods of contraception requiring the provision of specialized facilities and trained personnel.
4. Vasectomy is not effective immediately, and other contraception must be used until two consecutive negative sperm counts are obtained.

Counselling

Most couples seeking sterilization have been thinking about the operation for some considerable time. The counselling session should provide opportunities for information, explanation, discussion and advice and should enable a couple to decide what is in their own best interests. Many couples are quite certain of their wishes and the consultation should not be unduly prolonged unless doubt is expressed or perceived. The couple should be prepared to provide details about themselves, their circumstances and the reason for requesting sterilization. The counsellor should provide information about both procedures, and the implications and should cover:

a. description of operations and associated myths/misconceptions
b. failure rates
c. risks/side effects
d. which partner should be sterilized
e. alternative long-acting methods should be discussed.
   Some doctors and most lay people do not realize that depot medroxyprogesterone acetate, Norplant and the LNG-IUS are as effective, if not more effective, than female sterilization. They all also allow a change of heart
f. reversibility
g. possibility of wanting more children.

   Information sought from the couple should include:

a. reason for the request
b. relevant medical, gynaecological and obstetric histories
c. ages, occupations and social circumstances
d. numbers, ages and health of their children
e. previous and current contraception and any problems experienced
f. stability of the marriage and the possibility of its breakdown
g. quality of their sexual life.

   A leaflet which covers these points should be available for the couple to take away.
   Counselling for female sterilization is usually done by the general practitioner or family planning doctor who refers the woman to a gynaecologist who covers many of the points again. Some hospitals provide 'mail-order' female sterilization where all the counselling is done by the general

practitioner and the surgeon does not meet the patient until the operation. Vasectomy is often done under LA in a clinic setting or in the general practitioner's surgery. In some large family planning clinics, specially trained nurses do the counselling and only seek a medical opinion if there are contraindications, doubts or clinical problems. Sessionally employed surgeons operate on men who have been counselled by someone else. Locally agreed protocols should protect the surgeon from being faced with a patient he/she would prefer not to sterilize for whatever reason.

Effectiveness

Failure of female sterilization varies according to both the method used and the experience of the surgeon. The U.S. Collaborative Review of Sterilization demonstrated higher failure rates than had previously been reported. It has been suggested that the figures are misleading because they include a great many procedures performed by junior doctors in training. This, of course, is the reality in the UK. The 10-year cumulative pregnancy rate per thousand women was highest for spring clips at 36.5. The rates for bipolar diathermy were 24.8/1000 and for falope rings 17.7/1000. Cumulative pregnancy rates varied not only by the method of tubal occlusion but also by age at the time of sterilization with significantly higher failure rates among women aged 18–27 than those aged 34–44. The simplest way to explain these statistics is to tell women that they have a 1 in 200 chance of getting pregnant at some time after being sterilized.

Vasectomy is generally accepted as being more effective than female sterilization. In the Oxford/FPA study, Vessey et al (1982) reported a failure rate of 0.02 per HWY after vasectomy (1 in 2000).

The RCOG has recommended that a national register of sterilization failures would facilitate both national and local audit and allow couples to be given more accurate information about the procedures.

Reversibility

Couples should be advised that sterilization is intended to be permanent. Despite careful counselling, however, it is inevitable that a few couples will request reversal of their sterilization. This is most likely to happen when the marriage breaks down and one or other partner starts a new relationship. Although as many as 10% of couples regret being sterilized, only 1% of these will request reversal. Counselling for sterilization should include information on the success rates associated with reversal.

Reversal of female sterilization is more likely to be successful after occlusion with clips which have been applied to the isthmic portion of the tube since only a small section of tube will have been damaged. Patients should realize that reversal involves laparotomy, does not always work (microsurgical techniques are associated with around 70% success) and carries a significant risk of ectopic pregnancy (up to 5%). Reversal is unlikely to be available on the NHS in many parts of the UK.

Reversal of vasectomy is technically feasible in many cases with patency rates of almost 90% being reported in some series. Pregnancy rates are much less (up to 60%) perhaps as a result of the presence of anti-sperm antibodies.

Some laboratories now offer a sperm banking service to men prior to vasectomy. The availability of such services complicates counselling since the concept seems to contradict the advice that a couple should not consider vasectomy unless they are absolutely certain they want no more children.

Risks/benefits

Although sterilization operations do carry small but significant risks, the overall benefits in terms of effectiveness and convenience tend to outweigh these in well-motivated and adequately counselled couples. In a couple who have completed their family, the procedure avoids the need for continued motivation in contraceptive usage and the long-term side effects of effective reversible methods, such as the combined pill and IUD.

REFERENCES

Cale ARJ, Farouk M, Prescott RJ, Wallace IWJ 1990 Does vasectomy accelerate testicular tumour? Importance of testicular examinations before and after vasectomy. British Medical Journal 300: 370
Chi I-C, Jones DB 1994 Incidence, risk factors and prevention of poststerilization regret in women: an updated international review from an epidemiological perspective. Obstetrical and Gynecological Survey 49: 722–732
Gentile GP, Kaufman SC, Helbig DW 1998 Is there any evidence for a post-tubal sterilization syndrome? Fertility and Sterility 69: 179–186
Hieu DT, Tran TT, Tan DN, Nguyet PT, Than P, Vinh DQ 1993 31 781 cases of non-surgical female sterilization with quinacrine pellets in Vietnam. Lancet 342: 213–217
Hillis SD, Marchbanks PA, Tylor LR, Peterson HB 1998 Higher hysterectomy risk for sterilized than nonsterilized women: findings in the U.S. Collaborative Review of Sterilization. The U.S. Collaborative Review of Sterilization Working Group. Obstetrics and Gynecology 91: 241–246
Massey FJ, Bernstein GS, O'Fallon WM et al 1984 Vasectomy and health: results from a large cohort study. Journal of the American Medical Association 252: 1023–1029
McDonald SW 1997 Is vasectomy harmful to health? British Journal of General Practice 47: 381–386
Miracle-McMahill HL, Calle EE, Kosinski AS, et al 1997 Tubal ligation and fatal ovarian cancer in a large prospective cohort study. American Journal of Epidemiology 145: 349–357
Moller H, Knudsen LB, Lynge E 1994 Risk of testicular cancer after vasectomy: a cohort study of over 73 000 men. British Medical Journal 309: 295–299
Nirapathpongporn A, Huber D, Kieger JN 1990 No-scalpel vasectomy at the King's birthday vasectomy festival. Lancet 335: 894–895
Peterson HB, Xia Z, Hughes JM, Wilkox LS, Tylor LR, Trussel J for the U.S. Collaborative Review of Sterilization Working Group 1996 The risk of pregnancy after tubal sterilization:

findings from the U.S. Collaborative Review of Sterilization. American Journal of Obstetrics and Gynecology 174: 1161–1170

Peterson HB, Howards SS 1998 Vasectomy and prostate cancer: the evidence to date. Fertility and Sterility 70: 201–203

Royal College of Obstetricans and Gynaecologists (RCOG) 1999 Male and female sterilisation. Evidence-Based Clinical Guidelines No 4. RCOG, London

Strader CH, Weiss NS, Daling JR 1988 Vasectomy and the incidence of testicular cancer. American Journal of Epidemiology 128: 56–63

Vessey MP, Lawless M, Yeates D 1982 Efficacy of different contraceptive methods. Lancet i: 841–842

Appendix 7.1

STERILIZATION OF THE FEMALE BY LAPAROSCOPY

For a pregnancy to start, an egg must combine with a sperm. This usually takes place in one of the fallopian tubes which join the ovaries to the womb. All methods of female sterilization block the tubes.

The operation we intend to carry out is called laparoscopy. A short general anaesthetic is required. Through a one-inch-long cut below the navel (tummy button), an instrument is passed through the abdominal wall. This allows careful inspection of the womb, tubes and ovaries. If they appear normal, another small instrument is passed through a separate, even smaller incision. This allows the tubes to be blocked with small clips or rings or by means of a very small electric current.

Complications are rare and recovery rapid so that you will usually be allowed home the same day as your operation. Some patients experience pain in the region of the shoulders or vaginal bleeding for some days after the operation, but this need not cause any concern. Very rarely, some unsuspected abnormality will be seen or will occur at the time of operation so that a more major operation is necessary, but it must be emphasized that this is very unusual.

You will be sterile from the time of the operation and it is safe to resume intercourse as soon as you have completely recovered from the operation. Apart from the fact that you can no longer conceive, neither your periods nor your desire for sex will be affected. Once sterilization has been performed, it is permanent and does not require to be repeated after a number of years. Reversal of the operation, which is occasionally requested, is difficult.

Failure of the operation permitting further pregnancy is rare but does occasionally occur. Therefore, if at any time after operation your period is more than 2 weeks late you should consult your family doctor as soon as possible.

Appendix 7.2

MALE STERILIZATION

You have expressed an interest in having a vasectomy. You and your partner will be given an appointment to find out more about the procedure before a date is arranged for your operation. This information leaflet tells you about the operation, the effectiveness and side effects. It is designed to give you the facts and to help you decide whether this is to be your chosen method of contraception. It is not meant to sound off-putting but it tells you about the possible complications. You will have the opportunity to discuss the information and to ask questions when you come to the clinic for your vasectomy counselling appointment. All methods of contraception carry some risk and it is up to you to decide which method is most acceptable. We hope that this information sheet will help you in making your decision.

What is a vasectomy?

A tube called the vas deferens carries sperm from each testis into the penis. Vasectomy is the cutting or blocking of both these tubes to prevent the passage of sperm (see below). The vas are cut just above the testis. Vasectomy does not interfere with the production of seminal fluid so you will not notice any difference in the amount of fluid you produce when you ejaculate – the fluid simply will not contain sperm. The operation is done under local anaesthetic and takes less than half an hour. A small cut is made in the skin in the middle or on each side of the scrotum and the vas which lies just beneath the skin can then be cut or blocked. The skin may be closed with a stitch or tape or simply left to heal without any closure.

How effective is vasectomy?

Vasectomy is not 100% effective but one of the advantages of the procedure is that its efficacy can be tested. It takes some weeks for all the sperm that remain in the vas (tube) to disappear

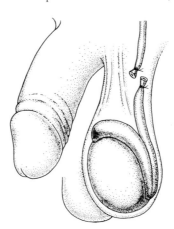

Vasectomy

and the rate at which this happens depends on how often you have intercourse. You will be asked to send a specimen of seminal fluid to the laboratory 12 weeks after your operation and again at 16 weeks. In most cases, both samples will be free of sperm and we will let you know that your operation is complete. In some cases, it takes more than 16 weeks for the sperm to clear and you will be asked to continue to send samples every 4 weeks until two consecutive samples are free of sperm. In up to 2% of cases (2 in 100 men), sperm continue to appear and you will be advised to have the vasectomy explored, usually under general anaesthetic in hospital. **Until you have been told that your operation is complete, you or your partner should continue to use another method of contraception.**

In 1 in 1000 cases the vasectomy fails at a later date – the two ends of the vas heal with time and rarely the canal re-opens (so-called 'late recanalization'). If this happens, your partner may become pregnant despite you having had two sperm-free samples and being told that your operation was complete. Late re-canalization may happen some years after you have had your vasectomy. By comparison, sterilization in the female fails in around 3 per 1000 cases.

Are there any problems?

Complications can be divided into those which might occur immediately after the vasectomy and those which do not occur for some years.

Immediate complications

All surgical operations carry some risk and vasectomy is no exception but the problems are usually minor.

Between 5 and 10% of men experience minor local problems after the procedure. Once the local anaesthetic has worn off (after about 2 hours), you will probably feel some discomfort which is usually helped by taking a mild painkiller (paracetamol or aspirin). Most men notice a certain amount of swelling and bruising around the operation site which lasts a few days. Sometimes the site can become infected and you may require antibiotics. If you notice persisting pain, swelling or redness you should contact your general practitioner. Occasionally, a moderate amount of bleeding occurs and the blood slowly collects at the base of the scrotum causing a large swelling or haematoma. 1 in 100 men requires hospital treatment for this complication and although this can be a rather frightening event, it does not cause any long-term problems.

Long-term consequences

In 10–15% of men, leakage of sperm from the cut end of the vas causes some inflammation and occasionally small painful lumps (sperm granulomas) may appear. Very rarely the pain may last for years after a vasectomy but further surgery usually cures the problem.

A large amount of research has been carried out on the long-term effects of vasectomy in order to establish whether the procedure has any effect on general health. While there seems to be no good evidence for any serious long-term effects, a number of studies have raised the possibility of there being a link between prostate cancer and vasectomy.

Cancer of the prostate is relatively common in men although rare below the age of 65. In Scotland about 650 men die from the disease each year compared with about 2700 men dying from lung cancer and about 1300 women who die from breast cancer. The cause of prostate cancer is not known but it is in some way dependent on the male hormone testosterone.

Most cancers are associated with certain risk factors, e.g. men who have worked with some chemicals are much more likely to develop bladder cancer than those who do not. We do not know what risk factors are related to prostate cancer.

Does having a vasectomy increase your chance of later developing cancer of the prostate? A lot of medical research has investigated the possibility of a relationship between vasectomy and prostate cancer. A number of large studies in China and in the USA have suggested that there is no link between vasectomy and the risk of prostate cancer. Indeed, in the Chinese study, men who had a vasectomy were healthier than those who had not but prostate cancer is rare in Chinese men. Recently, however, two more studies from America have suggested that there may be a link and that 20 years after a vasectomy your risk of developing prostate cancer may be almost double that of men of the same age who have not had a vasectomy. The risk of a man in Scotland developing prostate cancer is around 1 in 2000. If the American studies are correct this means that if you have a vasectomy, your risk increases to 1 in 1000. Cancer of the prostate is a relatively benign condition and although 1 in 25 men aged 74 years will have a tumour of the prostate, the vast majority will live to a ripe old age and die of other causes.

The World Health Organization (WHO) held a meeting of experts in 1991 to discuss the issue. The experts decided that, despite many years of research, there is no known biological reason for vasectomy causing prostate cancer. It is hard to see how vasectomy might affect the risk of prostate cancer. It is more likely that for some reason men who decide to have a vasectomy have some characteristics which also make them more likely to develop prostate cancer although we do not know what these characteristics might be. WHO recommends that more research should be done but that family planning policies should not be changed.

One or two small studies have also suggested a link between vasectomy and testicular cancer. Again there is no obvious physiological basis for such a link and it is possible that men who have recently had a vasectomy may be more likely to examine themselves and so find a lump in the testis.

What does this mean for you? All methods of contraception carry some risk. When you decide on a family planning method you weigh up the risks and benefits for you and your partner. Long-term use of the contraceptive pill carries a small risk for women as does female sterilization. On the whole, whatever the method, using contraception is probably safer than either having a baby or having an abortion. Moreover, apart from the health risks involved, individual couples must consider what an unplanned pregnancy would mean to their lives. While you and your partner have to decide for yourselves whether or not to choose a vasectomy, many couples may consider that the small risk of problems is acceptable when balanced with the benefits of an extremely effective method of contraception.

Can vasectomy be reversed?

Yes, but reversal is not always successful. It requires an intricate operation and even if the cut ends of the vas are successfully united and sperm can get through, fertility may not be normal. The operation may not be available from the National Health Service so if you were to request reversal you might have to pay for it. You should not have a vasectomy if you think that you might at some time want to have the operation reversed.

Practical details

This information leaflet is being sent to you before your appointment for counselling. You should expect to be in the clinic for about half an hour for this consultation. It is helpful if your partner accompanies you as she may also have some questions. Unfortunately, we do not have crèche facilities and you may find it difficult to concentrate if you are being distracted by your children so we strongly recommend a baby-sitter if you can find one!

If you decide to go ahead with a vasectomy, you will be given a date for the operation. You should remember to shave the scrotum and the skin around the base of the penis before you come to the clinic. This is best done in the bath the night before the operation.

After the operation you will have a short rest before going home. You will probably be in the clinic for less than 1 hour. You should rest at home for the remainder of the day and will probably find it comfortable to wear either an athletic support (jock strap) or a pair of well-supporting underpants for a couple of days.

Most men return to work the following day but you should avoid lifting heavy weights or doing other heavy manual work for 3 or 4 days. It is not sensible to arrange unavoidable commitments or energetic holidays immediately following the operation.

We hope that you have found this information leaflet helpful. When you come to the clinic you will be asked to sign a copy saying that you have read and understood the information and been given the opportunity to ask questions. The signed copy will be kept in your record; this copy is for you to keep.

I have read the information leaflet and have had the opportunity to ask questions.

I understand that we should continue to use some other method of contraception until I have been informed that the vasectomy is complete.

I understand that the operation does not work in a small number of cases and therefore must be re-done, and that very rarely the procedure may fail some time after having apparently been successful initially.

I understand that vasectomy cannot always be successfully reversed and that should I wish a reversal the operation may not be available from the National Health Service.

I understand that up to 10% of men experience minor complications such as bleeding, haematoma formation and infection, and that such complications occasionally require treatment in hospital.

I understand that there have been some concerns raised about the long-term effects of vasectomy but that present knowledge suggests that these are not significant.

Signature ....

Date ....

8

Emergency contraception

Anna Glasier

Risk of pregnancy   201
Methods   202
  Ethinyloestradiol and
    levonorgestrel   202
  Levonorgestrel   202
  Intrauterine devices   202
  Oestrogens   203
Mode of action   203
  Hormonal regimens   203
  Intrauterine devices   203
Effectiveness   203
Indications   205
Contraindications   205

Side effects   207
  Hormonal   207
  Intrauterine devices   207
New prospects   207
  Danazol   207
  Anti-progesterones   208
Clinical management   208
  Assessment   208
  Management of postcoital
    intrauterine device insertion   209
Information for users   209
Follow-up   210
Use and availability   210

When the first edition of this book was published in 1985, emergency contraception (EC) was still a 'well-kept secret'. The next 15 years saw a burgeoning interest in the topic and in the years since the most recent edition (1995), a new and better hormonal method has reached the market which before long is likely to be available off prescription. Added to the WHO list of essential drugs in 1996, EC is now recognized as an essential component of contraceptive choice.

RISK OF PREGNANCY

The risk of pregnancy differs depending on the day in the cycle when intercourse occurs. Intercourse which occurs more than 6 days before ovulation will not result in pregnancy. The risk of pregnancy increases from around 8% 6 days before ovulation to 36% on the day of ovulation (Wilcox et al 1995). The risk of pregnancy following intercourse on the day after ovulation may be zero and is certainly no more than 12%. It appears that sperm survive in the reproductive tract capable of fertilization for up to 6 days after intercourse. Most women find it difficult to recall exactly the date of their last menstrual period (LMP). Cycle length varies from month to month and ovulation does not always reliably occur on the same day each cycle. While it may be tempting to take physiology into account and withhold EC when there appears to be no genuine risk of conception (e.g. after intercourse on day 24 in a cycle which is usually 28 days in length), this is probably not in the woman's best interests.

202 HANDBOOK OF FAMILY PLANNING

METHODS
Ethinyloestradiol and levonorgestrel

The first method of EC to be licensed in the UK (in 1984) was Schering PC4. It consists of a combination of 100 µg ethinyloestradiol (EE) and 500 µg levonorgestrel (LNG) given twice, with the first dose taken within 72 hours of intercourse and the second 12 hours after the first. Often called the Yuzpe regimen after the gynaecologist who first described the method, Schering PC4 is relatively expensive (£1.60 in October 1999) and many clinics make up their own much cheaper supplies using combined oral contraceptive (COC) pills containing the same type and dose of hormones (e.g. Ovran). Although the COC is not licensed for this purpose, the practice is widespread and provided the pills are placed in a container with instructions for use, this would appear to be medicolegally acceptable. Recent guidelines suggest, however, that no drug should be issued by nurses if it is being used for a purpose for which it is not licensed.

Levonorgestrel

LNG 0.75 mg taken twice with the two doses separated by 12 hours and the first within 72 hours of intercourse is as effective (perhaps more effective) as Schering PC4 but is better tolerated because of the absence of oestrogen. One licensed product, Levonelle-2 (Schering) is currently available in the UK.

Intrauterine devices

Postcoital intrauterine device (IUD) insertion is sometimes used as an alternative to hormonal EC if there are contraindications to high-dose steroids or if a woman presents more than 72 hours after intercourse. IUD insertion may be used for up to 5 days after the calculated earliest day of ovulation (i.e. up to day 19 in a woman with a 28-day cycle). Thus, if intercourse occurs before ovulation, the IUD may be inserted more than 5 days after intercourse and may be used for multiple exposure (repeated episodes of intercourse). It is probably effective beyond 5 days after ovulation, but extending the time limits risks contravening the 1967 Abortion Act. IUD insertion is an invasive procedure, not always acceptable to women requesting postcoital contraception (PCC) who are often young and nulliparous. The IUD is particularly useful for women who wish to continue with the method for long-term contraception.

Oestrogens

High-dose oestrogens given over 5 days were used in early trials of hormonal EC and proved very effective but were associated with a high incidence of nausea and vomiting. When an association between high-dose oestrogens and vaginal adenosis and malignancy was recognized the approach was abandoned, although it is still used occasionally in Holland (EE 5 mg daily for 5 days). There is no evidence that the regimen is more effective than the Yuzpe regimen and there is really no place for oestrogen alone today.

MODE OF ACTION

Hormonal regimens

The exact mode of action of the hormonal regimens is not known. There is good evidence that the Yuzpe regimen inhibits or delays ovulation. Biochemical and histological changes in the endometrium have been described following the administration of the Yuzpe regimen but the findings are inconsistent and many experts agree that the changes may be insufficient to impair implantation. The observation in early studies that high-dose oestrogen was associated with increased risk of ectopic pregnancy led to the suggestion that tubal motility may be altered but this is not supported by any experimental evidence (see Glasier 1997 for review).

There are even fewer data on the mode of action of LNG alone although studies are ongoing. It probably inhibits ovulation and may have more of an effect on endometrial receptivity than the Yuzpe regimen. It may also alter the characteristics of cervical mucus, impairing sperm transport and preventing fertilization of an egg which is ovulated within a few days after treatment.

Intrauterine devices

The IUD diminishes the viability of ova, the number of sperm reaching the fallopian tube and their ability to fertilize the egg. However, since it is so often used effectively days after the act of intercourse, postcoital IUD insertion almost certainly acts by inhibiting implantation.

EFFECTIVENESS

The efficacy of EC is difficult to measure accurately. Most women are not absolutely sure of the date of their last period and ovulation does not always occur on the same day each cycle. It is likely that many women have had more than one act of unprotected intercourse when they use EC and some of them will have already conceived.

Pregnancy may also be due to another act of intercourse which occurred after EC had been used. In recent years, attempts to estimate the efficacy of EC have based estimates of expected pregnancy rates on data collected from women who were actively trying to conceive and who kept diaries of menses and intercourse.

Effectiveness rates are therefore only *estimates* as there have never been any placebo-controlled trials. With this caveat, it is estimated that the Yuzpe regimen will prevent around 75% of pregnancies (Trussell et al 1998), LNG around 85% (Task Force on Postovulatory Methods of Fertility Regulation 1998), and the IUD over 95% of pregnancies (Trussell and Ellertson 1995). Recent data from WHO (Piaggio et al 1999) suggest that both hormonal regimens become less effective with time, even within the 72-hour window (Fig. 8.1).

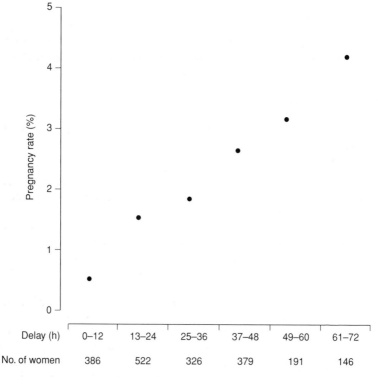

Delay (h)	0–12	13–24	25–36	37–48	49–60	61–72
No. of women	386	522	326	379	191	146

Figure 8.1 The effect on pregnancy rates of delaying use of emergency contraception. (Reproduced with permission from Piaggio G et al 1999 Timing of emergency contraception with levonorgestrel or the Yuzpe regimen. Lancet 353:721.)

INDICATIONS

EC may be used in the following circumstances:

1. After unprotected intercourse.
2. After 'accidents' with a barrier method, e.g. burst condom or diaphragm removed within 6 hours of intercourse.
3. If one or more COC pills have been missed *at the beginning or end of a packet* so that the pill-free interval is prolonged beyond 7 days, it is appropriate to give hormonal EC.

   For women who have forgotten to take one or more COC at other times, the risk of conception occurs some days after the missed pills when ovarian follicular development, freed from inhibition by the oral contraceptive, is sufficient to allow ovulation to occur. Pregnancy should be prevented if the rules for missed pills are followed (p. **52**). If more than three pills have been forgotten or if pill-taking seems so erratic as to render the method ineffective, then EC is indicated.
4. If more than two progestogen-only pills (POP) have been forgotten, EC may be offered.
5. Occasionally women are so insistent that they need EC that even if it seems unnecessary (e.g. after one missed pill), it is sometimes easier to give it than to withhold it. Hormonal EC will do no harm and under these circumstances serves to relieve anxiety.

CONTRAINDICATIONS

There really are no contraindications to hormonal EC. Situations which require some thought before prescribing EC include:

1. *Pregnancy*. It is not necessary to perform a routine pregnancy test for women presenting for EC. If pregnancy is suspected clinically, it should be excluded, not because of concerns about teratogenesis but because neither method will dislodge an already implanted embryo.

2. *Multiple exposure*. If there has been unprotected intercourse more than once in a cycle, conception may have already occurred by the time EC is given. Obviously if a woman has already conceived, EC will not work. If she has not and is refused EC, then she risks conceiving from the act of intercourse which has just occurred.

There is no evidence that either hormonal EC is teratogenic but direct evidence is hard to come by. Indirect evidence is reassuring. The increased risk of fetal malformation associated with COC or POP use during early pregnancy is, if any, extremely small. Furthermore, the timing of EC use, before organogenesis begins, makes it unlikely that either hormonal method would be teratogenic. However, there is a background incidence of fetal malformation and a perfect baby can never be guaranteed. In our clinic, we advise women of the data that exist and inform them that we do not believe that the continuation of a pregnancy, in the event of EC failure, is contraindicated. Given this information, a woman should be allowed to decide for herself whether she wishes to use EC or not.

3. *Contraindications to oestrogen therapy (Yuzpe regimen only)*. In reality an acute exposure to oestrogens, albeit in high doses, is highly unlikely to be dangerous even for women in whom COC would be contraindicated. Pregnancy, particularly if unwanted, is usually even more strongly contraindicated for them – if such a woman is genuinely at risk of conception, there are very few instances in which the method need be refused, provided she understands the risks. A very recent thromboembolic event or an attack of classical migraine with neurological disturbance at the time of presenting for EC might be regarded as genuine contraindications; diabetes or hypercholesterolaemia would not. The biggest concern for most doctors is the risk of venous thromboembolism (VTE). The data are as follows and are reassuring:

a. The exposure to this higher dose of oestrogen is acute whereas the risks of the COC are associated with long-term use.
b. In a study of the direct effects of Schering PC4 on clotting factors, no effect was identified.
c. Schering PC4 was licensed in 1984 and by July 1996 (when the data were last reviewed) had been used more than 4 million times. Few adverse events had been reported to the Committee on Safety of Medicines. 115 reports of 159 reactions (some women having more than one), included 61 pregnancies.
   Only three cases of venous thrombosis had been reported, and in none was the relationship between EC and the event clear cut.
d. In a study done using the general practitioner research database in the UK (Vasilakis et al 1999), over 73 000 women who had between them received over 100 000 prescriptions for Schering PC4 were reviewed. No women had a venous thrombotic event within 60 days of using EC. The study concluded that the use of Schering PC4 was not associated with an increased risk of VTE.

4. A history of ectopic pregnancy is not regarded as a contraindication to hormonal EC.

5. *Pelvic inflammatory disease*. The IUD is not recommended for women with a history of recent pelvic inflammatory disease (although these histories can often be rather vague). Nor is it recommended for someone who is HIV positive.

SIDE EFFECTS
Hormonal

1. *Nausea and vomiting*. These occur with both hormonal methods but are much commoner with the Yuzpe regimen because of the high dose of

oestrogen. In trials in which women were asked to record side effects, nausea was said to occur in 50% of women and vomiting in up to 20%. In a routine clinic setting, spontaneous complaints of side effects are much less frequent and the incidence of nausea and vomiting may have been overemphasized.

Nausea and vomiting may however decrease compliance. Some clinics routinely provide an anti-emetic with Schering PC4 (e.g. domperidone 10 mg to be given with or just before each dose). Some clinics supply two extra tablets (six in all), the spare ones to be taken if vomiting occurs within 2 hours of either dose. To avoid nausea and vomiting, vaginal administration of EC is recommended by some, but there are no data to suggest the correct dose.

Where LNG alone is available, it will probably be the treatment of first choice as the risk of nausea and vomiting is much lower.

2. *Breast tenderness.*

3. *Disturbance of menstruation.* Women often complain that the subsequent period is heavier and sometimes more painful than normal. It may also be early or late but women using EC should be advised that it is most likely to arrive at the expected time.

4. *Dizziness, tiredness and headache.*

Intrauterine devices

1. Insertion may be difficult and painful, particularly in nulliparous women.
2. Women should be counselled about the risk of infection as for routine IUD insertion.

NEW PROSPECTS

Danazol

Danazol is a semi-synthetic steroid preparation which is strongly gestogenic and widely used for the treatment of endometriosis. It has been tested as an EC. However, there is some doubt about its efficacy and interest in it has waned.

Anti-progesterones

Progesterone is a prerequisite for implantation and anti-progestational hormones given in early pregnancy induce menstrual bleeding and abortion. Studies have demonstrated that the anti-progesterone mifepristone (RU

486) is a highly effective EC with significantly fewer side effects than combined oestrogen–progestogen. In initial studies involving almost 600 women treated with a single dose of 600 mg mifepristone, there were no pregnancies; however, up to 42% of women experienced a delay in the onset of menstruation of more than 3 days (Glasier et al 1992, Webb et al 1992). A recent study from WHO (Task Force on Postovulatory Methods of Fertility Regulation 1999) demonstrated an efficacy of greater than 85% for three doses of mifepristone (600 mg, 50 mg and 10 mg) with no significant difference between them in terms of efficacy but less delay in the onset of next menses with the 10 mg dose. The side effect profile has been excellent in all three studies. Further trials are underway including a double blind randomized comparison of mifepristone and LNG. Since mifepristone is known to inhibit implantation, it is likely to be a more effective EC than either Yuzpe or LNG; however, the politics surrounding its use as an abortifacient jeopardizes its development as a contraceptive of any sort. The confusion over the mechanism of action and the widespread belief that EC is the same as an abortion has been exacerbated by the use of mifepristone for EC.

CLINICAL MANAGEMENT

Assessment

History

While it may be difficult to break with the tradition of taking a full medical and reproductive history, in practice it is only really necessary to exclude ongoing pregnancy and to determine by direct questioning which would be the best method of EC for an individual woman. When EC becomes available off prescription, then complicated protocols for provision in a clinic will seem illogical.

1. Pregnancy can be excluded by determining the date and normality of the last menstrual period. A pregnancy test is only necessary if indicated by the clinical history.
2. The most appropriate method of EC depends on the time elapsed since intercourse took place. Within 72 hours, hormonal methods may be used. Beyond 72 hours, an IUD can be offered up to 5 days after the earliest estimated day of ovulation.
3. Past history of or current contraindications to oestrogen suggest that LNG would be a better choice if it is available.
4. Current drug therapy may influence the choice of method. The Faculty of Family Planning and Reproductive Healthcare (Kubba and Wilkinson 1998) recommend in their current guidelines that women using drugs which are thought to interfere with the efficacy of the COC (e.g.

rifampicin, certain anticonvulsants) should take three tablets of Schering PC4 twice although there is no evidence to support this recommendation. No dose-finding studies of either Schering PC4 or LNG have been performed to date. We have no idea what is the lowest effective dose required and it is quite possible that the dose currently used is more than adequate even for women on enzyme-inducing drugs.

5. Method of contraception, if any, being used and the reason for presentation, e.g. burst condom. This information is necessary only in order to discuss how the need for EC might be effectively prevented in the future.

Most of this information can be collected by self-administered questionnaire.

Examination

1. Most providers, from force of habit, record the blood pressure (BP). Women with elevated BP should not be denied EC but should be encouraged to return to the clinic so the BP can be checked under less stressful circumstances.
2. Pelvic examination. Routine pelvic examination is not necessary and may deter women – particularly young women – from returning to the clinic. It is, however, indicated if there is any suspicion of pregnancy. If pregnancy is suspected and if the uterus is not enlarged, a pregnancy test should be done before treatment is given.

Management of postcoital intrauterine device insertion

Once the decision has been taken to offer an IUD, insertion should be performed according to the usual routine (Ch. 4). Screening for sexually transmitted infections should be performed if time and access to laboratory facilities allow. If not, IUD insertion should be covered by broad-spectrum antibiotics.

INFORMATION FOR USERS

Many clinics give standard information sheets which outline the points covered below and advise the timing of the second dose of pills. Verbal or written information should also cover:

1. The way in which EC acts. It should be stressed that it may inhibit implantation since to some women this may be morally unacceptable.
2. The possibility of failure.
3. The risk of teratogenesis.
4. The possible side effects.

5. The effect on the timing and character of the next menstrual period. Since the onset of vaginal bleeding is reassuring to women keen to avoid pregnancy, it is important to counsel patients about this. It should be made clear that EC does not work by 'bringing on a period'.
6. If the need for EC has arisen as a result of unprotected intercourse, a conventional (i.e. non-emergency) method of contraception should be discussed and, if appropriate, provided. Women who plan to use COC or the POP are often advised to wait until the first day of menses before they start the pill. This is not necessary and some pregnancies which are attributed to failure of EC are in fact the result of unprotected intercourse later in the cycle. If women wish, they can start their pills the day after they use EC.
7. It is quite unnecessary to ask women to sign a consent form before prescribing EC; indeed, it may deter them from returning, should it ever be necessary again.

FOLLOW-UP

Not all doctors arrange routine appointments after prescribing EC. It is good practice to offer follow-up but not to insist on it. Women should be informed that EC does not always work and that *if their period does not come or if it is lighter or shorter than normal, they should return to the clinic so that pregnancy can be excluded.*

Follow-up also permits further discussion about contraception and sexual behaviour which may not have been absorbed at the earlier consultation.

Women should be encouraged to return for EC should the need arise again. Repeated use of EC carries no risk. Accidents with barrier methods do happen and women who have been prescribed the contraceptive pill sometimes do not take it for long or never even start it. Many women are embarrassed about needing EC and do not feel able to admit to a second accident. If it is made clear that some women do need to use EC more than once in a lifetime, more women would use the method when it was required.

USE AND AVAILABILITY

Knowledge about EC has improved tremendously over the last 10 years and most women in the UK now know of its existence. They are less well informed about the time limits.

Women attending family planning clinics or consulting their general practitioner about contraception should be informed about EC. Users of barrier methods should be told about it, just as women on the pill are advised what to do when they make mistakes with pill-taking.

Women presenting with an unplanned pregnancy should also be informed about EC for future use. We provide a small laminated card, the size of a credit card which fits into a purse (Fig. 8.2). The card gives general information about EC on one side and details of local availability on the other.

Hormonal EC must be used within 72 hours of intercourse, and is probably more effective if it is used as soon as possible. At the time of writing, it still has to be prescribed by a doctor in the UK. The greatest need for EC is often at weekends when clinics and general practice surgeries are closed and on a Monday morning when they are at their busiest. Many people, particularly the young, often find it difficult to approach their general practitioner for EC and not all hospital accident and emergency departments will supply it. For these reasons, and recognizing the potential of EC for reducing unwanted pregnancies, many people feel that EC should be made available off prescription. This seems more likely to happen now that LNG has become available since it is easier to make the case on the grounds of safety. Indeed LNG was licensed in France in 1999 for sale in pharmacies off prescription. It will always be argued that making EC more easily available will risk women abandoning other more reliable methods of contraception, will increase promiscuity and will encourage and increase unsafe sex. If EC were available off prescription, undoubtedly a few women would use it in place of a regular method of contraception. EC is less effective than all existing artificial methods of contraception so these women will be at increased risk of pregnancy. They are also at increased risk of sexually transmitted infection.

For the vast numbers of women who would use EC appropriately, easier access would be of enormous benefit. We have recently demonstrated (Glasier and Baird 1998) that women given EC to keep at home, use it correctly, appropriately and do not abandon more reliable methods. They may also be less likely to have an unwanted pregnancy. Reassured by these data, the British Pregnancy Advisory Service now offers supplies to women (at a cost of £10 for one course of Schering PC4) which they can keep at home. Further studies are ongoing and it is likely that by the time the next edition of this book is being prepared, EC will be available in the UK from pharmacies without a prescription.

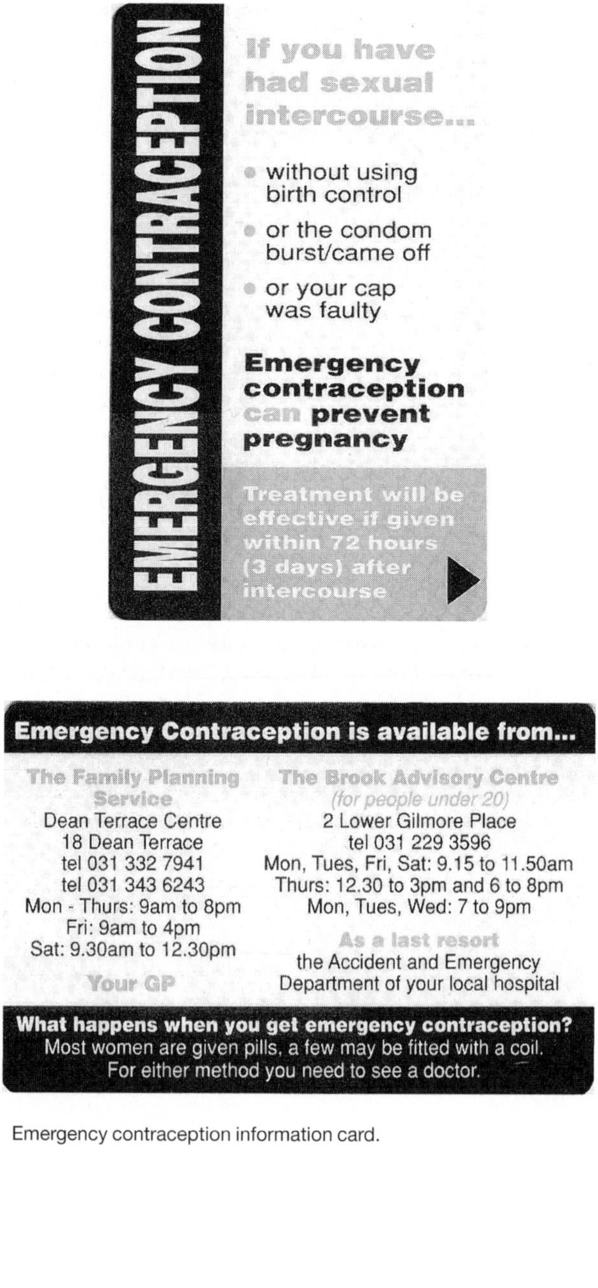

EMERGENCY CONTRACEPTION

If you have had sexual intercourse...

- without using birth control
- or the condom burst/came off
- or your cap was faulty

Emergency contraception can prevent pregnancy

Treatment will be effective if given within 72 hours (3 days) after intercourse

Emergency Contraception is available from...

The Family Planning Service
Dean Terrace Centre
18 Dean Terrace
tel 031 332 7941
tel 031 343 6243
Mon - Thurs: 9am to 8pm
Fri: 9am to 4pm
Sat: 9.30am to 12.30pm

Your GP

The Brook Advisory Centre
(for people under 20)
2 Lower Gilmore Place
tel 031 229 3596
Mon, Tues, Fri, Sat: 9.15 to 11.50am
Thurs: 12.30 to 3pm and 6 to 8pm
Mon, Tues, Wed: 7 to 9pm

As a last resort
the Accident and Emergency
Department of your local hospital

What happens when you get emergency contraception?
Most women are given pills, a few may be fitted with a coil.
For either method you need to see a doctor.

Figure 8.2 Emergency contraception information card.

REFERENCES

Glasier A 1997 Emergency post-coital contraception. New England Journal of Medicine 337: 1058–1064

Glasier A, Baird DT 1998 The effects of self-administering emergency contraception. New England Journal of Medicine 339: 1–4

Glasier A, Thong KJ, Dewar M, Mackie M, Baird DT 1992 Randomised trial of mifepristone (RU 486) and high dose estrogen–progestogen as an emergency contraceptive. New England Journal of Medicine 327: 1041–1044

Kubba A, Wilkinson C 1998 Recommendations for clinical practice: Emergency contraception. Faculty of Family Planning and Reproductive Healthcare of the Royal College of Obstetricians and Gynaecologists, London, CSC 1/98

Piaggio G, Von Hertzen H, Grimes DA, Van Look PFA 1999 Timing of emergency contraception with levonorgestrel or the Yuzpe regimen. Lancet 353: 721

Task Force on Postovulatory Methods of Fertility Regulation 1998 Randomised controlled trial of levonorgestrel versus the Yuzpe regimen of combined oral contraceptives for emergency contraception. Lancet 332: 428–433

Task Force on Postovulatory Methods of Fertility Regulation 1999 Comparison of three single doses of mifepristone as emergency contraception: a randomised trial. Lancet 353:697–702

Trussell J, Ellertson C 1995 Efficacy of emergency contraception. Fertility Control Reviews 4(2): 8–11

Trussell J, Rodriguez G, Ellertson C 1998 New estimates of the effectiveness of the Yuzpe regimen of emergency contraception. Contraception 57: 363–369

Vasilakis C, Jick SS, Jick H 1999 The risk of venous thromboembolism in users of postcoital contraceptive pills. Contraception 59: 79–83

Webb AMC, Russel J, Elstein M 1992 Comparison of the Yuzpe regime, danazol and mifepristone in oral post-coital contraception. British Medical Journal 305: 927–931

Wilcox AJ, Weinberg CR, Baird DD 1995 Timing of sexual intercourse in relation to ovulation – effects on the probability of conception, survival of the pregnancy and sex of the baby. New England Journal of Medicine 333: 1517–1521

9

Adolescent reproductive health

Audrey H. Brown

Global perspectives   215
UK perspectives   216
Teenage pregnancy   217
  Statistics   217
  Causes of teenage pregnancy   219
  Outcome of teenage
    pregnancy   220
  Strategies to reduce teenage
    pregnancy   221
Sex education   222
  Content of sex education   223

Training the teachers   224
Contraception for teenagers   225
  Combined oral contraception   225
  Condoms   226
  Other barrier methods   227
  Progestogen-only pill   227
  Long-acting progestogen
    methods   227
  Intrauterine device   228
  Emergency contraception   228
Confidentiality for under-16s   228

The World Health Organization (WHO) defines 'health' as 'a state of complete physical, mental and social well-being and not merely the absence of disease or infirmity'. The adolescent years of our lives span the transition period from the carefree years of childhood to the achievement of responsible adulthood. Adolescence is generally accepted to cover the years from 10 to 19, and thus adolescent reproductive health concerns the physical, social and emotional needs of young people. Adolescents have different problems from adults, and thus sexual health and family planning programmes aimed at young people must be geared specifically to their needs, rather than adapted from existing adult-orientated programmes. Young people need to gather the knowledge and develop the skills necessary to enable them to avoid unplanned pregnancies, to protect themselves against sexually transmitted infections (STIs) and to grow into sexually healthy adults.

GLOBAL PERSPECTIVES

In October 1999, the world population reached 6 billion, and at the current growth rate will reach 7 billion within the next 12 years. The current generation of 10 to 19 year olds now numbers over 1 billion, and will form the largest group in history to make the transition from childhood to adulthood. These young people are growing up in a world which is greatly different to that experienced by their parents and grandparents. As many societies worldwide move toward greater urbanization and industrialization, obtaining an education becomes a central feature to securing a stable position within the new society. Indeed, in most countries of the world, over 70% of children are now educated to primary school standard. Worldwide, adolescent girls are now two to three times more likely to get a basic education than did their mothers. None the less, disparities in opportunity still exist, with girls in many developing countries being less likely to receive a secondary education than boys, and those living in rural areas being particularly disadvantaged.

As girls become better educated, they become more empowered to make decisions about marriage and childbearing. Women who achieve at least a basic education are less likely to marry during the adolescent years than those without a basic education. Across Sub-Saharan Africa and Latin America, women without a basic education are three times more likely to be married before the age of 18. Such differences are also apparent in the developed world. In the USA, 30% of those with less than 10 years education will marry before the age of 18. This contrasts with those women with over 10 years of education, where early marriage occurs in less than 10%.

Similar education-related differences are seen in relation to age at birth of first child. In Sub-Saharan Africa, around half of all girls with less than 7 years education will give birth before the age of 18, whereas only one-fifth of those with over 7 years education will do so. Again such differences are mirrored in the developed world. In the USA, one-third of girls with less than basic education will give birth before the age of 18, compared to only 5% of those with above-basic education. As education levels have increased worldwide, many of today's young women are less likely to give birth during adolescence than were those of their mothers' generation.

None the less, we must not become complacent. Adolescent childbirth remains commonplace. The proportion of women giving birth under the age of 18 years varies from around 1% in Japanese society, to over 50% in parts of Africa. Adolescent births account for over 14 million births, or just over 10% of all births worldwide each year. A woman in the developing world who gives birth before the age of 18 will have an average of seven children; if she delays childbearing until her early 20s, she will have five or six children; and if she postpones childbirth until her late 20s, she is likely to have only three or four children. Programmes to improve education and delay childbearing amongst the current adolescent population are likely to have a major impact on global population growth, and on the daily lives and aspirations of our young people.

UK PERSPECTIVES

There are currently over 7 million adolescents in the UK, accounting for around 12% of the total population. Both physical and behavioural changes have had a major impact on the reproductive wellbeing of the young people of this country. Young people now mature physically at an earlier age, probably as a result of improved nutrition throughout the childhood years. The average age of menarche in the UK is now 13 years, at least 2 years earlier than that recorded in the early part of this century. Likewise, the onset of male puberty has also fallen by several years through the course of this century. Thus young people are physically capable of reproducing at a younger age. However, we cannot assume that psychological and emotional maturation has followed a similar pattern of earlier onset. Young people may not yet be mentally equipped to cope with the consequences of this earlier sexual maturation.

The sexual behaviour of adolescents also appears to have changed over the latter half of this century. Johnson et al (1994) report on a series of interviews carried out in 1990–1. Of those women aged 16 to 19 years at the time of interview, 18.7% report sexual activity before the age of 16. This contrasts sharply with a cohort of women aged 55 to 59 years at the time of interview, where less than 1% report becoming sexually active prior to their 16th birthday. Even higher levels of sexual activity have been reported in other studies. Graham et al (1996) studied school pupils in South East Scotland aged 14 and 15, and found a sexual activity rate of 32.7% in girls, and 27.5% in boys. Pupils from less academically achieving schools were more likely to be sexually active. In 1992, Mellanby et al questioned girls aged 16.5 to 17.5 years, and reported that 54% were sexually active (Mellanby et al 1993). Half of those had become sexually active before their 16th birthday. In addition, those who had become sexually active before the age of 16 were more likely to have had sex without contraception than those who had delayed sexual intercourse until after 16 years (64% vs 35%).

This increase in adolescent sexual activity has implications for two important areas of sexual health, namely rates of teenage pregnancy and of STIs. Data from the Public Health Laboratory Service, published by Nicoll et al in 1999, show worrying rates of STIs among 16 to 19 year olds in England and Wales, with implications for the future reproductive health of this population. In 1996, 2272 new cases of gonorrhoea were diagnosed in this age group, 1377 cases occurring in young women and 895 in men of the same age. These numbers represented an increase of 34% in women and 30% in men over the preceding year. Similarly, rates of chlamydial infection were found to have increased by 16.5% in women and 17.9% in men, and of genital warts by 12.2 and 12.8% respectively. These rises in rates of infection were greater than those reported for any other age group, leading to calls that sexual health promotion should be prioritized for young people.

TEENAGE PREGNANCY
Statistics

Births to teenage women account for around 10% of all births in the UK. It is the highest teenage conception rate in Western Europe, seven times higher than that in the Netherlands, four times higher than France and three

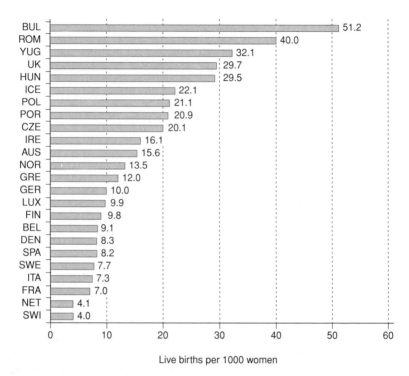

Figure 9.1 Live births per 1000 women aged 15 to 19 years in European countries ranked by order, 1996 (reproduced with kind permission from the Health Promotion England).

times that in Germany. In the UK in 1996, the annual birth rate amongst women aged 15 to 19 years was almost 30 per 1000 women (Fig. 9.1). In 1994, the annual rate of termination of pregnancy was 20 per 1000 in women of that age group. The conception rate in women aged 16 to 19 years has decreased slightly during the 1990s, and the overall pregnancy rate in this age group (includes births, terminations of pregnancy and spontaneous pregnancy losses attending hospital) is now 56.8 per 1000 women. This figure is likely to be an underestimation of the true pregnancy rate, as many women with an early spontaneous pregnancy loss will not attend hospital. A similar trend is seen in Scotland during the 1990s (Fig. 9.2).

The UK government has highlighted teenage pregnancy as an area of major concern. In 1992, the Health of the Nation white paper identified a reduction in the rate of teenage pregnancy as a key objective. A target was set to reduce the conception rate in girls under 16 years by at least 50%, from the 1989 rate of 9.5 per 1000, to no more than 4.8 per 1000 by the year 2000. Early indications would suggest that this target has not been met.

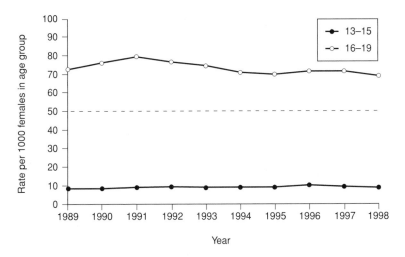

Figure 9.2   Teenage pregnancy rates in Scotland, 1989-98, by age group at conception (reproduced with kind permission from Information and Statistics Division, Scotland).

Causes of teenage pregnancy

Although around 30% of teenage girls are likely to be sexually active before the age of 16, only 1% of these girls will become pregnant by this age. Factors other than sexual activity must therefore determine whether or not a sexually active teenager becomes pregnant.

Teenage pregnancy is linked to social deprivation, with the highest rates of teenage pregnancy reported in the most socially deprived areas. In 1993, Smith reported on teenage pregnancies within the Tayside area of Scotland occurring over a 11-year period. He found that pregnancy rates were up to eight times higher in the areas of maximum socio-economic deprivation, compared to rates in the more affluent areas. In addition, the outcome of the pregnancies differed between areas. In the most deprived areas of the region, only one in four pregnancies ended in abortion, whereas in the most affluent areas, around two out of every three pregnancies were terminated. This is unlikely simply to reflect ability to pay for abortion services, as virtually all abortions carried out in Scotland are funded through the National Health Service. In 1992, Wilson et al reported similar socio-economic correlations in English regions, with higher teenage pregnancy rates and lower proportions of pregnancies ending in abortion in deprived northern regions compared to more prosperous south-eastern regions. Teenage mothers are more likely than their older counterparts to be unemployed and living in subsidised housing, even when other confounding variables such as level of education and social class are accounted for.

Factors in the teenager's immediate family also influence the likelihood of early childbirth. If the teenager's mother herself, or an older sister had a pregnancy in the teenage years, the risk of teenage pregnancy is increased. In addition, if the teenager is raised in a single-parent household, there is a higher risk of teenage pregnancy, with a relative risk of teenage pregnancy of 1.7 for those raised by a lone mother and 2.0 for those raised by a lone father. Children who have been looked after in local authority care, who have been absent from school either through truancy or exclusion, and children who have run away from home or are homeless are all more likely to experience teenage pregnancy. Attitudes towards sexuality within the family and within society in general also play an important role. If parents are open and informative about sexuality, teenagers are more likely to delay the onset of sexual intercourse and less likely to experience teenage pregnancy. In a wider perspective, societies which have an open and permissive attitude towards sex and sexuality actually have lower teenage conception rates.

For young people to avoid unplanned pregnancy (and also STIs), they must be able to access contraceptive and sexual health services. A direct relationship has been shown between the distance from a youth-orientated health clinic and the risk of teenage pregnancy (Clements et al 1998). Work carried out in Hull (Konje et al 1992) revealed that 92% of pregnant women aged 16 or under had never used any form of contraception. Clinics aimed at young people must have a wide remit, offering not only contraceptive services, but also information, support and advice about sexual health and sexuality in general. Such clinics should be needs led, and should be available in locations and at times convenient for young people.

Of course, not all teenage pregnancies are unintended. Some teenagers will plan to become pregnant, perhaps because they see a lack of future alternatives, such as higher education and a rewarding career. Other teenagers express ambivalence about pregnancy, and do not use reliable contraception, taking the approach 'if it happens, it happens'. The Social Exclusion Unit, which is attached to the Cabinet Office of the UK government has recently addressed the issue of teenage pregnancy (Social Exclusion Unit 1999). It has developed a strategy to reduce teenage conceptions, by introducing new health service standards for provision of contraceptive advice for young people, by developing guidelines for health professionals working with young people and assessing the options for making contraceptive services more accessible and attractive to young people. It has also addressed the social exclusion of teenage parents, and has set a goal to get more teenage parents back into education, training or employment.

Outcome of teenage pregnancy

Half of all pregnancies among under-16s and one-third of pregnancies among 16 to 19 year olds end in termination of pregnancy. Although serious complications following therapeutic abortion are rare in the UK, up to 5% may experience retained products of conception, necessitating further evacuation of the uterus, and around 1% may develop post-termination pelvic infection. Psychiatric problems are not increased following termination of pregnancy, but some women will experience emotional stress consequent to feelings of guilt and regret. However, there is no evidence that therapeutic abortion carries any greater health risks for teenagers than for adults.

Those teenagers who continue their pregnancy to term are likely to have a different experience of pregnancy from their older counterparts. 33% of adolescents giving birth are lone parents. Those under-20s who are married at the time of the birth have a higher risk of marriage breakdown, and over 20% will become single parents. Konje et al (1992) reported a series of pregnant teenagers aged 16 and under, and compared them to a cohort of pregnant women in their 20s. The teenagers were significantly more likely to book for antenatal care in the third trimester of their pregnancy. During pregnancy, they were more likely to develop the complications of anaemia, urinary tract infection and pregnancy-induced hypertension. Providers of antenatal care should offer care programmes targeting teenagers and their families. This may take the form of home-based care, particularly for teenagers who are reluctant to attend hospital-based clinics. Parenting skills can be taught, and support can be provided for the young woman and her family during and after pregnancy. Some local authorities have special education units which allow young mothers to continue their education after the birth of the baby, and provide child care whilst the mother is in class.

Several authors have reported increased perinatal mortality and prematurity in offspring of teenage mothers. There are additional future health concerns for the children of teenage mothers, with higher rates of sudden infant death syndrome and increased hospital admissions following accidental injuries. These children also demonstrate more developmental delay in the pre-school years. They are more likely to become teenage parents themselves in the future. Teenagers who become pregnant are more likely to drop out of school, and therefore fail to achieve their full educational potential. Their employment prospects are reduced, leading to increased reliance on welfare and a life in poverty and poor housing. These factors of course all have an impact on the future life and aspirations of the child of the teenage parent.

Strategies to reduce teenage pregnancy

Reducing poverty

Teenage pregnancy rates are highest in areas of socio-economic deprivation. The Child Poverty Action Group states that over 4 million children currently live in relative poverty in the UK. Strategies which decrease poverty and improve the socio-economic prospects of the families of young people are likely to decrease teenage pregnancy rates.

Improving contraceptive provision

Services offering contraception should be tailored to meet the needs of young people, with local expansion of dedicated young people's facilities. Work carried out in Wessex in the UK (Clements et al 1998) showed that the distance at which a young woman lives from a youth-orientated family planning clinic is directly proportional to her chance of becoming pregnant. Clinics should be located in places which young people can access without embarrassment, and should be open at times convenient for them. Emergency contraception (EC) should be made more readily available, and teenagers should be informed about its use. An integrated service offering sexual and general health services for young people should be provided, and the service should be well advertised.

Targeting high-risk groups

Certain groups of young people are more likely to have a pregnancy during their teenage years, and thus can be selected for targeting. These groups might include young people in local authority care, young homeless people, young people in areas of socio-economic deprivation, and young people who are themselves the children of teenage parents.

Increasing education

School-based sex education plays a key role in reducing teenage pregnancy. The timing of this education is paramount, and needs to be initiated early in adolescence. Sex education programmes are more likely to be successful when there is an integrated approach between school and health service. Health service staff can be involved in the delivery of sex education, and schools can organize group visits to clinics to establish familiarity and boost the confidence of teenagers who may wish to access the service.

SEX EDUCATION

Sex education should enable young people to develop into sexually healthy persons, who are able to make informed choices about their current and future sexual life. It should equip young people not only with the necessary facts, but also develop their skills in applying this knowledge in the context of their day-to-day lives. As such, sex education will encompass not only the learning of 'hard' biological facts, but also the issues of ethics, faith, morality and personal values. Sex education shares many features with other areas of education. It should be appropriate to the needs of young people, and should be appropriate to the culture in which they live. It must be based on factually correct information, and should develop over time from simple concepts through to complex issues. The learning environment should encourage discussion and exploration of appropriate themes.

Content of sex education

To make a sexually successful transition from childhood to adulthood, the young person will need to develop knowledge and skills in key areas of reproductive health:

- Relationships, both social and sexual.
- Negotiation within a relationship, including the 'right to say no'.
- Sex and sexual behaviour.
- Taking responsibility for their own health, and sharing responsibility for the health of others.
- Fertility and contraception.
- Pregnancy including outcomes and options.
- STIs.
- Practising safer sex.
- Parenting skills.

By teaching sex education to young people, we can expect that we will eventually have beneficial effects on society in general by reducing prejudices and assumptions about sexuality and creating a positive sexual climate.

The 1993 Education Act legislated for the first time that sex education must be taught to all secondary school pupils in the UK. The government defines sex education as 'the physical, emotional and social aspects of an individual's development as a male or female, personal relationships, responsible attitudes and appropriate behaviour'. It does not, however, define the nature of 'responsible' attitudes or clarify what 'appropriate' behaviour entails. There is as yet no nationally agreed and evaluated sex education programme for schools to use. The content and structure of sex education are therefore often at the discretion of individual schools and school governors. Sex education has been shown to be more effective when given before young people become sexually active. We know that 20–30% of young people experience sexual intercourse before the age of 16, and it is therefore imperative that sex education is initiated early enough. Many workers in this field have suggested 'the earlier the better', although there is no legislation requiring sex education to begin prior to secondary school.

Sex education has traditionally been taught in schools by science teachers. This approach tends to concentrate inevitably on the biological aspects of sex, and neglects the development of the personal and social skills which are central to sexual health. More schools are now moving to teach sex education within the broader context of personal and social development classes, which will draw on knowledge gained across the curriculum. Sexuality will be encountered in many areas of the curriculum, e.g. reproduction in biology classes, sexual relationships in novels studied in English, over-population problems in geography and moral values in religious education. Personal and social development classes can act as a forum to consolidate this knowledge, and explore key issues further.

Training the teachers

Teachers will need training themselves if the value of sex education in schools is to be maximized. Teachers involved in sex education should be motivated volunteers for the task, rather than appointed by order. Teachers will require in-service training themselves to adequately prepare for the task. This training should allow teachers the opportunity to:

- Discuss the political and moral issues surrounding sex education, and consider parental concerns.
- Explore personal values and feelings about human sexuality.
- Become familiar with the facts about reproduction, STIs, contraception and safe sex.
- Develop guidelines for dealing with sensitive or controversial areas.
- Develop different teaching methods which may be used, e.g. role play, drama.
- Increase personal confidence and self-esteem.

Of course, young people get information about sex from many other important sources, including parents, peers, health professionals and the media. Parents often feel ill-equipped to discuss sex and sexuality with their children, perhaps lacking the language or indeed the knowledge to introduce the subject. Many parents will themselves have had little, if any, sex education, and have learned as they 'go along'. Involving parents in the development of school-based sex education programmes may help to improve parent confidence. As sex education is developed and improved, perhaps the teenagers of today will be the better-equipped parents of tomorrow.

Health professionals who are involved with the care of young people should be aware of sexual health issues, and should promote a positive and approachable attitude. Evidence suggests that a 'joined-up' approach works best, and there should be an integration between the health and education services. This may, e.g., involve family planning staff taking part in the sex education programme, or providing a clinic on school premises.

Young people often cite their peers as one of the main sources of information about sexual health, even although they recognize that the information is not always accurate. Young people feel more comfortable discussing sexual matters with their friends than with teachers, parents or health professionals. Several workers have reported on the success of peer-based sex education projects, and consideration should be given to including this type of approach in programmes.

A vast section of the media is aimed at the teenage population, and young people will often use resources such as magazines and television programmes as sources of information. Producers of such material for the teenage market have a responsibility to ensure that the information presented is factually accurate, and does not sensationalize sex. Unfortunately, this is not always the case. Many health education groups produce literature aimed at the adolescent population. Such literature should be evaluated to ensure that it is of interest to young people and is understood by them.

Lastly, there is much moral and political opposition to sex education. Anti-sex education campaigners have claimed that sex education has led directly to a demise in the sexual health of young people by encouraging promiscuity and decreasing the age of first sexual intercourse. However, research would indicate that the reverse is in fact the case. WHO (Baldo 1994) reviewed this area and found that sex education actually led to a delay in the onset of sexual activity and increased the adoption of safer sex practices.

CONTRACEPTION FOR TEENAGERS

The majority of young people will become sexually active in their teenage years. The median age of first sexual intercourse has fallen over the past four decades to 17 for both sexes. Teenagers therefore have a greater need than ever before for access to acceptable and reliable forms of contraception, if they are to avoid unplanned pregnancies. Sexually active teenagers are also at risk from STIs, particularly chlamydial infection, and providers of contraceptive services must consider this when providing advice. No one contraceptive method is likely to provide maximum protection against both unplanned pregnancy and STI, and a combination of methods may be indicated. No one method is going to suit every teenager, and contraceptive advice and choice should therefore be tailored to the needs of the individual.

Combined oral contraception

Combined oral contraception (COC) is an extremely reliable form of contraception, and is often the method of choice for young women where protection against unplanned pregnancy is of paramount importance. However, the efficacy of this method relies on the woman remembering to take her pill correctly, and being aware of situations in which contraceptive efficacy may be lost. Some young women will lead chaotic lifestyles which are non-conductive to reliable pill-taking. In such circumstances, a change to a less user-dependent method will be indicated. Unplanned pregnancies often occur at the start of a new relationship, prior to reliable contraception being instituted. Often the woman has previously been on COC, but stopped the method when her last relationship ended, and has not yet restarted COC. Young women could be encouraged to stay on their pill between relationships. Health concerns have often led to women 'taking a break' from the pill. Unplanned pregnancies can then occur during the breaks. Young women should be reassured that there is no evidence to suggest any health benefits in short pill-free breaks, and should again be encouraged to remain on the pill if they have an ongoing need for reliable contraception. Some young women may not want their parents to know that they are sexually active, and may therefore worry about the pill packet being discovered. Such women may prefer an 'invisible' method such as an injectable contraceptive.

Young women may be reluctant to use COC because of fears about weight gain. However, advice can be given about maintaining a healthy diet and exercise regimen to ensure this does not become a problem. Concern has also been expressed about the risk of breast cancer when COC is used early in reproductive life, i.e. in the years between menarche and the birth of the first child. However, teenage women can none the less be reassured that their absolute risk of breast cancer is almost negligible.

COC offers many non-contraceptive benefits, which may offer additional attraction to young women. There is a reduction in menstrual bleeding and in dysmenorrhoea. There is also a reduction in anaemia, which will be of importance in developing countries. COC will benefit young women with acne, and can reduce hirsutism. In addition, there is protection against functional ovarian cysts, benign breast disease and ovarian malignancy. COC, although reducing the risk of pelvic inflammatory disease, does not offer any protection against STI, and adolescents using this method should be advised about other strategies to ensure safe sex.

Condoms

Male condoms are central to the practice of safe sex, and their use should be encouraged even when the adolescent is using another method of birth control such as COC (the 'Double Dutch' approach). Condoms have the advantage of being readily available to young people in chemist shops, in supermarkets and from condom machines. Young people have reported that they feel more comfortable accessing condoms through these outlets (Harden and Ogden 1999) than from traditional sources of contraceptives – such as family planning clinics – perhaps because they feel less stigmatized.

Condoms are available free from family planning services, but unfortunately, general practitioners are unable to provide condoms. In Lothian, a 'C-card' system operates which provides free condoms from a variety of community outlets such as student unions on production of an identity card. This system is widely utilized by young people. Condoms have a higher failure rate when used by teenagers, presumably because of user inexperience. Sex education programmes could play a role here by allowing young people to become confident in putting on a condom – the 'condom on a banana' class.

Like male condoms, the female condom offers protection against HIV and other STIs, and is available from family planning services and from commercial outlets. The Femidom is not popular amongst adolescents, perhaps because of concerns about its appearance and worries about noise during sex. However, it may have a role in safe sex when the young woman is unable to negotiate male condom use.

Other barrier methods

Diaphragms and caps are very seldom used by teenagers. They are unlikely to offer an acceptable level of protection against either pregnancy or STIs for this group of clients.

Progestogen-only pill

The progestogen-only pill (POP) has a higher failure rate amongst adolescents when compared to older users, and requires a high degree of discipline in regular pill-taking. It is certainly not suited to those with even moderately chaotic or unpredictable lifestyles. It is unlikely to be chosen by teenagers as a method of contraception. It will occasionally be used by young women in whom COC is contraindicated. It would be prudent in this circumstance to recommend contraceptive back-up with a barrier method.

Long-acting progestogen methods

Depot medroxyprogesterone acetate (DMPA; Depo-Provera) is popular amongst teenage girls. It is even more effective against unplanned pregnancy than COC, and is ideal for those who forget to take the pill. The frequent amenorrhoea is often seen as an added bonus amongst teenagers, when reassured about the reason for the lack of menses and about the low likelihood of pregnancy. DMPA can lead to weight gain and acne in some users, which may make it unacceptable. Like COC, it will offer no protection against STIs, and concurrent condom use should be encouraged. The 3-monthly visits to the clinic for the injection provide an ideal opportunity for the health professional to reinforce the safe sex message.

The 5-year progestogen implant, Norplant, was a relatively popular method amongst adolescents who did not have plans for childbearing in the near future. The single capsule progestogen implant, Implanon, has now become available, provides contraception for 3 years, and should prove to be an acceptable method to many, after adequate pre-insertion counselling.

Intrauterine device

The intrauterine device (IUD) is unlikely to be a suitable method of contraception for the adolescent. Teenagers tend to have shorter relationships, and are therefore more likely to have multiple sexual partners over the lifespan of an IUD. Women under the age of 20 are more likely to be infected with *Chlamydia trachomatis* than their older counterparts. In addition, it may be more difficult to fit an IUD in the adolescent woman, as she is likely to be nulliparous and may have a small uterine cavity. None the less, it is sometimes necessary to fit an IUD as a post-coital method of contraception in the adolescent. In such circumstances, it is prudent either to screen for chlamydial infection at the time of fitting, or to offer anti-chlamydial antibiotics. The young woman may decide to keep the IUD as her ongoing method of contraception, and the safe sex message should then be strongly reinforced and the use of condoms encouraged.

Emergency contraception

Adolescents will require EC when they have had intercourse without contraception, or when their usual method of contraception is known to have failed. Graham et al (1996) reported a study carried out among 14 and 15 year olds in Edinburgh. Although 93% of pupils were aware of EC, knowledge of correct time limits was poor. Reassuringly, however, girls who had been sexually active were the most likely group to know the correct time limits (56.2% answered correctly). Disappointingly, only 11.9% of sexually active boys knew the time limits. Recent work by WHO (1998) has shown that EC is more effective the earlier it is taken. Young people therefore need firstly to be aware of the existence of EC, and secondly need to know how to obtain a supply quickly. EC needs to be widely promoted amongst adolescents, and suppliers should ensure easy and rapid access, perhaps by offering no appointment 'walk-in' services for EC. The case should be pushed for EC to be made available 'over-the-counter'.

CONFIDENTIALITY FOR UNDER-16s

Many young people are reluctant to consult doctors about sexual matters, as they are afraid that their confidentiality will be broken. Almost 75% of under-16s interviewed expressed concern that a request for contraception would not be treated confidentially. These fears will deter young people from accessing the sexual health services which they require.

The General Medical Council states that:

Patients are entitled to expect that the information about themselves or others which the doctor learns during the course of a medical consultation, investigation or treatment, will remain confidential. An explicit request by a patient that the information should not be disclosed to particular people, or indeed to any third party, must be respected save in the most exceptional circumstances, for example where the health, safety or welfare of someone other than the patient would otherwise be at serious risk.

Doctors owe the same duty of confidentiality to those under the age of 16 as to those over 16. Young people under the age of 16 are able to consent on their own behalf for any procedure or treatment, provided that in the doctor's opinion they are capable of understanding the nature and consequences of the procedure. 'Procedure' includes the provision of contraception. Young people should be reassured that they can expect confidentiality from their doctor. The doctor has a duty to encourage the young person to involve his or her parents in the decision-making process, but will respect the wishes of the young person if parental involvement is declined. Some young people may be reluctant to consult their family doctor for contraceptive or sexual health advice, as they may have known this doctor since childhood. They should be made aware that they can choose to register with another doctor solely for contraceptive services. Young people must feel certain that the consultation will remain confidential, or for many the fear that someone will 'tell' will be so great that they will not attend the clinic until it is too late, presenting with an unplanned pregnancy or an STI.

Today's adolescents are tomorrow's adults. Good practices learned in adolescence will be maintained into adult life. We can help our young people make a successful transition into adulthood by providing effective and appropriate sexual health services, and equipping them with the knowledge and skills to reach their full potential as sexual beings.

REFERENCES

Baldo M 1994. Does sex education lead to earlier or increased sexual activity in youth? World Health Organization Global Programme on AIDS, Geneva
Clements S, Stone N, Diamond I, Ingham R 1998. Modelling the spacial distribution of teenage conception rates within Wessex. British Journal of Family Planning 24: 61–71
Department of Health 1992 Health of the nation: a strategy for health in England. HMSO, London
Graham A, Green L, Glasier AF 1996. Teenagers' knowledge of emergency contraception: questionnaire survey in south east Scotland. British Medical Journal 312: 1267–1269
Harden A, Ogden J 1999. Sixteen to nineteen year olds' use of, and beliefs about, contraceptive services. British Journal of Family Planning 24: 141–144

Johnson AM, Wadsworth J, Wellings K, Field J 1994. Sexual attitudes and lifestyles. Blackwell Science, Oxford

Konje JC, Palmer A, Watson A, Hay DM, Imrie A 1992. Early teenage pregnancies in Hull. British Journal of Obstetrics and Gynaecology 99: 969–973

Mellanby A, Phelps F, Tripp JH 1993. Teenagers, sex, and risk taking. British Medical Journal 307: 25

Nicoll A, Catchpole M, Cliffe S, Hughes G, Simms I, Thomas D 1999. Sexual health of teenagers in England and Wales: analysis of national data. British Medical Journal 318: 1321–1322

Smith T 1993. Influence of socioeconomic factors on attaining targets for reducing teenage pregnancies. British Medical Journal 306: 1232–1235

Social Exclusion Unit 1999. Teenage pregnancy. HMSO, London

Wilson SH, Brown TP, Richards RG 1992. Teenage conceptions and contraception in the English regions. Journal of Public Health Medicine 14: 17–25

World Health Organization Task Force on Postovulatory Methods of Fertility Regulation 1998 Randomised controlled trial of levonorgestrel versus the Yuzpe regimen of combined oral contraceptives for emergency contraception. Lancet 352: 428–433

10

Legal aspects of family planning

Alan D. G. Brown

Age of consent and Gillick
  competence   232
Confidentiality   232
Medical negligence, the Bolam
  principle and Bolitho
  criterion   233
Consent to treatment   234
Extended role of the nurse   235

Litigation and family planning
  methods   237
Female sterilization   237
Vasectomy   240
Termination of pregnancy   241
Intrauterine devices   242
Hormonal contraception   243
How to reduce litigation risk   246

In the last few decades, opinion polls have been published in the UK concerning the esteem the British public has for the professions. Doctors have consistently topped the list ahead of policemen and teachers, with journalists and Members of Parliament commanding least respect. In spite of these findings, medical litigation continues to rise causing considerable concern and adding enormous expenditure to healthcare. In 1995–96, the cost of National Health Service (NHS) litigation was £200 million and it was forecast to rise by 25% annually (National Audit Office 1995–96). However, in 1997–98, health authorities and hospital trusts were asked to set aside £1.3 billion to settle negligence claims, but it was expected a further £1 billion would be needed for cases still to be notified (Murray 1998)

The reasons for spiralling litigation include improved medical outcomes which increase patients' expectations, so when results are poor or problems arise detailed explanation and compensation are demanded. Potentially large payments and their attendant publicity also encourage a litigious culture.

Gynaecologists and doctors working in family planning are at the forefront of medicolegal issues and James (1994) and Clements and Huntingford (1994) showed that among the commonest gynaecological claims were those relating to fertility regulation, particularly sterilization and termination of pregnancy. These findings confirmed a study by Brown (1985) which reviewed nearly 400 gynaecological complaints in which 63% of problems related to some aspect of contraception with the majority being sterilization errors. Knowledge of legal aspects of family planning will forewarn and, hopefully, prevent healthcare professionals from being involved in these anxiety-provoking situations.

AGE OF CONSENT AND GILLICK COMPETENCE

From 16 years of age in the UK, a girl can give consent to sexual relations and is presumed to have the capacity to decide on health issues. Children under 16 may also have that capacity provided they understand the nature, purpose and possible consequences of medical treatment or non-treatment. In 1974, the UK Department of Health and Social Security (DHSS) published advice concerning family planning provision. For a girl under 16 years, information need not be given to her parents and the doctor could decide on her management, having first discussed with the teenager the benefit of involving her family. If the girl declined to involve her parents or guardian, the practitioner could provide contraception on the grounds that it was in her best interests. In 1982, Mrs Victoria Gillick, a mother of daughters under 16, legally challenged this advice. She lost but won in the Appeal Court where the judges considered that parents' interests were greater than those of the child. Subsequently, however, the House of Lords ruled the DHSS circular was lawful and underage girls could give consent on contraception (including abortion) without parental knowledge, provided there was the capacity to understand (Gillick v. West Norfolk and Wisbech Area Health Authority 1985). Thus the concept of the 'Gillick competent' under 16 years old was established.

When a competent child refuses help, a person with parental responsibility may authorize medical care, except in Scotland. There are differences in the laws within the UK and the important legislations are: in England and Wales – the Family Law Reform Act 1969 and Children Act 1989; in Scotland – Age of Legal Capacity (Scotland) Act 1991 and Children (Scotland) Act 1995; and in Northern Ireland – Age of Majority Act 1969. When a young person or an adult is not competent to give or withhold consent, there should be consultation with those who have responsibility for the individual, experienced clinicians, a medical defence organization, and legal advice concerning possible court authorization. For example, in the guidelines on male and female sterilization published in 1999 by the Royal College of Obstetricians and Gynaecologists (RCOG) it is stated:

If there is any question of the patient not having the mental capacity to consent to a procedure which will permanently remove their fertility, the case should be referred to court for judgement.

CONFIDENTIALITY

A General Medical Council (GMC) Guidance on Confidentiality (1995) states:

Patients have a right to expect that you will not disclose any personal information which you learn during the course of your professional duties, unless they give permission. Without assurances about confidentiality patients may be reluctant to give doctors the information they need in order to provide good care.

Issues of confidentiality are of particular concern to young people. Allan (1991) found that about 75% of girls under 16 were concerned that the general practitioner would inform their parents about their contraceptive requests. The GMC (1995) also states:

> You must respect requests by patients that information should not be disclosed to third parties, save in exceptional circumstances (for example, where the health or safety of others would otherwise be at serious risk); ... If you decide to disclose confidential information, you must be prepared to explain and justify your decision.

Thus if a practitioner decides to disclose information against the child's wishes, the practitioner should, with rare exceptions, inform the child of his or her intentions. The overriding consideration must be what is, in the practitioner's view, the best interest of the child (Schütte 1997).

Concerning sexual abuse, the GMC (1995) advises:

> If you believe a patient to be a victim of neglect or physical or sexual abuse, and unable to give or withhold consent to disclosure, you should usually give information to an appropriate responsible person or statutory agency, in order to prevent further harm to the patient. In these and similar circumstances, you may release information without the patient's consent, but only if you consider that the patient is unable to give consent, and that the disclosure is in the patient's best medical interest.

A useful review of general legal issues in fertility regulation has been published by Gupta and Bewley (1998).

MEDICAL NEGLIGENCE, THE BOLAM PRINCIPLE AND BOLITHO CRITERION

A health professional owes a duty of care to the patient, i.e. has to take reasonable steps to avoid foreseeable harm. When a complication occurs, that duty of care may have been breached but in law a negligence claim will not succeed unless it is proved that there was resultant damage. An example is the placement of a clip for female sterilization on the round ligament instead of the fallopian tube which results in a pregnancy. It is also necessary for the plaintiff (complainant) to show that the defendant's (doctor's) action fell below the standard of care which should be reasonably expected. The Bolam principle states:

> A doctor is not negligent if he acts in accordance with a practice accepted as proper by a responsible body of medical men skilled in that particular art even if there is another body of opinion which takes a contrary view.
>
> *Bolam v. Friern Hospital Management 1957*

If a dispute reaches court, the judge may have difficulty when competent medical experts from each side have genuinely-held opposing views. In these circumstances it is likely the doctor will prevail, because an expert has agreed that the action taken would be supported by a 'responsible body of medical opinion' according to the Bolam test. However, a ruling from the House of Lords in the case of Bolitho v. City and Hackney Health Authority (1997) is relevant and binding throughout the UK. In this case, the doctors from both sides had contrary views concerning the clinical management.

In a unanimous decision in favour of the defendants, Lord Browne-Wilkinson held that in the Bolam definition the adjective 'responsible' required the court to be satisfied that the expert opinions expressed had a 'logical' basis, i.e. were evidence-based and not outdated opinions. Thus when weighing up medical risks and benefits the experts must address these issues and reach defensible conclusions. If it was proved that an expert opinion was not logical, the court would reject it as not responsible or reasonable. In the Bolitho appeal, the Lords considered the defendant's expert opinion was logical and therefore it was accepted. This judgment may make claims more difficult to defend but it will prevent experts giving outdated and unsupported opinions.

CONSENT TO TREATMENT

Consent has three legal components:

1. Voluntariness – a willingness to undergo a procedure.
2. Capacity – to understand what is involved.
3. Knowledge – sufficient information to make a balanced judgment.

If one of these elements is omitted, there is not valid consent. The standard operation consent form used in the UK usually includes only general statements, but when signed it is documentary evidence that some discussion has occurred. Invariably, however, it is proof only of the patient's voluntariness.

In 1990, the Department of Health published 'A Guide to Consent for Examination and Treatment'. This states:

A patient has the right under common law to give or withhold consent prior to examination or treatment.... This is one of the basic principles of health care. Subject to certain exceptions the doctor or health professional and/or health authority may face an action for damages if a patient is examined or treated without consent.

Patients are entitled to receive sufficient information in a way that they can understand about the proposed treatments, the possible alternatives and any substantial risks, so that they can make a balanced judgment.

The accompanying circular noted that:

Written consent should be obtained for any procedure or treatment carrying a substantial risk or side effect. If the patient is capable, written consent should always be obtained for general anaesthesia, surgery, certain forms of drug therapy – for example cytotoxic therapy, and therapy involving ionising radiation.

Thus in obtaining consent, e.g. for male or female sterilization, patient information must include the small failure rate, because although it is uncommon, an unexpected pregnancy and the associated costs of bringing up a child constitute a 'substantial risk' which requires discussion with the person.

The GMC advice on consent (1998a) states:

You must use the patient's case notes and/or consent form to detail the key elements of discussion, including the nature of information provided, specific requests by the patient and details of the scope of consent given.

In practice, the patient's records are the most appropriate place for these issues to be recorded (see female sterilization). The GMC also recommends who obtains patient consent:

If you are the doctor providing treatment or undertaking an investigation, it is your responsibility to discuss it with the patient and obtain consent, as you will have a comprehensive understanding of the procedure or treatment, how it is carried out, and the risks attached to it. Where this is not practical, you may delegate these tasks provided you ensure that the person to whom you delegate is suitably trained and qualified and has sufficient knowledge of the proposed investigation or treatment, and understands the risks involved.

Satisfactory consent requires explanation from an appropriately trained practitioner, discussion and a contemporaneous record in the patient's notes. Explanatory leaflets are helpful and advisable but they do not replace the consultation with the patient.

EXTENDED ROLE OF THE NURSE

A major advance in healthcare has been the concept of the nurse's extended role to take maximum advantage of his or her skills. This allows better use of limited resources so that with appropriate training and protocols, nurses are able to manage routine clinical situations and allow medical staff to concentrate on complex problems.

However, the law on nurse-prescribing is confusing and it has been necessary to interpret old legislation in the light of significant advances in patient care (Doherty 1997). The Medicines Act 1968 allows only doctors, dentists and veterinary surgeons to prescribe drugs, which means nurse-prescribing would be unlawful. However, Section 50 2 (b) suggests that a nurse can administer medicines if the nurse is acting in accordance with the request from an appropriate practitioner. It states:

No person shall administer any such medicinal products unless he is an appropriate practitioner or a person acting in accordance with the directions of an appropriate practitioner.

Further confusion surrounded the interpretation of the word 'administer' which was broadly defined.

In 1992, the UK Council for Nursing, Midwifery and Health Visiting issued guidance on the Standards for Administration of Medicines. Paragraph 6.12 referred to protocols and states:

... and where it is the wish of the professional staff concerned that practitioners in a particular setting be authorised to administer on their own authority certain medicines, a local protocol having been drawn up between medical practitioners, nurses, midwives and the pharmacist.

This suggests it is lawful for nurses to administer prescription-only substances. Also in 1992, the Medicinal Products; Prescribing by Nurses Act appeared, but there was still no clarification concerning which drugs could be prescribed by nurses, midwives or health visitors. Because of the uncertainties, the UK Government asked Dr June Crown to chair a review group to examine arrangements throughout the country. Her report was published as the Review of Prescribing, Supply and Administration of Medicines in 1998. This review concerned group protocols which were defined as:

a specific written instruction for the supply or administration of named medicines in an identified clinical situation. It is drawn up locally by doctors, pharmacists and other appropriate professionals, and approved by the employer advised by the relevant professional advisory committees. It applies to groups of patients or other service users who may not be individually identified before presentation for treatment.

These protocols had evolved to provide timely access to treatment and reduce patient waiting times, and also to make appropriate and effective use of professional skills and resources.

The main Crown Report recommendations were that the current safe and effective practice of using group protocols which were consistent with the criteria laid down should continue, and all other protocols should be reviewed in the light of the criteria. Also the law should be clarified to ensure that health professionals who supply or administer medicines under approved group protocols are acting within the law. The important criteria were that protocols should take into account patient convenience and choice, also that patient safety was not compromised and there should be arrangements for professional responsibility and accountability.

Guidance was published by the Royal College of Nursing (1998) which stressed the importance of a multidisciplinary team to construct and audit protocols, and also that:

all protocols must be agreed by local clinical managers, and lines of professional accountability must be specified and agreed by all those involved in the use of the protocol. Finally, the employer of people providing care under the protocol must approve its use.

Thus the nurse practitioner role is now well established and worries of the profession and the defence organizations concerning the legality of nurses administering drugs is being addressed.

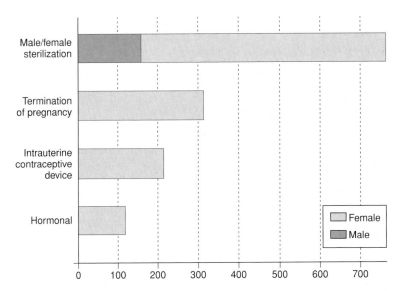

Figure 10.1   Family planning-related claims against the Medical Protection Society 1974–1999.

LITIGATION AND FAMILY PLANNING METHODS

Between 1974 and mid-1999, the Medical Protection Society (MPS), one of the major UK medical defence organizations, opened 1417 files concerning complaints against their members involved in family planning (Fig. 10.1). This database is limited but sufficient broadly to categorize areas of concern. There were 770 incidents relating to sterilization (mainly female), 318 relating to termination of pregnancy and 216 intrauterine device complications, with 113 events relating to hormonal contraception. A detailed analysis of these cases serves to illustrate common causes of litigation in the field of fertility regulation.

Female sterilization

In all gynaecologically-related litigation, failed sterilization accounts for most claims and these often attract large financial settlements. Figure 10.2 details claims referred to the MPS relating to 615 cases of female sterilization. In 475 women (77%), pregnancy resulted from failed surgery.

In the Royal College of Obstetricians and Gynaecologists (RCOG) evidence-based clinical guidelines on male and female sterilization (1999), a major recommendation was that trainees should perform at least 25 supervised laparoscopic tubal occlusions before operating without supervision. For all surgeons regardless of experience or seniority it is advisable, when

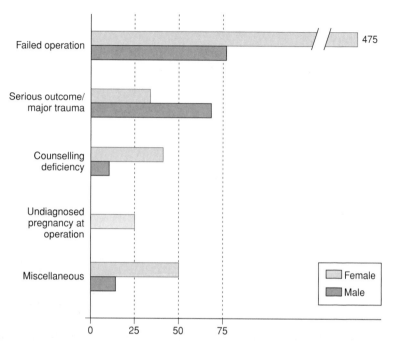

Figure 10.2 Sterilization-related claims against the Medical Protection Society 1974–1999.

possible, to have the procedure checked by another doctor/gynaecologist and so recorded in the operation note. The RCOG advised that tubal occlusion may be performed at any time in the menstrual cycle, but reliable contraception should continue until the next menstrual period so that a luteal phase pregnancy is avoided; also routine uterine curettage to prevent pregnancy should not be done.

Major trauma at gynaecological laparoscopy happens infrequently and in this series there were 31 (5%) incidents. Laparotomy was necessary for 15 bowel and five urinary tract injuries, and four major haemorrhages. There were two deaths, one each from bowel perforation and peritonitis, and one patient had brain damage following intra-operative cardiac arrest. These events highlight the risks of female sterilization, the need for skilled surgery and advice concerning potential problems, as well as the safety of vasectomy (see below).

Deficient counselling is a frequent criticism and there were 42 (7%) complaints including 25 women who were sterilized without consent and 10 who claimed that the prospect of failure was not mentioned. There is now general agreement that many issues need to be addressed when counselling a woman for sterilization; therefore, based on clinical practice, medicolegal experience and RCOG guidelines, the following points should be discussed and recorded in the patient's notes:

1. Current contraception (e.g. IUD – to be removed at operation).
2. Permanence intended (reversals have variable outcomes).
3. Purchaser/Health Board may not pay for reversal.
4. Failure rate small (approximately 1/200 lifetime risk).
5. If fails, small ectopic risk.
6. Vasectomy considered (approximately 1/2000 failures after two azoospermic samples).
7. Seek advice if thinks pregnant/missed period.
8. Not associated with heavier periods when done after age of 30.
9. Usual method is day-case laparoscopy using clips or rings.
10. a. Surgical risks are small (often related to obesity/previous surgery).
    b. If a problem, proceed to laparotomy.

When this checklist has been completed, the standard hospital consent form is less relevant as it usually contains non-specific statements about risks; nevertheless, all hospitals require it to be signed. Also, as stated before, concise explanatory leaflets to be studied at home are useful and advisable, but they do not replace patient counselling.

Among the MPS files there were 27 (4%) cases involving sterilization undertaken in the presence of a pregnancy which went undiagnosed. Surgery of any type should not be performed when a period has been missed, even by 24 hours, because of the possible risk of pregnancy. A detailed menstrual history is essential and when there is doubt, a pregnancy test is required; even if this is negative, the patient should be warned an early gestation cannot be excluded, and if amenorrhoea persists postoperatively a pregnancy test is necessary (Brown 1997). The 51 (8%) miscellaneous complaints included failure to remove an intrauterine contraceptive device (7), retained foreign bodies (including two swabs) and 15 cases of patients suffering from pain, bleeding or infection after surgery.

In four cases of failed sterilization, three mentally handicapped children and one with a cleft palate were born. Outcomes such as these increase the size of financial awards and in a recent English High Court ruling, a mother was given £1.3 million because of the child's severe mental and physical handicaps (Johnstone 1999). When a healthy child is born after negligent sterilization, the compensation in the last 15 years has usually included large sums to take into account the costs of education (Brahams 1999). Recently, the House of Lords ruled against claiming costs of bringing up an 'unwanted' healthy child resulting from failed surgery (Times Law Report 1999). The case concerned a man who had a vasectomy and yet, in spite of negative sperm counts, his wife became pregnant and a normal child was delivered. One judge, Lord Hope, stated: 'This is economic loss of a kind which must be held to fall outside the ambit of duty of care' owed to the couple by the hospital and laboratory staff. Lord Clyde commented:

... the expense of child rearing (as) ... wholly disproportionate to the doctor's culpability has been recognised in the American jurisprudence as one factor supporting the rule of limited damages.

The judges allowed the mother to claim up to £10 000 for pain, distress and loss resulting from the unwanted pregnancy. This important decision is likely now to reduce significantly future compensation when a healthy child results from failed sterilization. However, in these two recent cases, some of the logic (which differentiates between a healthy and a disabled child when determining compensation) is obscure. Lord Slynn concluded:

... it is not fair, just or reasonable to impose on the doctor or his employer for the consequential responsibilities, imposed on or accepted by the parents to bring up a 'healthy' child. ... If a client wants to be able to recover such costs he or she must do so by an appropriate contract.

This argument implies that no compensation should be paid when a child is handicapped and, as Brahams (1999) argues, where is the line drawn between a healthy and a handicapped child?

Vasectomy

Vasectomy also attracts a disproportionate amount of litigation. Among the MPS files were 155 complaints about vasectomy (Fig. 10.2). A total of 78 (50%) procedures failed and pregnancy followed. Most failures occur soon after surgery and were due to faulty technique or unprotected intercourse before azoospermia had been established. The main complications in this series were haematoma, infection and/or pain (in 59–38%), with haematoma being the commonest. Serious consequences included testicular atrophy (7) – mostly from haematoma, orchidectomy (2), ileo-inguinal nerve trauma (1) and testicular artery thrombosis (1). The need for good training, supervision and skilled surgery is again highlighted and the RCOG guidelines (1999) recommend that 10 supervised procedures should be done by a trainee before operating alone.

Counselling inadequacies accounted for nine (6%) complaints with failure to warn of complications and confusion over postoperative sperm counts the commonest problems. A counselling checklist of discussion points, as recommended for female sterilization, would help to reduce this type of complaint. For example, the RCOG guidelines (1999) recommend that women should be informed that vasectomy has a lower failure rate and less operative risk.

The 14 miscellaneous claims included granuloma formation, a needle left in the scrotum and advising vasectomy on spurious medical grounds.

Termination of pregnancy

Major morbidity following medical and surgical termination of pregnancy (TOP) occurs in less than 1% of cases (Grimes and Cates 1979, Royal College of General Practitioners/RCOG 1985, UK Multi-Centre Trial 1990), but vacuum aspiration is associated with a greater incidence of morbidity requiring treatment compared with medical abortion (Henshaw et al 1994, Cameron et al 1996). Among the MPS cases there were 318 complaints involving TOP (Fig. 10.3). The commonest were incomplete and failed procedures accounting for 81 (25%) and 79 (25%) cases respectively. These figures indicate that inappropriately experienced surgeons were frequently operating, and with very early and late gestations good technique is essential to ensure the pregnancy is not missed completely or significant tissue retained. Measures to prevent operation failure include inspection of products of conception with histological confirmation if necessary; also ultrasonography after the procedure if there is doubt whether the abortion is complete. A detailed operation record, particularly by trainees, is preferable to the often vague and unsatisfactory comment 'routine procedure performed'.

Uterine perforation occurred in 66 (21%) of cases with bowel damage in 15 women and bladder damage in one patient. Perforation occurs more easily in the soft, gravid uterus and when it is suspected, laparoscopy is necessary to ensure there has been no other trauma. Litigation is more likely to succeed when these steps are not taken and the diagnosis is delayed. Postoperatively, if there are excessive symptoms of pain, bleeding or

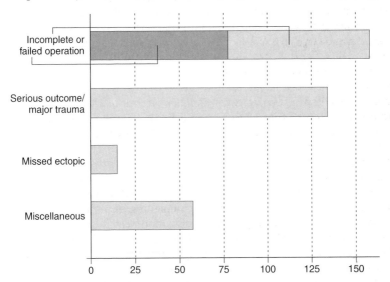

Figure 10.3 Termination of pregnancy-related claims against the Medical Protection Society 1974–1999.

pyrexia, uterine perforation and intra-abdominal trauma should be considered and appropriate clinical measures taken, and consultation with senior colleagues is advised.

Significant infection was seen in 19 claims and hysterectomy was necessary in 18 (6%) cases. As the incidence of sexually transmitted infection in termination patients is about 5–10% (Southgate et al 1989, Cameron et al 1996), it is good practice to screen, particularly for chlamydia (Chief Medical Officer's Expert Advisory Group 1999). If this is not done and postoperative infection occurs which leads to litigation, the doctor could not be defended. Missed ectopic pregnancy occurred in 14 (4%) women. There were 8 (3%) serious outcomes, including four maternal deaths and brain damage in two women. Neonatal brain damage was diagnosed in two failed terminations which continued to delivery. Uterine perforation leading to massive haemorrhage or septicaemia was the main cause of maternal death.

There were 57 (18%) miscellaneous complaints relating to TOP. They included retained foreign bodies (swabs or forgotten intrauterine devices); inadequate counselling; subsequent infertility; and termination without consent. In five cases in each category, claims were raised because termination had been refused or the patient was not pregnant at operation. Detailed counselling and documentation are again essential preoperatively to ensure the patient fully understands the consequences of termination. With changes in medical methods, e.g. reduction in prostaglandin dose and different administration routes, it is probable that morbidity and acceptability will improve and the need for surgical techniques will be reduced (Cameron and Baird 1998). Finally, it is advisable to arrange a follow-up appointment after abortion to ensure that there have been no adverse sequelae and confirm that adequate contraception is being used.

Intrauterine devices

Problems with intrauterine devices (IUDs) accounted for 216 complaints referred to the MPS (Fig. 10.4). Of these, 34 (16%) and 45 (21%) concerned insertion and removal complications respectively. Eleven IUDs were inserted when there was already an undiagnosed pregnancy. In 25 women an IUD was not removed before a second insertion (14) or at sterilization (11). In eight cases infertility resulted from failure to remove an IUD.

In 58 (27%) procedures the uterus was perforated with associated bowel or bladder damage in five women. Two hysterectomies were needed because of an IUD in the broad ligament or causing infection, and four perforations occurred at attempted IUD removal.

Infection was noted in 26 claims with two episodes of actinomycosis (one requiring colostomy) and four women blamed their subsequent infertility on the sepsis. The 10 counselling deficiencies included six women who became pregnant after IUDs were removed without their knowledge. In the

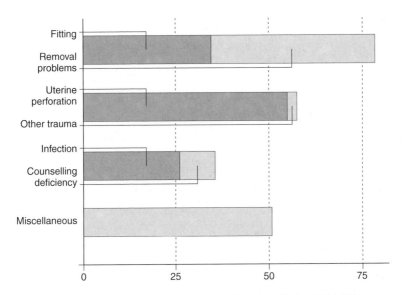

Figure 10.4   IUD-related claims against the Medical Protection Society 1974–1999.

51 miscellaneous cases, there was misdiagnoses of three ectopic pregnancies and two cervical carcinomas, and in four women request for an IUD was refused and pregnancy ensued.

IUD use requires detailed counselling which should include a gynaecological history, particularly concerning the presence of menorrhagia, previous pelvic infection and ectopic pregnancy, and whether or not there is a stable sexual relationship. Points to be covered include the small risk of failure, expulsion, heavy periods and infection (see Ch. 4). The mode of action should be explained (Spinnato 1997). This discussion should be recorded in the notes as proof of valid consent being obtained. The RCOG (1996) recommends that prior to IUD insertion the patient should be screened for sexually transmitted infection, or alternatively antibiotics should be administered at the time of insertion.

Hormonal contraception

Complaints concerning hormonal contraception accounted for 113 (8%) cases among the MPS series (Fig. 10.1). The subdermal implant, Norplant, featured in 58, and 55 involved combined oral contraception (COC) of which there were 21 counselling problems (invariably resulting in pregnancy) and 20 thrombotic/thromboembolic complications. Emergency contraception and injectables accounted for seven and four claims respectively with three miscellaneous issues.

Subdermal implants

The 58 complaints about Norplant related to irregular bleeding, hair loss, allergies, and insertion/removal difficulties as well as pain and scarring. The saga surrounding this long-acting subdermal implant typifies the contraceptive industries' difficulties with introducing badly needed new technology (Ch. 18) (Boonstra et al 1999). Norplant was marketed in the UK in 1993 after clinical trials had proved its reliability, with the commonest side effects being menstrual disturbance, acne and headaches; side effects similar to those seen with the progestogen-only pill. To minimize anticipated problems the distributors, Hoechst Marion Roussel, set up training programmes concerning counselling and insertion/removal techniques.

Initial enthusiasm for the method was not maintained because of frequent, adverse criticisms reported in the press. In 1995, the Norplant Action Group was set up to seek compensation for users complaining of side effects and removal problems. Most complainants were state-funded through the UK Legal Aid system, but this support was withdrawn when it was decided the poor chance of success and small size of each claim did not justify the high trial costs. Thereafter, all 275 actions were dropped in 1999 when the manufacturers voluntarily withdrew the product from the market (see also Ch. 3).

This 'boom-and-bust' phenomenon of contraceptive innovations mirrored Norplant's introduction to the US market in 1991 (Boonstra et al 1999). By 1994 about 1 million American women were using the method, but problems were highlighted in the media and by 1995 over 50 000 claims had been filed: as a result Norplant's sales plummeted. This experience caused the manufacturers of the second-generation, two-capsule version to drop launch plans despite approval by the US Food and Drug Administration.

However, in 1999 in the UK, a single-rod progestogen-only contraceptive implant (Implanon) was launched (Ch. 3). This preparation promises to provide a highly effective and acceptable alternative to existing hormonal contraceptives, but appropriate counselling of potential users will be essential if litigation history is not to be repeated.

Combined oral contraception

The benefits to health and well-being from COC far outweigh the side effects and infrequent complications. Nevertheless, before prescribing COC, detailed assessment including medical/family history and relevant examination is essential to identify major risk factors (Ch. 2). The 21 inadequate counselling claims handled by the MPS concerned when to take COC and circumstances requiring additional contraception, e.g. vomiting or diarrhoea, and drug interactions with antibiotics, barbiturates and anticonvulsants.

There were 20 complaints related to arterial and venous thrombotic episodes. There are regular press reports about inappropriate COC use leading to serious outcomes. In a recent court case, a 38-year-old obese woman who smoked was inappropriately prescribed the low-dose COC. She suffered a major cerebrovascular accident with long-term hemiparesis, a changed personality and loss of memory. She received nearly £500 000 in damages (Trueland 1999).

Epidemiological studies show an association between COC and increased risk of venous thromboembolism (Ch. 2).

Delayed diagnosis of adverse events is common so when there is sudden development of severe chest pain, breathlessness or headache accompanied by loss of vision/speech or collapse, a venous thromboembolic episode must be considered. In five COC claims the outcome was death, with four resulting from pulmonary emboli and one from cerebral thrombosis.

Emergency contraception

There were seven complaints notified to the MPS; six practitioners refused to prescribe it and all cases resulted in pregnancy. The remaining claim followed inaccurate advice and twins were delivered. With increased knowledge and acceptance of emergency contraception, these difficulties should not recur.

Injectables

The long-acting intramuscular progestogen-only method, depot medroxyprogesterone acetate (DMPA), accounted for four complaints in the MPS series. There was an embolus causing loss of sight (1), an injection was given when there was an undiagnosed pregnancy (1) and two episodes of poor counselling. Routine counselling should include discussion of bleeding problems during and after cessation of treatment (particularly if given in the immediate puerperium), the delayed return of fertility and possible reduction in bone mineral density with long-term use (see Ch. 3).

Other complaints

The miscellaneous complaints relating to hormonal contraception included one patient prescribed hormone replacement therapy (HRT) for contraception. In a recent case, two general practice partners appeared before the GMC Professional Conduct Committee for the same complaint and other errors which included not informing the patient of herpes virus in her cervical smear, altering records and drug abuse of one of the doctors. The charges were found proved except the prescription of HRT for contraception, and both doctors were found guilty of serious professional misconduct

(General Medical Council 1998b). The Chairman, when announcing the determination of the committee concerning one doctor, commented on note-keeping:

Clear and accurate patient records showing relevant clinical findings, decisions made, information given to patients and any drugs or other treatments prescribed are an essential part of good practice. Without such records patient care is put at risk. The committee are very concerned at the manner in which you amended a patient's records. Any such amendments should have been made in an appropriate manner so that the original entry could still be read and the date and nature of the amendment was clear.

HOW TO REDUCE LITIGATION RISK

1. Accurate and thorough documentation is vital. A complete record which is contemporaneous, legible, dated and signed enhances a practitioner's defence when litigation occurs compared with inadequate notes and memory of events which frequently happened years before. If it was not documented, lawyers will assume it was not done.
2. Good communication and rapport are very important, so when there is a complication, a full explanation should be given in addition to immediate and skilled care to correct the problem. An apology is not an admission of liability.
3. Successful outcomes invariably are the product of teamwork which is essential in all healthcare. Nurse-prescribing is an appropriate example involving multidisciplinary development of high quality protocols, regular audit and good communication. As a result, mutual respect develops to the benefit of all.
4. Satisfactory consent requires appropriate explanation/discussion and a record in the patient's notes. In addition, concise written information is advised but it does not replace patient counselling.
5. For trainees, good teaching, supervision and appropriate delegation are essential. Knowing when to seek advice (early rather than late) is a prerequisite to developing a satisfactory standard of care.
6. Skilled surgery should be preceded by detailed preoperative assessment which includes consulting the patient and the patient's records to ensure the correct procedure is planned and relevant consent has been obtained.
7. The concept of clinical freedom is acknowledged but it can involve outdated or idiosyncratic care. The mandatory process of clinical governance has been introduced to the NHS and should be accepted and implemented. It may be defined as 'the corporate responsibility of clinicians and managers for ensuring quality of services'. This includes competent patient care using evidence-based

practice when possible and regularly updated guidelines, also clinical audit and risk management, and the professional development of all staff.
8. Good practice is about well-developed clinical skills, judgement, experience and common sense.

Acknowledgement

The author is grateful to the Medical Protection Society, in particular Dr John D. Hickey, Medical Director, and Mr Keith Haynes, Head of Risk Management Services, for making available the MPS database on family planning litigation.

REFERENCES

Allan I 1991 Young people's experience and views of family planning projects and services. Family planning projects and pregnancy counselling projects for young people. Policy Studies Institute, London, p 84–106
Bolam v. Friern Hospital Management Committee 1957 1WLR 582; 1 All ER 871
Bolitho v. City and Hackney Health Authority 1997 4 All ER 771: 3 WLR 1151
Boonstra H, Duran V, Weaver K 1999 Norplant and the boom-and-bust phenomenon. IPPF Medical Bulletin 33(5): 3–4
Brahams D 1999 Commentary – End of compensation for unwanted healthy children. Lancet 354: 1924
Brown ADG 1985 Accidents in gynaecological surgery – medico-legal. In: Chamberlain GVP, Orr CJB, Sharp F (eds) Litigation and obstetrics and gynaecology. Royal College of Obstetricians and Gynaecologists, London, ch 8, p 81
Brown ADG 1997 Pitfalls in sterilisation procedures. Protection matters. The Medical Protection Society, London, 6: 1–3
Cameron S, Baird DT 1998 Comparison of complications and morbidity following medical and surgical methods of abortion. In: O'Brien PMS (ed) Yearbook of obstetrics and gynaecology. RCOG Press, London, ch 6, p 394
Cameron ST, Glasier AF, Logan J, Benton L, Baird DT 1996 Impact of the introduction of new medical methods on therapeutic abortions at the Royal Infirmary of Edinburgh. British Journal of Obstetrics and Gynaecology 103: 1222–1229
Chief Medical Officer's Expert Advisory Group 1999 *Chlamydia trachomatis* – executive summary. Department of Health, London
Clements RV, Huntingford PJ 1994 Introduction. In: Clements RV (ed) Safe practice in obstetrics and gynaecology – a medico-legal handbook. Churchill Livingstone, Edinburgh, ch 1, p 3
Crown J 1998 Review of prescribing, supply and administration of medicines; a report on the supply and administration of medicines under group protocols. Department of Health, London
Department of Health 1990 A guide to consent for examination and treatment. HC(90)22. Department of Health, London
Doherty C 1997 An outline of legal issues. Conference report – The enhanced role of the family planning nurse. Brook Advisory Centres, London, ch 2, p 25
General Medical Council (GMC) 1995 Guidance on confidentiality. GMC, London, p 2–6
General Medical Council (GMC) 1998a Seeking patients' consent: the ethical considerations – guidance to doctors. GMC, London, p 1–19

General Medical Council (GMC) 1998b Extracts from minutes of Professional Conduct
    Committee: Bourne S J, Shantikumar M. GMC, London 10–13 Nov
Gillick v. West Norfolk and Wisbech Area Health Authority 1985 3 All ER 402–437
Grimes DA, Cates W 1979 Complications from legally-induced abortion: a review. Obstetrical
    and Gynaecological Survey 34: 177–191
Gupta S, Bewley S 1998 Medico-legal issues in fertility regulation. British Journal of Obstetrics
    and Gynaecology 105: 818–826
Henshaw RC, Nadji SA, Russell IT, Templeton AA 1994 A comparison of medical abortion
    (using mifepristone and gemeprost) with surgical vacuum aspiration: efficacy and early
    medical sequelae. Human Reproduction 9: 2167–2172
James CE 1994 Medico-legal aspects of obstetrics and gynaecology. In: Studd JWW (ed)
    Yearbook of obstetrics and gynaecology. RCOG Press, London, p 69–77
Johnstone H 1999 'Sterile' mother wins £1.3 m over disabled child. The Times Nov 26
Murray I 1998 NHS faces £2.3 bn bill for negligence payouts. The Times July 21
National Audit Office 1995–1996 NHS Summarised Accounts
Royal College of General Practitioners and the Royal College of Obstetricians and
    Gynaecologists Joint Study Group 1985 Induced abortion operations and their early
    sequelae. Journal of the Royal College of General Practitioners 35:175–180
Royal College of Nursing (RCN) 1998 Guidance for nurses on the supply and administration
    of medicines under group protocol arrangements. RCN, London
Royal College of Obstetricians and Gynaecologists (RCOG) Study Group 31 1996 Prevention of
    pelvic infection. RCOG Press, London, p 1–6
Royal College of Obstetricians and Gynaecologists (RCOG) 1999 Male and female sterilisation
    – evidence-based clinical guidelines summary No. 4, RCOG Press, London, p 1–8
Schütte P 1997 Confidentiality. Medical Defence Union, London, p 6
Southgate L, Treharne J, Williams R 1989 Detection, treatment and follow up of women with
    Chlamydia trachomatis infection seeking abortion in inner city general practices. British
    Medical Journal 299: 1136–1137
Spinnato JA 1997 Mechanism of action of intrauterine contraceptive devices and its relation to
    informed consent. American Journal of Obstetrics and Gynaecology 176: 503–506
Times Law Report 1999 No damages for cost of bringing up a child. McFarlane v. Tayside
    Health Board. The Times Nov 26
Trueland J 1999 £468 750 damages for woman on pill who had a stroke. The Scotsman Dec 14

11

Therapeutic Abortion

David T. Baird

Legal aspects   250
Counselling   251
Information counselling   252
Assessment   253
Referral   253
Techniques of abortion   254
  Early first trimester
    (up to 9 weeks)   254
  Late first trimester
    (9 to 14 weeks)   257

Mid-trimester   258
Complications   259
  Early   259
  Late   260
Follow-up   260
  Contraception   261
Conclusion   261
Appendix   263
  Patient information
  sheet   263

Abortion occurs in every country in the world. The World Health Organization has calculated that approximately 50 million pregnancies are terminated by abortion each year. Even in those countries where abortion is illegal, many women attempt to terminate an unwanted pregnancy illegally (e.g. in Brazil) or travel abroad to a country with more liberal laws (e.g. from the Republic of Ireland to England). Illegal abortions are often performed in unsanitary conditions by unqualified people and as a result are a considerable cause of morbidity and mortality. It is estimated that 100–200 000 women die each year as a result of the complications of abortion (Segal and La Guardia 1990, Fathalla 1992). In contrast, abortion performed using modern methods in optimum conditions is an extremely safe procedure, and legalization of abortion is always followed by a drop in maternal deaths presumed to be due to the reduction in the complications of illegal abortions.

After the Abortion Act was passed in 1967, there was a rapid rise in the number of abortions notified in England and Wales and Scotland (Fig. 11.1) reaching a plateau of 110 000 per year in 1978 (Botting 1991). Since then, there has been a gradual rise in the numbers each year but much of this can be explained by demographic changes. The rate of abortion varies according to the woman's age and many of the girls born during the 'baby boom' of the mid-1960s have until recently been at the age of maximum risk of abortion. The abortion rate in Britain (9–14 per 1000 women aged 15 to 45 years) is relatively low compared to many other developed countries and probably reflects a wide acceptance of contraception and a comprehensive network of family planning services.

Women become pregnant without planning to do so either because of lack of forethought or contraceptive failure. Although the timing may be inconvenient, many will choose to have the baby but some will want an

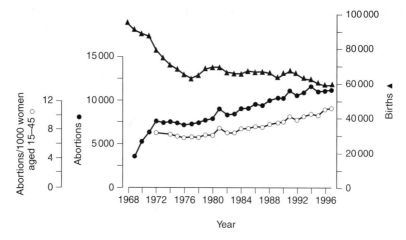

Figure 11.1   Abortions and Births in Scotland 1969–1997.

abortion. Abortion should never be considered as a method of contraception; however, failures occur with any method and without access to abortion, the ability of women to regulate their fertility and plan their families is impaired. It is important, therefore, that anyone involved in providing contraceptive services should be aware of the legal indications and different methods of therapeutic abortion available.

LEGAL ASPECTS

It is illegal in the UK to induce an abortion except under specific indications as defined by law. Many couples are under the mistaken belief that there is 'abortion on demand'. The conditions of the 1967 Abortion Act as amended in 1990 state that abortion can be performed if two registered medical practitioners, acting in good faith, agree that the pregnancy should be terminated on one or more of the following grounds:

1. The continuance of the pregnancy would involve risk to the life of the pregnant woman greater than if the pregnancy were terminated.
2. The termination is necessary to prevent grave permanent injury to the physical or mental health of the pregnant woman.
3. The pregnancy has *not* exceeded its 24th week and that the continuance of the pregnancy would involve risk, greater than if the pregnancy were terminated, of injury to the physical or mental health of the pregnant woman.

4. The pregnancy has *not* exceeded its 24th week and that the continuance
   of the pregnancy would involve risk, greater than if the pregnancy were
   terminated, of injury to the physical or mental health of the existing
   child(ren) of the family of the pregnant woman.
5. There is a substantial risk that if the child were born it would suffer from
   such physical or mental abnormalities as to be seriously handicapped.

Modern methods of inducing abortion are now so effective and safe that
almost always it is safer for the woman to have an abortion than to continue
with the pregnancy. That is not to say that abortion should be recommended
always, but a doctor should think very carefully before refusing to recommend abortion for a woman who is convinced that her mental and/or physical health or the welfare of her children would be better preserved by
ending the pregnancy.

There are differences in the law as it applies to abortion between different
parts of the UK.

In England and Wales, it is illegal to attempt to induce abortion except
under the 1967 Abortion Act even if the woman is not pregnant. The *inten-
tion* to induce abortion is sufficient.

In Scotland, no criminal charge of inducing abortion can be sustained
unless the prosecution can prove that the woman was pregnant.

The 1967 Abortion Act does not apply to Northern Ireland where abortion
is only legal under exceptional circumstances, e.g. to save the life of the
mother.

The law concerning abortion is the subject of continuing debate within
the UK. Although a vociferous lobby would wish to make abortion illegal or
severely restrict its application, Parliament, reflecting the view of the majority, have repeatedly confirmed their support for the current law. In 1990, the
law was amended to reduce the upper limit from 28 to 24 weeks gestation
reflecting earlier fetal viability owing to advances in neonatal care. An
exception was made in the case of a fetus with severe congenital abnormality incompatible with life, e.g. anencephaly, when there is no upper
limit (Section 5).

COUNSELLING

Faced with the news of an unintended pregnancy, many women are emotionally devastated. They may well have conflicting feelings about the pregnancy, e.g. to continue with the pregnancy may present insoluble problems
and seem quite impractical, whereas to have an abortion may seem abhor-
rent. It is important to provide a sympathetic hearing in order to allow the
woman to explore her own feelings.

Early in the consultation, a doctor should indicate that the doctor's role is
to provide information and to help the woman decide what is best for her

within the constraints of the law. The law recognizes that some doctors have ethical objections to abortion and, hence no doctor is required to counsel or treat a woman requesting an abortion against his or her moral principles. However, if such a doctor is consulted by a woman requesting an abortion, referral of the woman to another colleague who does not hold similar views is obligatory.

The aim of counselling, therefore, is to help the woman to:

1. Determine her real wishes.
2. Decide on the best course of action.
3. Take responsibility for her own decision.
4. Understand how she came to have an unwanted pregnancy so that she can plan to avoid another.

Information counselling

It is important that the woman be provided with sufficient information so that she can make up her mind. This includes:

1. Alternatives to abortion, i.e. keeping the baby or having it adopted. In this respect, the following questions are relevant:
   a. Is her husband/partner supportive?
   b. If her partner has deserted her, does she have supportive parents, relatives, or friends?
   c. What are her financial resources?
   Information about maternity grants, leave, social security payments should be made available.
2. Details of the method of abortion (Appendix 11.1).
3. Arrangements by which abortion will be performed. Ideally she should be referred to a National Health Service (NHS) hospital free of charge, but in some parts of the UK it may be necessary for her to pay for an abortion through the private sector or through a charitable organization.
4. The likely complications and long-term side effects of the abortion.
5. Future contraception.

The majority of women make up their minds as to what they want within a few days of learning that they are pregnant. Some, however, remain ambivalent and may require more extensive professional counselling, taking into account psychological, social and medical factors. Women with severe medical conditions which could worsen in pregnancy, e.g. pulmonary hypertension, or with psychiatric disorders, require particularly careful assessment of the relative risks of continuing with the pregnancy. Expert medical or psychiatric advice is required in such cases.

ASSESSMENT

After it has been decided that there are grounds for abortion and the woman has been fully counselled, it is important to make a careful assessment.

1. A pregnancy test must always be performed to confirm that the woman is definitely pregnant. Arranging the test, obtaining the result and discussing it with the woman should be achieved with as little delay as possible.
2. The stage of gestation should be determined by pelvic bimanual examination as well as by menstrual history. A pelvic ultrasound scan is unnecessary unless there is real doubt about the gestation, e.g. irregular menstrual history or obesity making pelvic examination unreliable, or if ectopic pregnancy is suspected.
3. A complete medical history is necessary paying particular attention to conditions such as heart or respiratory disease which may influence the choice of method of abortion.
4. Optimally, swabs should be taken routinely for microbiological examination and, if possible, antibiotic therapy started before abortion is performed. There is now good evidence that infection with *Chlamydia trachomatis* is a significant cause of subsequent infertility because of tubal disease. In some populations, the incidence of infection with *Chlamydia*, gonorrhoea and other organisms may be so high, e.g. more than 10%, that routine administration to everyone of a broad-spectrum antibiotic such as doxycycline or erythromycin before abortion may be a cost-effective way of reducing pelvic infection.
5. Blood should be collected for measurement of haemoglobin concentration and blood group determined.
6. As fetal red cells pass into the maternal circulation during all methods of abortion, women who are rhesus negative should be injected with anti-D immunoglobulin prior to or within 48 hours of the abortion to prevent the development of rhesus isoimmunization.

REFERRAL

Most women seeking an abortion in the UK consult their general practitioner in the first instance. Others prefer to approach a family planning clinic or pregnancy advisory service directly. Once the decision has been made, the woman should be referred to a gynaecologist as quickly as possible.

Provision for abortion varies throughout the UK. In Scotland and North-East England, over 90% of abortions are performed in NHS hospitals while in other areas of England, the majority are carried out in private clinics or by charities. The incidence of complications of abortion is directly related to the period of gestation so that an efficient referral system such as exists in

Lothian is optimal, although a few days reflection between decision and having the pregnancy terminated is desirable (Glasier and Thong 1991).

TECHNIQUES OF ABORTION

In the last 10 years, there have been several advances in the techniques to induce abortion so that safe and effective methods are now available at all stages of gestation. There has been an increasing use of medical methods since mifepristone was licensed in 1991 (Fig. 11.2). The optimum method depends on gestation, parity, medical history and the woman's wishes. It is usual to divide abortions into first trimester (up to 12 weeks amenorrhoea) when the uterus can be safely evacuated by vacuum aspiration (VA) and second trimester (12 to 24 weeks) when cervical preparation or medical methods are required. However, a more logical classification in keeping with the newer methods is as discussed below.

Early first trimester (up to 9 weeks)

Women seeking abortion at this early stage of pregnancy can be offered a choice of two equally effective methods, VA and medical abortion. VA has the advantage that the abortion is completed in a single visit and, if general anaesthesia is used, there is no pain or discomfort and the woman is unaware of the events at the time of abortion. Some women choose the med-

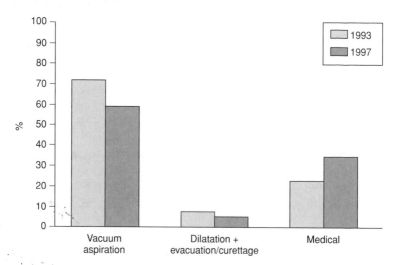

Figure 11.2 Percentage of abortions performed by different methods in Scotland.

ical method because they feel more in control of the situation and it avoids passing instruments into the uterus under general anaesthesia.

Vacuum aspiration

The most frequently used method is VA under local or general anaesthesia. Before 6 weeks gestation, it is possible to insert a small (4 mm) catheter and, using a hand-held syringe (Fig. 11.3), complete the abortion without dilatation of the cervix because the negative pressure together with the scraping movement of the catheter tip disintegrates the fetus which is tiny at this gestation. This technique is sometimes referred to as 'menstrual extraction'. Beyond 6 weeks it is usually necessary to dilate the cervix in order to insert a larger curette (up to 12 mm) through the cervix and the contents of the uterus are usually aspirated using a mechanical pump.

In the UK, the operation is mainly performed using general anaesthesia, although in many countries, e.g. USA, local paracervical block appears to be sufficient.

VA at this stage of pregnancy is an extremely safe and effective procedure with a very low incidence of complications.

Failure is more likely to occur in very early pregnancy (i.e. within 2 weeks of the missed menstrual period), probably because at this stage it is possible to miss the tiny fetus with the curette. For this reason, it may be better to defer the operation until after this time or to use medical methods.

The mortality from VA in the first trimester is less than about 1 per 100 000, i.e. considerably less than the maternal mortality from continuing pregnancy. Complications which include damage to the cervix, uterine perforation and post-abortion infection are rare (Frank 1985).

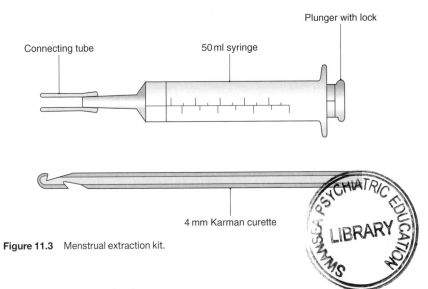

Plunger with lock

Connecting tube

50 ml syringe

4 mm Karman curette

Figure 11.3   Menstrual extraction kit.

Medical abortion

Abortion can be induced medically in the first 9 weeks of pregnancy. Although a number of substances which could induce abortion had been known for many years, it was the discovery of the antigestogen mifepristone or RU 486 in 1980 which made medical abortion a practical reality (Baird 1992). Mifepristone (Mifegyne) is a synthetic steroid chemically similar to norethindrone (the gestogen in one of the first combined oral contraceptives) which blocks the biological action of progesterone by binding to its receptor in the uterus and other target organs. Following withdrawal of the effect of progesterone, the uterus contracts and bleeding from the placental bed occurs followed by abortion 2 to 5 days later.

Initial trials showed that the rate of complete abortion was only 60% necessitating VA on the remaining women who had an incomplete abortion or ongoing pregnancy. However, subsequently it was shown that the rate of complete abortion could be increased to over 95% if a prostaglandin was given 36 or 48 hours after the administration of mifepristone.

In the UK, mifepristone is currently licensed for the induction of abortion up to 9 weeks gestation given as a single oral dose of 600 mg (3 tablets) followed 48 hours later by 1 mg vaginal pessary of cervagem (Gemeprost). Cervagem is a synthetic derivative of the naturally occurring prostaglandin E, which causes strong contraction of the uterus. It also causes softening and dilatation of the cervix and is widely used for preparation of the cervix prior to VA and dilatation and evacuation (D&E) in the second trimester. There is now substantive evidence that the dose of mifepristone can be reduced to 200 mg and that an alternative prostaglandin, e.g. misoprostol, is equally as effective and cheaper than cervagem.

Contraindications. Medical abortion is not a suitable method for all women in early pregnancy, and it is important to take a careful medical history and to counsel the woman accordingly (Table 11.1). Mifepristone binds to the glucocorticoid receptor and blocks the action of cortisol. Thus, any patient on corticosteroids or who has suspected adrenal insufficiency should not be given mifepristone. Prostaglandins can cause bronchospasm – asthma is therefore an absolute contraindication to medical methods.

Table 11.1   Contraindications to medical abortion

Absolute	Relative
Adrenal insufficiency	Heavy smoker
Ectopic pregnancy	>35 years
>9 weeks gestation	Obesity
Asthma	Hypertension (diastolic >100 mmHg)
Cardiac disease	
Heavy smoker – older than 35 years	
On anticoagulants or bleeding disorder	

Side effects. There are very few side effects following administration of mifepristone (Baird and Thong 1998). Although for legal reasons the tablets must be taken in the presence of a doctor or nurse in a hospital or approved place, it is only necessary to observe the woman for about 10 minutes after swallowing the tablets before she goes home. After 48 hours, she returns to hospital for insertion of the cervagem pessary into the vagina. The fetus is usually aborted in the next 4 hours and this is accompanied by bleeding and pain. The bleeding is usually described as being like a heavy period although rarely (less than 1% of cases) there may be very heavy bleeding requiring resuscitation.

Most women experience period-like pains although there is great variability in degree, with some needing no analgesia while others (about 10–20%) may require opiates. Bleeding usually continues for about 10 days after the abortion although the total amount of blood lost (around 80 mL) is similar to that occurring at the time of VA.

Late first trimester (9 to 14 weeks)

At this stage of pregnancy, the method of choice is VA. Although abortion can be induced by antigestogens and prostaglandins, the incidence of incomplete abortion is higher than before 9 weeks and many women require subsequent surgical evacuation of the uterus. It is necessary to dilate the cervix prior to passing a curette of sufficient diameter to suck out the fetal parts. Forcible dilatation of the cervix, especially in young nulliparous women, may damage the cervix resulting in bleeding or long-term cervical incompetence (Frank et al 1987).

A variety of methods are available to soften and dilate the cervix prior to VA including hygroscopic bougies, prostaglandins and mifepristone.

Bougies. Lamicel or Dilapan are hygroscopic rods which are placed in the cervix several hours prior to surgery and, by taking up water, swell to several times their original diameter and dilate the cervix. Because they require to be inserted by a doctor several hours prior to surgery, they are usually used only in more advanced pregnancies (over 14 weeks) when considerable cervical dilatation is required prior to D&E.

Prostaglandin. Prostaglandins such as cervagem and misoprostol have a short action and will achieve adequate dilatation in only 3 hours.

Mifepristone. This is equally effective at preparing the cervix but takes longer.

Although VA is an extremely safe operation, the blood loss and other complications rise as gestation advances. It is important, therefore, to refer the women for abortion promptly after the decision to terminate the pregnancy has been made.

Mid-trimester

Because termination of pregnancy is more difficult and has more complications after 14 weeks, every effort should be made to reduce the number of mid-trimester abortions. Some gynaecologists are very reluctant to perform mid-trimester abortions except for life-threatening conditions. However, women who are least able to cope with an unwanted pregnancy often first present at this time. In addition, screening for congenital abnormalities such as neural tube defects is usually performed after the 14th week and it may therefore be after the 20th week before severe fetal abnormality is discovered. Thus, it may well be necessary to induce abortion in the mid-trimester. At this stage of pregnancy, abortion may be induced either surgically or medically.

Dilatation and evacuation

D&E is the method of choice in the USA, but in the UK its use is confined largely to gynaecologists in private practice (Francome and Savage 1992). It may be necessary to dilate the cervix up to a diameter of 20 mm before the fetal parts can be extracted using special instruments.

In skilled hands, D&E is a safe procedure but requires careful training of the operator if complications such as haemorrhage and perforation of the uterus are to be avoided. D&E has the advantage that the woman is unaware of the procedure which can be performed as a day case. There is evidence from the USA that women prefer D&E to medical methods although many nurses and doctors find it disturbing.

Medical methods

The alternative medical methods involve inducing uterine contractions so that the fetus is expelled from the uterus.

1. In the past, a variety of substances such as hypertonic saline, urea, and Rivanol were injected into the amniotic sac or through the cervix into the extra-amniotic space. Often they were combined with the intravenous infusion of oxytocin or prostaglandins to induce uterine contractions. Such methods were relatively inefficient and the woman underwent a prolonged labour, in some cases of greater than 48 hours, when the risk of infection was increased. Moreover, there was a risk of cardiovascular collapse as a result of inadvertent injection of prostaglandin or hypertonic solution directly into a blood vessel. For these reasons, although they are still used in some places, they are not to be recommended if more effective methods involving mifepristone and prostaglandins are available.

2. The use of mifepristone as pretreatment has been a major advance in the management of mid-trimester abortion by shortening the interval between administration of the prostaglandin and abortion of the fetus to 6 to 8 hours (Rodger and Baird 1990). 600 mg mifepristone is given 36 hours before insertion of a 1 mg cervagem pessary into the vagina or infusion of prostaglandin E_2 into the extra-amniotic space. The prostaglandin is repeated at intervals of 3 or 6 hours until expulsion of the fetus occurs. Most women require opiate analgesia to relieve the pains of uterine contractions and in a minority (about 10–20%) it is necessary to evacuate the uterus of the placenta in whole or in part.

In spite of the disadvantages, induction of abortion by medical means with prostaglandins alone or preferably in combination with mifepristone is a very effective method of abortion associated with a very low incidence of complications. Because it requires less surgical experience, the potential for serious complications is probably less than for D & E and, hence, it will continue to be used in many parts of the world.

COMPLICATIONS

Early

Persistence of placental and/or fetal tissue. This is the commonest complication following abortion. Incomplete or missed abortion is commoner after medically induced abortion in the first trimester and up to 5% of women will require surgical evacuation of the uterus within the first month. However, it should be emphasized that incomplete abortion and ongoing pregnancies also occur after VA with the incidence rising as the gestation increases.

The occurrence of bleeding and presence of residual trophoblastic tissue in the uterus at 2 weeks after a medical or surgical abortion are not in themselves indications to evacuate the uterus. Although an ultrasound scan of the uterus and the measurement of human chorionic gonadotrophin in plasma may be helpful in diagnosing an ongoing pregnancy, the decision as to whether evacuation of the uterus is indicated should be made on clinical grounds, i.e. continued heavy or persistent bleeding from a bulky uterus in which the cervix is still dilated.

The majority of women with an incomplete or missed abortion will pass the residual tissue with time if they are prepared to be patient. Previous teaching that all women with an incomplete abortion had a high risk of intrauterine infection until the uterus was evacuated, probably stemmed from the time when many incomplete abortions resulted from clandestine attempts to terminate the pregnancy under conditions which were far from optimal. Minor complications such as lower abdominal pain, vaginal bleeding and passage of clots or trophoblastic tissue are relatively common and usually only require reassurance.

Established pelvic infection. Such infection with pyrexia, abdominal pain and offensive vaginal discharge is rare (around 1%) following all methods of abortion particularly if women are screened for pathogens in the vagina, e.g. *Chlamydia* and gonorrhoea and treatment with antibiotics started prior to abortion.

Urinary infection, cervical and vaginal lacerations and perforation of the uterus. These are rare complications.

Late

There are very few late complications from abortion if the women have been carefully counselled.

Guilt or regret. Many women feel tearful and emotional in the weeks following the abortion but these feelings usually pass rapidly although occasionally fleeting memories may be triggered by some event.

Psychiatric disease. There is no evidence of an increase in the incidence of serious psychiatric disorder following abortion although relapse can occur in those with pre-existing psychiatric disease. In contrast, the incidence of depression, suicide and child abuse is higher in women who have continued with the pregnancy because abortion was refused (Matejcek et al 1985).

Infertility. Post-abortion infection is a significant cause of tubal disease and hence infertility, particularly following illegal abortion. However, as indicated above, with modern methods performed under optimal conditions, the incidence of infection is very low.

Pregnancy complications. Damage to the cervix or perforation of the uterus can predispose to cervical incompetence, preterm delivery and/or uterine rupture. However, a large prospective trial carried out by the Royal College of General Practitioners and the Royal College of Obstetricians and Gynaecologists showed that previous induced abortion had no effect on outcome in subsequent pregnancies (Frank et al 1987).

FOLLOW-UP

A follow-up visit at about 2 weeks is desirable for all women irrespective of the timing or method of abortion.

This visit is absolutely essential after administration of prostaglandin for those (about 30%) who have not passed the fetus and/or placental tissue in the few hours after the administration of the prostaglandin. Although the incidence of ongoing pregnancy is low (less than 1%), it will be necessary to evacuate the uterus because of incomplete or missed abortion in about 2–5%. Those women with ongoing pregnancies should be strongly advised to have VA because the development of the fetus could be compromised.

Follow-up can be undertaken by the general practitioner, family planning clinic or abortion service. Careful coordination of these services is essential to ensure that any ongoing pregnancies are identified promptly and to treat any complications.

Contraception

The fact that a woman has had an abortion is an indication that she probably requires a review of her method of contraception (if any). It is difficult during the emotionally stressful events surrounding the abortion for a woman to make a reasoned judgement about future methods of fertility control.

Decisions about permanent irreversible methods such as sterilization are better left for some months when the events of the abortion can be seen in perspective. However, ovulation returns fairly rapidly after abortion (20 to 60 days) and contraceptive precautions must be taken early if a further unwanted pregnancy is to be avoided. The method of contraception advised will vary depending on circumstances and needs of the couple.

Hormonal contraception. This can be started immediately following the abortion, although it is probably wise to delay starting it immediately after *medical* abortion if fetal or placental tissue has not been passed following prostaglandin administration. Otherwise, there is always the remote risk that high doses of hormones may be given to a woman who changes her mind and chooses to continue with the pregnancy. This risk must be balanced against the risk of the individual woman's becoming pregnant again in the weeks following abortion owing to lack of effective contraception. A reasonable compromise is to advise against intercourse for the 2 weeks between the abortion and the follow-up visit. At the same time, condoms can be supplied in the event of weakening of resolve. All hormonal methods, including injectables and implants, can be started at this time without risk of the woman already being pregnant.

IUDs. An IUD may be inserted immediately following the abortion, under the same anaesthetic if surgical abortion is chosen. Following medical abortion, it is probably preferable to wait until the 2-week follow-up before IUD insertion. However, there are no data to suggest that immediate insertion has any additional risks in women in whom products of conception have been identified at the time of prostaglandin administration.

Barrier methods. Any of these may be started immediately but the diaphragm should be checked at follow-up to ensure that the user does not need a different size.

CONCLUSION

Abortion should never be regarded as a method of contraception. Indeed, the request for termination of an unplanned pregnancy is evidence of a lack of knowledge of contraception, failure to use an effective method or failure of the method. Good family planning seeks to reduce the number of unplanned pregnancies and evidence suggests that abortion rates are lowest in those countries with a comprehensive system of sex education and contraceptive services. The occurrence of an abortion is an indication to review the method of contraception and consider whether change to another method, which would suit the needs of the woman better, should be made.

REFERENCES

Baird DT 1992 Medical termination of pregnancy. In: Edwards CR, Lincoln DW (eds) Recent advances in clinical endocrinology and metabolism, vol 14. Churchill Livingstone, Edinburgh, p. 83–94
Baird DT, Thong KJ 1998 Advances in methods of inducing abortion. In: Otteson B, Talbor A (eds) New insights in gynaecology and obstetrics. Parthenon, London, p 193–200
Botting B 1991 Trends in abortion. Population Trends 64. HMSO, London, p 19–29
Fathalla MF 1992 Reproductive health in the world: two decades of progress and the challenge ahead. In: Khanna J, Van Look PFA, Griffin PD (eds) Reproductive health: a key to a brighter future. World Health Organization, Geneva, p 3–31
Francome C, Savage WD 1992 Gynaecologists' abortion practice. British Journal of Obstetrics and Gynaecology 99: 153–157
Frank P 1985 Sequelae of induced abortion. In: Porter R, O'Connor M (eds) Abortion: medical progress and social implications. Ciba Foundation Symposium 115. Pitman, London, p 67–79
Frank PI, Kay CR, Scott LM, Hannaford PC, Haran D 1987 Pregnancy following induced abortion: Maternal morbidity, congenital abnormalities and neonatal death. British Journal of Obstetrics and Gynaecology 94: 836–842
Glasier AF, Thong KJ 1991 The establishment of a centralised referral service leads to earlier abortion. Health Bulletin 49: 254–259
Matejcek Z, Dytrych Z, Schüller V 1985 Follow up study of children born to women denied abortion. In: Porter R, O'Connor M (eds) Abortion: medical progress and social implications. Ciba Foundation Symposium 115. Pitman, London, p 136–146
Rodger MW, Baird DT 1990 Pretreatment with mifepristone (RU 486) reduces interval between prostaglandin administration and expulsion in second trimester abortion. British Journal of Obstetrics and Gynaecology 97: 41–45
Segal SJ, La Guardia KD 1990 Termination of pregnancy – a global view. Baillière's Clinical obstetrics and gynaecology 4: 235–247

APPENDIX 11.1

PATIENT INFORMATION SHEET

Abortion has been legal for many years but must be done in an approved place and with the agreement of two doctors who believe that you have good reasons for not wanting to continue with your pregnancy. If you are less than 9 weeks pregnant, there are two alternative ways of doing the abortion. The following information may help you decide which method you prefer. Remember that you only have a choice if you are less than 9 weeks pregnant.

Vacuum aspiration

This is the commonest method and is not normally used in this hospital at more than 12 weeks of pregnancy. Once the gynaecologist has agreed to your request for an abortion, you will be given a date to return to hospital usually just for the day.

After being admitted to the ward, you may have a tablet or pessary inserted into the vagina. This, as it dissolves, will soften the cervix (neck of the womb). The abortion procedure itself takes about 5 minutes and is done under a general anaesthetic, i.e. while you are asleep. The cervix is stretched open, a thin plastic tube is inserted into the uterus (womb) and the pregnancy is carefully sucked out. After you wake up from the anaesthetic, you may feel a little tearful but this and any period-like discomfort you may have will soon pass and you will be allowed home later the same day. Vacuum aspiration is a very safe procedure but all operations carry a small risk. However, the abortion is over in a single procedure and you are not aware of what is happening.

Medical abortion

Having agreed to your request for an abortion, the doctor will arrange for you to attend the ward on two separate occasions. At the first visit – which may be immediately after you have seen the doctor today – you will be given tablets of a drug called Mifegyne (RU 486). Once you have swallowed these tablets, you can leave the hospital.

2 days later, you will come back for the second part of the treatment. During these 2 days, you can behave entirely normally and go to work as usual.

You may have some light bleeding but it is very unlikely that the abortion will take place.

When you go back to the hospital, you will stay on the ward for about 6 hours.

You will not be asked to get undressed or to get into bed. A small pessary is put into the vagina which causes the uterus to contract and expel the pregnancy. You will probably have some period-like pains which may be strong enough for you to be given a painkiller and you will have some vaginal bleeding. It is likely that the abortion will occur during the time you are in hospital but the fetus is tiny at this stage of the pregnancy and you will not experience anything much different from your normal period.

Medical abortion can only be used if you are less than 9 weeks pregnant and is not available to you if you are over 35 years of age and smoke heavily, or suffer from asthma or heart disease. Provided that you are suitable for a medical abortion, the main advantage is that you do not need to have an anaesthetic or an operation.

After the abortion

Whichever method is used, you will bleed for up to 2 weeks, although this will not be heavy. You must see a doctor within a month after the abortion to check that all is well and that you have sorted out some contraception.

You will have an opportunity to discuss any questions you have with the doctors and other staff during the consultation.

12

Screening and reproductive health promotion

Sally Hope

Screening   265
Breast cancer   268
  Breast self-examination   268
  Breast awareness   269
  Routine breast examination   269
  Mammography   269
  Special groups   270
Weight   270
Domestic violence   271
Sexually transmitted
  infections   271
Urinary incontinence   272
Cholesterol   272
Smoking   272
Cervical cancer   272
  Risk factors for cervical
    cancer   273

Cervical intraepithelial neoplasia
  and carcinoma in situ   274
Prevention of invasive cervical
  cancer   275
Taking a cervical smear   276
Choice of spatula   276
Management of abnormal
  smears   278
Carcinoma of the ovary   278
  Ovarian cancer screening   278
  Routine pelvic examination   279
Other screening
  procedures   279
  Blood pressure   279
  Pre-pregnancy screening   279
  Tests that do not need to be
    done   279

SCREENING

Screening is, by definition, the examination of asymptomatic individuals in an attempt to discover early disease or the predictors of disease. The screening test must be acceptable, reliable and economically possible within the resources of the healthcare service of the country concerned. The screenable disease must be amenable to treatment and there must be an advantage in treating the disease at a stage before the patient would otherwise present. This all seems simple but screening programmes are fraught with controversy. The basic concept is well supported by the medical profession and by the general public: people want to remain well and healthy. However, all the many strands of screening now require an evidence-based approach. It is clear that well-meaning doctors and nurses have in the past toiled in vain, carrying out procedures that are now no longer thought to be worthwhile.

    The other fundamental conflict is that many women are falsely reassured by screening, believing that if they have been checked by a health professional, nothing could possibly go wrong in the future. Evidence-based patient choice now places the responsibility on the patient herself to decide whether or not she wants a particular test, but this poses a huge burden on the healthcare professional to explain all the pros and cons, and short-falls of that particular test. Moreover, in general practice there is pressure of a financial nature to coerce women to agree to health screening in order to achieve payment targets for that practice. The health professional needs to be sensitive to all these issues.

The family planning consultation offers an excellent opportunity for screening and for promoting health. This chapter will outline screening procedures and health promotion issues that the healthcare professional might discuss with a woman. Open questions in a consultation allow a woman to raise issues that particularly concern her or areas of family history that would be irrelevant to another woman. Women may have been coming to the same clinic for 20 to 30 years. During that time their health needs and the appropriate screening measures will change as they age, and information or technologies related to specific diseases become more refined. Screening is dynamic, and not static.

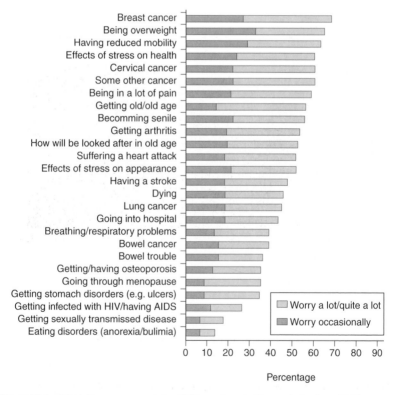

Figure 12.1 What do women worry about? (Reproduced with permission from McPherson A, Waller D (eds) 1997 Women's health, 4th edn. Oxford University Press, Oxford.)

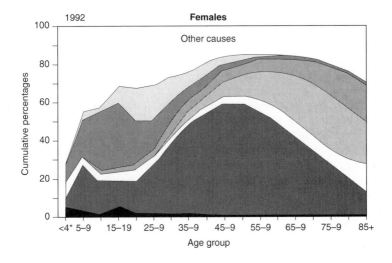

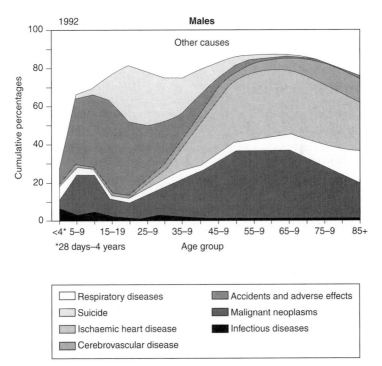

Figure 12.2 Causes of death by age and sex, England and Wales 1992. (Reproduced with permission from Mortality Statistics 1992 Office for National Statistics © Crown Copyright 1999.)

A final strand of this complex tapestry of health is the woman's own health beliefs and fears. For example, most women fear they will die of breast cancer and perceive it as a very real threat (Fig. 12.1), whereas actuarial figures reveal that 50% of women will die of heart attacks and strokes and only 8% of breast cancer (although breast cancer deaths do occur at a younger age) (Fig. 12.2). Unless a woman's fears and misconceptions are addressed, very little of the value of health promotional activity will be understood by the individual. For example, 16-year-old girls do not perceive smoking as a problem, but are terrified their parents will find out that they are on the pill. They do not worry about the risks of smoking, as they want to appear cool and stay thin. If they had to choose, they would rather give up the pill than cigarettes. The most effective health promotion any healthcare professional can do in any clinic is to assist people to stop smoking.

BREAST CANCER

In the UK, 1 in every 12 women will develop breast cancer at some time in their lives. Each year in the UK some 26 000 women are newly diagnosed and some 16 000 die from it (Fig. 12.3). There is immense confusion about breast screening.

Breast self-examination

More than 90% of breast cancers are detected by the woman herself. This led in the early years to women being encouraged to do breast self-examination

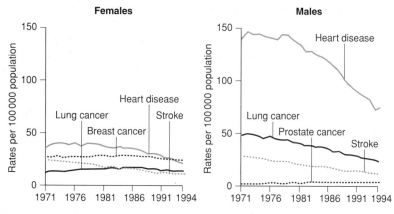

Figure 12.3   UK death rates for people aged under 65 by gender and selected cause of death. (Reproduced with permission from Surveys in Social Trends 1996 Office for National Statistics © Crown Copyright 1999.)

(BSE), a monthly palpation performed by a woman at the same time each month in a routine manner, on the premise that the earlier the lump was found the better was the prognosis. Unfortunately, BSE has never consistently demonstrated a reduction in mortality from breast cancer. Additionally, it has inevitably produced a high number of false positives, where women have found benign lumps, causing immense unnecessary anxiety. The Advisory Committee of the Department of Health in the UK has recommended that BSE should not be promoted as a screening procedure (Department of Health 1998).

Breast awareness

BSE was replaced by the concept of breast awareness where women are advised to be conscious of what is normal for them about the feel and look of their breasts throughout the menstrual cycle and to seek help if they notice anything different. Women should be aware of their breasts in everyday activities such as bathing and dressing (Mant 1992). This can be discussed in the family planning consultation and instruction given.

Routine breast examination

The Department of Health in the UK has stated that there is no evidence to support the efficacy of breast examination by health professionals of well women without symptoms, as it is liable to give false reassurance and discourage breast self-awareness. The committee advise that palpation of the breasts by either medical or nursing staff should not be included as part of a routine health screening for women. There are some studies showing that nurses working in specialist breast units with appropriate educational training in breast palpation are competent to detect abnormalities where there is a full range of facilities necessary for immediate access to breast cancer diagnoses. Further studies are underway in this specialist area.

There is no evidence that it is essential for a doctor to examine a woman's breasts before prescribing the combined oral contraceptive pill or hormone replacement therapy for the first time, other than for medicolegal reasons. However, the pros and cons of breast awareness should always be discussed (Chs 2 and 17).

Mammography

Randomized controlled trials have shown the value of mammography (Day 1991). Women over the age of 50 years undergoing mammographic screening have decreased mortality for breast cancer. It has been demonstrated that women are more likely to attend mammographic screening if there has been a brief discussion prior to the screening invitation with a healthcare professional (Austoker et al 1997).

The current UK guidelines at present are that all women between the ages of 50 and 64 should be screened routinely every 3 years. There will be an initial two-view radiographic examination with a subsequent single oblique view if required. There is no routine screening for under-50 year olds, and women over 65 may be screened on request but not more often than 3-yearly.

It is interesting to note that in one study 81% of women who had mammography claimed to experience discomfort (actual pain in 46% and severe pain in 7%). Of the women questioned on this discomfort, 60% said that a cervical smear or venepuncture was more uncomfortable (McIlwaine 1993).

Special groups

Women with a strong family history

Women with a strong family history of breast cancer under the age of 50 affecting a first-degree relative can be offered screening outside the national guidelines. This service varies greatly from region to region. In some areas, there are specialist genetic clinics, and in other regions, breast specialists advise and screen these high-risk women.

Women with symptoms

A woman with a breast lump must be examined and referred as appropriate.

Women with breast cancer

Women with breast cancer will generally be given more frequent mammograms and follow-up than the standard 3-yearly recall but this will be at the discretion of the clinician looking after that particular woman.

WEIGHT

Other than worrying about breast cancer, women are concerned about being overweight. In a survey for the BBC Radio 4 programme *Woman's Hour*, 33% of women in the UK over the age of 16 were concerned about being overweight (McPherson and Waller 1997). Offering advice about healthy diet and exercise is an important health promotion issue but there is little evidence to show any efficacy. Most women do not appreciate that being extremely thin puts them at higher risk of future osteoporosis and Alzheimer's disease, and conversely if they are significantly overweight, they have a greater risk of breast cancer. A Swedish study found that the commonest reason for discontinuation of combined oral contraception (COC) was perceived weight gain (Larsson et al 1997).

DOMESTIC VIOLENCE

Screening for intimate partner violence in the healthcare setting has been widely advocated but efforts to assess its effectiveness and ensure adequacy of screening and advice for the battered woman are untested. Doctors and nurses rarely ask about it and women across the socio-economic classes are often too ashamed to talk about it. The women affected may present in the family planning consultation in urgent need of contraception or even termination of pregnancy.

Facilities and help for battered women vary enormously throughout regions and between urban and rural areas. It may be helpful to have general information posters in the waiting room which women can read and obtain information from without making it obvious to others that they need help. When asked how to screen for domestic violence, non-abused women typically suggested general screening questions whereas women who had been abused suggested specific screening questions asking about direct violence (McNutt et al 1999). Like all other screening subjects, if the healthcare professional involved is too busy or feels it inappropriate, the opportunity for screening will be missed (Larkin et al 1999). Community awareness campaigns have identified that domestic violence is an important social problem. However, most doctors have never received the education on any aspects of family violence and feel impotent to help.

Strategies for detection and management of the problem include understanding the dynamics of the family, careful enquiry about victimization, screening for risk factors such as previous violence and high alcohol intake, and assuring patient safety. Healthcare professionals should be aware of available services local to their area and facilitate referral. There should always be a reporting of incidences of family violence. Often the medical role is most useful by providing non-judgemental support and information about legal and social services to the victim confidentially (Elhassani et al 1999).

SEXUALLY TRANSMITTED INFECTIONS

Many women may confide during the family planning consultation that they are worried that they might have a sexually transmitted infection (STI) (see Ch. 13). Within Genito-Urinary Medicine Clinics, screening tests are well established but will vary in different regions. The prevalence of *Chlamydia* is currently around 10% in sexually active teenagers in the UK and potential screening programmes for this are under consideration.

URINARY INCONTINENCE

Urinary incontinence is an important and under-reported problem in women, often because of embarrassment. If the appropriate questions are asked, referral can be made to relieve the burden of this considerable problem which is often suffered in silence by middle-aged and elderly women.

CHOLESTEROL

In the USA, the College of Physicians recommends that young healthy adult men aged under 35 and pre-menopausal women under 45 should not be screened for elevated cholesterol concentrations because of concerns about costs and health risks associated with over-use of pharmacological therapy. Their recommendation was that these individuals should be given lifestyle advice. If a woman is particularly worried about a strong family history of hypercholesterolaemia this can be discussed, but all women should be offered advice about a healthier lifestyle (Davis et al 1998).

SMOKING

The single most important health prevention measure any healthcare professional can do is to help an individual stop smoking. Around 70% of smokers would like to stop if they could. Unfortunately, young women are continuing to smoke and doing so in increasing numbers. Ex-smokers can substantially restore their life expectancy to that of non-smokers, but if they do not stop, half of those who smoke will die prematurely (Peto et al 1994).

The essential features of the individual smoking cessation advice are:

1. Ask (about smoking at every opportunity).
2. Advise (all smokers to stop).
3. Assist (the smoker to stop).
4. Arrange (follow-up to monitor progress and/or additional support).

In the UK, the government intends to set up new specialist support services between 2000 and 2003 to give healthcare professionals assistance in helping individuals to stop smoking (Donaldson 1999).

CERVICAL CANCER

Cancer of the cervix is the fifth most common cancer in women in England and Wales. The national cervical screening programme has reduced the incidence of the most common form of cervical cancer, squamous cell carcinoma, but it cannot identify all cases. It is not designed to detect adenocarcinoma (Effective Health Care 1999). In 1994, there were still 1369 deaths from cancer of the cervix and 95% of these were in the over-35 age group. There is an interesting north/south English divide in cervical carcinoma mortality. The 20 district health authorities with the highest standardized mortality ratios for deaths with cancer of the cervix are all in the north of England. This may be linked with the risk factors for cervical cancer, or anomalies of health service provision over the UK. 5-year survival rates for cervical cancer are around 58% (Fig. 12.4).

Risk factors for cervical cancer

The cause of cervical cancer is not yet known. Risk factors include having first sexual intercourse at a young age (less than 20), having many sexual

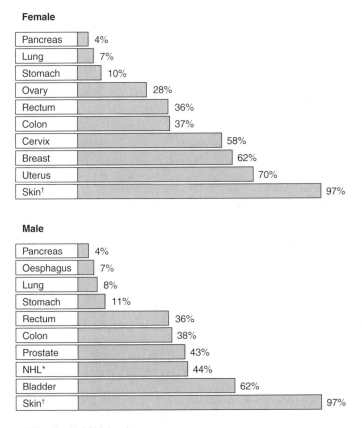

* NHL = Non-Hodgkin's lymphoma
† Excluding malignant melanoma

Figure 12.4 Survival: 5-year relative survival % in England and Wales 1981. (Reproduced with permission from CRC 1995 Scientific Yearbook.)

partners (or partners who have had multiple partners), being of lower social class, smoking, having STIs, and taking COC (Ch. 2). There is current interest in the role of the human papilloma virus (HPV) in the development of cervical cancer, especially types 16 and 18 which seem to be present in over 28% of invasive squamous carcinomas. In the future, it may be possible to select out the subgroup of women at higher risk of cervical cancer by detecting positive oncogenic HPV types and to offer them increased surveillance. Prophylactic vaccines against these viruses are an area of ongoing research. Smoking may separately enhance the carcinogenicity of certain viruses and COC may also be a weak co-factor.

Cervical intraepithelial neoplasia and carcinoma in situ

The majority of invasive cervical cancers are preceded by a neoplastic non-invasive process – cervical intraepithelial neoplasia (CIN) – which cannot be diagnosed by the naked eye but which may be detected by exfoliative cytology. Cervical cytology identifies cellular abnormalities but cannot diagnose the severity of the histological changes.

Three stages of CIN are recognized (Fig. 12.5):

1. CIN 1 – equivalent to mild dysplasia.
2. CIN 2 – equivalent to moderate dysplasia.
3. CIN 3 – equivalent to severe dysplasia and carcinoma in situ.

Reversion to normal can occur in CIN 1, especially in women under 30 years of age. Reversal to normal in cases of CIN 2 and CIN 3 is uncommon. In 1989, 17 818 women in England and Wales had carcinoma in situ and 85% of these were under 45 years old.

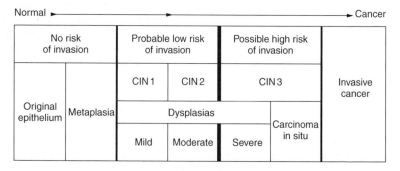

Figure 12.5   Three stages of cervical intraepithelial neoplasia (CIN).

Prevention of invasive cervical cancer

Since CIN is virtually 100% curable, cervical screening by cytological testing must rank as one of the most important screening procedures available to women. In countries with effective cervical screening programmes, the registration rates for cervical cancer are falling.

National screening programme

Screening for cervical cancer has been in place in the UK since 1967. It is currently under the control of a UK National Co-ordinator who administers both the breast and cervical screening programmes. At present, the programme offers screening to all women from the ages of 20 to 60 years who have been sexually active and who still have a cervix. Nationally, the screening interval recommended is 5 years although evidence shows a 10% decrease in incidence of carcinoma of the cervix if the screening interval is reduced to 3 years, which is why in many regions a 3-yearly recall system is in operation.

The general public's confidence in the National Screening Programme has been affected by a series of well-publicized 'scandals' in the UK national press, where errors occurred in reading smears or abnormal results were overlooked. Each woman needs to have the test explained, and arrangements made for how they will be informed of the result. It is the responsibility of the person taking the smear to instigate further investigation and follow-up, or check that it is happening. A computerized call and recall system is in place in most regions. However, the programme can only work well if it is given accurate information. Unhappily, human beings are not overly cooperative in such a scheme. Women move house not infrequently, and the majority change their name at least once, if not twice, during their lives. Inevitably some women will escape the call/recall net.

Opportunistic screening should be offered to women who have never had a smear or have not had a smear within the past 3 to 5 years. There are still a significant number of deaths in women over 65 years from cervical cancer and this has led to the argument that the smear-screening programme should be extended to woman up to the age of 69 years (Law 1999). Others argue that a woman who has had normal smears all her life, and no new sexual partner, need not have smears after the age of 55 years, as her likelihood of developing cervical cancer in these circumstances is extremely low. Although abnormal smears are uncommon under the age of 20, they have been reported in girls as young as 16. Individual girls should have cervical screening performed at a young age at the discretion of their healthcare adviser if their sexual history is suggestive of increased risk.

Taking a cervical smear

This requires adequate training. Nurses are often properly trained but doctors may only have been given minimal instruction when at medical school. There are now post-qualification and refresher courses in cervical smear training which are available every 3 years for health professionals. Many women feel anxious about having a cervical smear, particularly the indignity and discomfort of the procedure, as well as concern about the outcome.

The room for taking a cervical smear needs to have a strong and comfortable couch, with adequate lighting and be at a warm, pleasant temperature. There needs to be a supply of clean, sterilized specula of varying sizes to cope with different women, spatulas and cytobrushes, slides, fixative, non-leaking slide transportation boxes and a sharp pencil.

The commonest error in taking a smear is failing to take an adequate sample from the squamocolumnar junction, the area where neoplastic change occurs. In nulliparae, and in women past the menopause, the squamocolumnar junction may be well within the cervical canal and it is not always possible to sample this area.

Technique

The technique used is as follows:

1. Place the patient in the dorsal or left lateral position.
2. With good illumination, insert the speculum, lubricated only with water, and expose the cervix.
3. If the presence of an invasive carcinoma is suspected on clinical examination, refer the woman for urgent gynaecological assessment irrespective of the smear result.
4. Insert a wooden or plastic spatula into the cervical os and rotate through 360°(Fig. 12.6).
5. Spread the scrapings from the spatula thinly and evenly onto an indelibly-named glass slide (using a pencil not a ball-point pen).

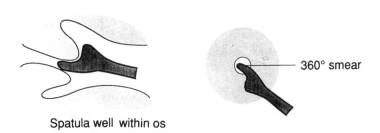

Spatula well within os

360° smear

6. Fix immediately with a spray or by immersing the slide for 10 to 15 minutes in equal parts of absolute alcohol and ether.
7. A pelvic examination may be performed if a doctor is undertaking the examination and it is clinically indicated although nurses are usually not trained to undertake this.
8. Complete all sections of the request form, which must accompany each smear to the laboratory.
9. Discuss when the woman may expect the result, and make arrangements for how she will receive it.
10. Explain what the result will mean and be available to discuss the implications of an abnormal result with the woman concerned.

Choice of spatula

The Aylesbury spatula is still the most popular as it seems as reliable as the rest and is the cheapest (Fig. 12.7). Endocervical brushes are very efficient at sampling the endocervical canal. They are not necessarily better than cervical spatulas at sampling the squamocolumnar junction so should not replace the spatula but be used in conjunction with it.

Indications for the use of an endocervical brush sampler:

1. No endocervical cells on a previous smear.
2. Previous cone biopsy.
3. A patient with symptoms whose cervix looks normal.
4. Requested by the cytolaboratory.

Management of abnormal smears

1. CIN 2 and CIN 3 should be treated once diagnosed.
2. CIN 1 may be treated or kept under close surveillance.

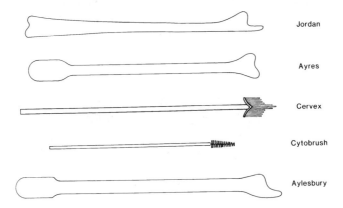

Figure 12.7
Types of sampling spatula.

Jordan

Ayres

Cervex

Cytobrush

Aylesbury

3. A woman should be referred for colposcopy the first time that she has a moderately or severely dyskaryotic smear.
4. A smear showing borderline nuclear or mildly dyskaryotic change should be repeated 6 months later and consideration given to colposcopic referral if it is not then normal.
5. There should be a minimum of two consecutive negative smears at least 6 months apart following a borderline or mildly dyskaryotic smear before surveillance is reduced to the frequency of a woman with no previous abnormality, preferably 3-yearly.
(See Duncan 1992 for further details.)

Doctors should be clear about the facilities for investigation and treatment available locally. Colposcopic examination and treatment services are widely available in the UK and the traditional cone biopsy will be avoided in the vast majority of women with abnormal smears. Local ablative treatments include cold coagulation, laser vaporization and excision by loop diathermy. Cone biopsy may still be necessary for a few women in whom the abnormal epithelium extends up the cervical canal and where its upper edge cannot be delineated.

CARCINOMA OF THE OVARY

Carcinoma of the ovary is the fourth commonest female cancer. It is uncommon in young women but often is undetected until presenting at a late stage of the disease with poor survival rates.

Ovarian cancer screening

A review of screening found that ovarian cancer can be detected in asymptomatic women, but there is as yet no evidence that this enhances survival (Bell 1998). It would be logical to assume that screening would be more appropriate for women at higher risk, but at present there is no clear evidence to support this. Women with one affected first-degree relative have a two to three times greater risk of ovarian cancer than the general population. When more than one relative is affected, the relative risk goes up to 11. About 14% of these women will develop ovarian cancer. The main genetic marker is BRCA1 mutation and is present in 5% of women with ovarian cancers diagnosed before the age of 70 years (Strutten et al 1997).

If a mass is detected on pelvic examination, the woman should be referred for a gynaecological opinion. It is usually possible to distinguish most benign cysts from malignant tumours by combining ultrasound examination with a CA125 serum level. If the woman has a strong family history of ovarian cancer, she should be referred for advice to an ovarian cancer screening clinic, if available locally. There are some prospective trials in progress at present, screening high-risk women in the UK.

Routine pelvic examination

Performing bimanual pelvic examination on asymptomatic low-risk women to 'check' for ovarian cancer is not helpful.

OTHER SCREENING PROCEDURES

Blood pressure

Blood pressure should be recorded as a baseline investigation in all women when attending for the first time in a family planning consultation. It is the single most important examination procedure in women using COC and should be checked regularly (p. **38**, pp **59–60**).

Pre-pregnancy screening

Many women attending a family planning consultation are considering stopping contraception to have a planned pregnancy. Pre-pregnancy health advice for women such as stopping smoking, getting fit, taking adequate levels of folic acid and screening for rubella should be readily available and there are many excellent books and leaflets on this (e.g. *Emma's Diary* from the Royal College of General Practitioners).

Rubella screening

A national mumps, measles and rubella vaccination programme is established in the UK for all babies and young children and has now replaced the immunization programme in teenage schoolgirls. A past history of infection or vaccination does not exclude the need for determining the current immune status and testing should be offered to women in a family planning consultation before they embark on a pregnancy. The accepted information is that women should not conceive within a month of vaccination although there is no evidence of teratogenicity with the vaccine.

Tests that do not need to be done routinely

There is no good evidence that routine weighing, urine testing or blood tests have any value in screening asymptomatic fit and healthy women.

REFERENCES

Austoker J, McPherson A, Clarke J, Lucassen A 1997 Breast problems. In: McPherson A, Waller Women's health, 4th edn. Oxford University Press, Oxford, p. 71–127
Bell R, Pettigrew M, Shotton T 1998 The performance of screening tests for ovarian cancer: results of a systematic review. British Journal of Obstetrics and Gynaecology 105: 1136

Davis SK, Ahn DK, Fortmann SP, Farquhar JW 1998 Determinants of cholesterol screening and treatment patterns. Insights for decision-makers. American Journal of Preventive Medicine 15(3): 178–186

Day NE 1991 Screening for breast cancer. British Medical Bulletin 47: 500–515

Department of Health 1998 Clinical examination of the breast. Calman K, Moores Y PL/CMO/98/1

Donaldson L 1999 Helping smokers stop. CMO Update 23. Department of Health p 5

Duncan ID (ed) 1992 National co-ordinating network NHS screening programme guidelines for clinical practice and programme management. National Co-ordinating Network, Oxford

Effective Health Care 1999 Management of gynaecological cancers 5(3) June: 5–8. Edited by The University of York and NHS Centre for Reviews and Dissemination. Royal Society of Medicine, London

Elhassani SB 1999 Domestic violence: An old and rapidly growing problem with few new solutions. Public Health Medicine 1: 12–17

Larkin GL, Hyman KB, Mathias SR, D'Amico F, MacLeod BA 1999 Screening for intimate partner violence in the emergency department: Annals of Emergency Medicine 33(6): 669–675

Larsson G, Blohm F, Sundell G, Andersch B, Milsom I 1997 A longitudinal study of birth control and pregnancy outcome among women in a Swedish population. Contraception 56: 6–16

Law M 1999 Upper age limits should be raised for cancer screening. Journal of Medical Screening 6: 16–20

McIlwaine G 1993 Satisfaction with NHS breast screening programme: Women's views. In: Austoker J, Patnick J (eds) Breast screening acceptability: research and practice. NHS BSP Publications, Sheffield, p 14–16

McNutt LA, Carlson BE, Gagen D, Winterbauer N 1999 Reproductive violence screening in primary care: perspectives and experience of patients and battered women. Journal of the American Medical Womens Association 54(2): 85–90

McPherson A, Waller D 1997 BBC Woman's Hour survey. Women's health and its controversies – an overview. In: McPherson A, Waller D (eds) Women's health, 4th edn. Oxford University Press Oxford, 1–21

Mant D 1992 Should all women be advised to practice regular breast self-examination. The Breast 1: 108

Peto R, Lopez AD, Boreman J et al 1994 Mortality from smoking in developed countries 1950–2000. ICRF and WHO. Oxford University Press, Oxford

Strutten JF, Gather SA, Russell P et al 1997 Contribution of all BRCA1 mutation to ovarian cancer. New England Journal of Medicine 338: 1125–1130

13

Sexually transmitted infections

Alexander McMillan

Prevalence   281
Genitourinary medicine
  clinics   281
Examination of the female
  patient   282
Bacterial infections   282
  Gonorrhoea   282
  Syphilis   287
  Non-specific genital
    tract and chlamydial
    infections   288
  Bacterial vaginosis   290
Protozoal infestation   292
  Trichomoniasis   292

Fungal infection   293
  Candidiasis   293
Viral infections   295
  Herpes simplex virus   295
  Human papilloma virus   298
  Human immunodeficiency virus   300
  Hepatitis B virus   307
  Hepatitis C virus   307
  Molluscum contagiosum virus   308
  Cytomegalovirus   308
Arthropod infestations   308
  Phthiriasis   308
  Scabies   308
Appendix   311

Doctors who provide contraceptive services deal with a young sexually active population, some of whom may be at risk of sexually transmitted infections (STIs). The family planning consultation may be the first opportunity for a young person to confide that he or she has acquired an STI. Many infections are symptomless but signs may be noted during routine examination.

Prevalence

The prevalence of sexually transmitted infections varies geographically, but Figure 13.1 illustrates the trends in their prevalence in the UK over the past 17 years. Gonorrhoea has declined since the early 1970s, while viral infections, particularly with human papilloma virus (HPV), and *Chlamydia* have become increasingly common. Bacterial vaginosis, a cause of vaginal discharge, is being recognized with increasing frequency although the incidence of trichomoniasis has fallen over the past 20 years.

GENITOURINARY MEDICINE CLINICS

Ideally, anyone in whom a sexually transmitted infections is suspected should be referred to a genitourinary medicine (GUM) clinic. In the UK, the Venereal Diseases Regulations (1916) allowed for the establishment of clinics for the diagnosis and treatment in confidence of STIs. Today, these clinics provide facilities for the collection of the most appropriate

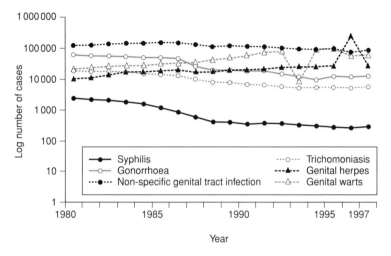

Figure 13.1 Numbers of cases of sexually transmitted infections in the UK 1980–1997, excluding HIV infection.

samples for microbiological examination. Trained counsellors who can assist with contact tracing are immediately available. As most departments are within hospitals, there is ease of access to additional diagnostic services. Referral to a GUM clinic is not always possible and therefore the family planning doctor or general practitioner may need to undertake appropriate investigations.

EXAMINATION OF THE FEMALE PATIENT

Appendix 13.1 outlines the examination for suspected STI. This schedule can of course be individually modified as required. The investigation of women with vaginal discharge is outlined in Figure 13.2. Co-existing infections are common and every effort should be made to exclude other infections when one is discovered.

BACTERIAL INFECTIONS

Gonorrhoea

Gonorrhoea is caused by *Neisseria gonorrhoeae*, small kidney-shaped Gram-negative cocci arranged in pairs. In adults, it is almost always sexually acquired. Although gonococcal vulvovaginitis may result from accidental contamination, in children the infection may indicate sexual abuse.

Although the prevalence of strains of *N. gonorrhoeae* that are relatively insensitive to antibiotics has been increasing for several decades, it was the discovery in 1976 of β-lactamase-(penicillinase) producing *N. gonorrhoeae* (PPNG) that caused concern. These organisms are endemic in South-East Asia and in West Africa but account for only a small proportion of strains in developed countries. In the UK, the prevalence of infection associated with PPNG has declined in the past few years.

Clinical features

In men

1. Most patients with urethral gonorrhoea develop symptoms 2 to 10 days after sexual intercourse with an infected partner. There is usually dysuria and a profuse mucopurulent urethral discharge but less severe urethritis is not uncommon. Up to 5% of men with urethral infections are symptomless (and hence represent a reservoir of infection).
2. Pharyngeal gonorrhoea, resulting from orogenital sexual contact, is mostly symptomless, but occasionally the patient complains of a sore throat.
3. Rectal infection, almost invariably acquired through homosexual anal intercourse, is often symptomless but there may be features of proctitis (anal discharge, pain, bleeding, tenesmus).
4. Epididymo-orchitis occurs as a complication in about 5% of men who have untreated urethral gonorrhoea.

Other complications, such as periurethral, prostatic and seminal vesicle abscesses and disseminated gonococcal infections are rare.

In women

1. Most women (about 80%) with uncomplicated gonorrhoea are symptomless. Some, however, complain of increased vaginal discharge and dysuria.
2. In the absence of concurrent infections, the only abnormal clinical finding may be a mucopurulent exudate from the cervical os.
3. Infection of the paraurethral glands may be manifest as mucopurulent exudate on gentle massage of the distal urethra through the vagina.
4. Pelvic inflammatory disease (PID) occurs as a complication in about 15% of women with untreated gonorrhoea, and its presentation may be acute, subacute or chronic.
5. Bartholinitis with abscess formation may develop in 10% of infected individuals, and, less commonly, disseminated gonococcal infection (presenting as a febrile illness with polyarthralgia and vasculitic skin lesions or as a septic arthritis) may result.

As in the male, pharyngeal and rectal gonorrhoea are usually symptomless.

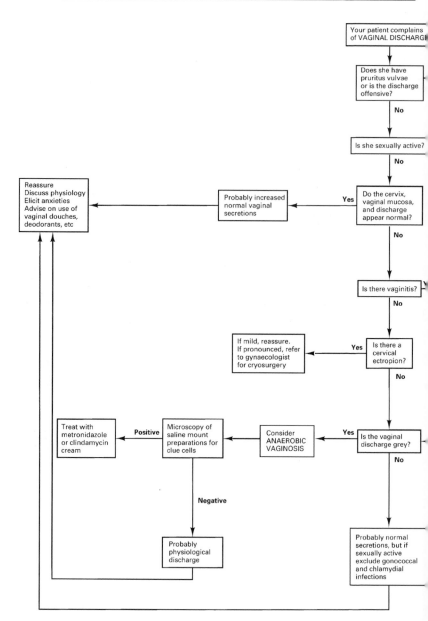

Figure 13.2 Investigation of vaginal discharge. (Reproduced with permission

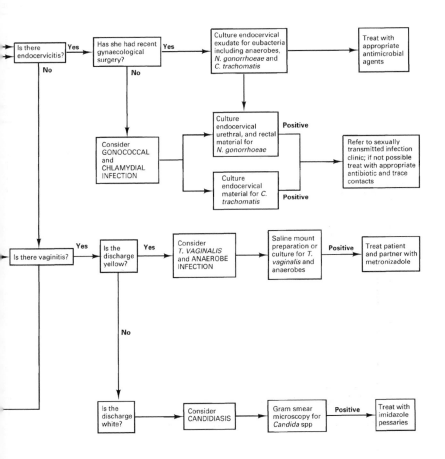

Millan A 1986 Vaginal discharge. British Medical Journal 293: 1357–1360.)

In prepubertal girls. The parents usually notice a discharge on the girl's underclothes, and on examination there is redness and swelling of the vulva and a purulent vaginal discharge. Other causes of vulvovaginitis include foreign bodies in the vagina (also threadworms), faulty hygiene or urinary infection.

Diagnosis

In men. For men with suspected urethral gonorrhoea, a smear of exudate is prepared on a microscope slide, using a plastic, disposable inoculating loop (Nunc Products, Denmark), fixed by passing gently over a spirit lamp flame and sent to the laboratory. Material, collected on an applicator stick tipped with cotton wool, should also be sent in the appropriate transport medium for culture (Appendix 13.1). For the diagnosis of rectal and pharyngeal gonorrhoea, culture of the appropriate material is essential.

In women (and young girls). Material for culture from women should be obtained from all possibly infected sites (endocervical canal, urethra, rectum, oropharynx and vagina in prepubertal girls). As a single set of cultures may fail to identify about 7% of infected women, culture-taking should be repeated once, about 1 week later.

Note. A high vaginal swab frequently yields negative results and is unreliable for the diagnosis of gonorrhoea. When facilities are limited, however, an endocervical swab at least should be taken. As gonococci may not survive in the transport medium, it is sometimes helpful to send appropriately fixed smears to the laboratory. Serological tests for gonococcal antibodies are useless for routine diagnosis.

Treatment

Although the choice of antimicrobial agent should depend on the sensitivity pattern of the gonococcal isolate, treatment often has to be commenced before this is known. A suitable drug can be selected easily with knowledge of the drug sensitivities of the strains in the community. In the UK, national guidelines have been developed for the treatment of gonorrhoea (Fitzgerald and Bedford 1996).

In geographical areas where PPNG strains are uncommon, the penicillins remain the drugs of first choice, but other antimicrobial agents may be used (Table 13.1). Where PPNG strains are more prevalent, β-lactamase stable antimicrobial agents must be used as first-line treatments. In the UK, such drugs should also be used in the treatment of individuals who have acquired their infection in areas where PPNG are common. To guarantee patient compliance, single-dose treatment should be given whenever possible. Pharyngeal gonorrhoea is much more difficult to treat with standard

Table 13.1   Some schedules for the treatment of uncomplicated gonorrhoea in adults

Antimicrobial agent	Dosage	Comments
Penicillins		
Amoxycillin	3 g stat orally*	
Ampicillin	2–3.5 g stat orally*	
Cephalosporins		
Ceftriaxone†	250 mg stat by i.m. injection	Hypersensitivity in penicillin-hypersensitive
Cefotaxime†	500 mg stat by i.m. injection	patients
Fluoroquinolones		
Ciprofloxacin†	250–500 mg stat orally	Avoid in pregnancy
Ofloxacin	400 mg stat orally	Avoid in pregnancy
Other		
Spectinomycin†	2 g stat by i.m. injection	

i.m., intramuscular.
* Use with 1 g of probenecid given orally.
† Useful in infections caused by β-lactamase-producing *N. gonorrhoeae*, but in some geographical areas, there is increasing prevalence of strains resistant to ciprofloxacin and spetcinomycin.

regimens; ceftriaxone (a single intramuscular dose of 250 mg), or ciprofloxacin (a single oral dose of 500 mg) may be effective.

As some 40% of patients with gonorrhoea have a concurrent chlamydial infection, many clinicians give simultaneous treatment for this (see below).

In patients with symptomless urethral infection, pharyngeal and rectal gonorrhoea, cultures should be repeated twice after treatment.

In all cases, contact tracing must be undertaken.

The possibility of sexual abuse must be considered in prepubertal children with gonorrhoea and the appropriate action taken to ensure the safety and future well-being of the child.

Syphilis

Syphilis, caused by *Treponema pallidum* ssp. *pallidum*, is uncommon in the UK (Fig. 13.1), but its incidence has increased in the countries of the former Soviet Union. It is most frequently acquired by sexual intercourse with an infected partner, but congenital infection also occurs. Serological screening for treponemal antibodies of all pregnant women has reduced the prevalence of congenital syphilis in developed countries. For a detailed description of the clinical features and diagnosis of syphilis, a standard textbook of sexually transmitted infections should be consulted.

Non-specific genital tract infection and chlamydial infections

The prevalence of non-specific (NSU) or non-gonococcal (NGU) urethritis has increased over the past 15 years. Although chlamydiae can be detected in the urethras of more than 55% of these men, the aetiology in other cases is uncertain. Anaerobes and mycoplasmas, including *Mycoplasma genitalium* and *Ureaplasma urealyticum*, may play some role.

Amongst adults, the oculogenital *Chlamydia trachomatis* is sexually transmitted, e.g. the organism can be detected in the cervices of about 80% of the sexual partners of men with chlamydial urethritis. Adult chlamydial ophthalmia is usually the result of autoinoculation of infected material from the genital tract.

Clinical features of chlamydial infection

In men

1. After an incubation period of about 3 weeks, men develop a mucoid or mucopurulent urethral discharge and dysuria of variable severity. At least 25% of infected men, however, are symptomless.
2. Proctitis may result from chlamydiae acquired through anal intercourse.
3. Epididymitis is the most common complication of untreated chlamydial infection.

In women

1. Most women with a chlamydial cervical infection are symptomless but some complain of increased vaginal discharge, and dysuria is an occasional feature.
2. There may be no specific signs. The cervix may appear normal or there may be an endocervicitis with mucopus exuding from the os.
3. PID may occur as a complication in up to 20% of women with an untreated chlamydial infection of the cervix with subsequent infertility and an increased risk of ectopic pregnancy. In general, the clinical features are less pronounced than those of gonococcal infection. The pelvic pain tends to be of lower intensity and fever is less frequent. Mild adnexal tenderness is usual.
4. Occasionally, perihepatitis is a complication: there is an acute onset of pain in the right hypochondrium, the pain being exacerbated by deep inspiration, nausea, anorexia and low-grade pyrexia. There is tenderness over the liver and a friction rub may be heard.

Chlamydiae probably play a part in the aetiology of reactive arthritis (including Reiter's disease) in both men and women.

Diagnosis

Until recently, the diagnosis of chlamydial infection depended on the detection of chlamydial antigen or on the isolation of the organism in tissue culture. The detection of specific DNA in genital secretions is now possible, and, as the sensitivity of tests such as the ligase chain reaction for chlamydial DNA greatly exceeds that of antigen detection, it is likely that such tests will eventually replace the current immunological methods. An additional advantage of the nucleic acid detection methods is their ability to detect DNA in urine of infected men and women, with sensitivities and specificities almost comparable to those using genital specimens. The local microbiology laboratory will advise on the system to be used.

1. For the detection of chlamydial antigen or DNA, cellular material should be obtained by inserting the cotton wool applicator stick supplied with the appropriate manufactuer's kit into the endocervical canal and rotating gently. As there is a risk of cross-contamination, particular care should be exercised in taking material for DNA tests.
2. When DNA detection methods are available, a first-voided specimen of urine, collected in a sterile universal container, may replace the endocervical specimen (in most women with chlamydial infection of the uterine cervix, there is concurrent urethral infection).
3. When material has been taken from the endocervical canal, there is little advantage in obtaining additional specimens from the urethras of women even when they complain of dysuria.
4. Where DNA detection methods are available, the examination of a first-voided specimen of urine is used for the diagnosis of infection in men. Elsewhere, it is necessary to use the cotton wool-tipped wire swab supplied with the kit by inserting it into the urethra to a distance of about 2–3 cm from the meatus.
5. As it is still necessary to obtain genital tract material for chlamydial culture for medicolegal purposes (such as in a rape case), such cases should be referred to a GUM clinic.

Treatment

Tetracyclines and the macrolides are equally effective in the treatment of adult chlamydial infections. In the UK, guidelines have been developed for the treatment of genital chlamydial infection (Central Audit Group in Genitourinary Medicine 1998).

Uncomplicated genital chlamydia infection can be treated with the following agents:

1. Doxycycline 100 mg twice per day for 7 days.
2. Azithromycin 1 g stat.
3. Ofloxacin 200 mg twice per day for 7 days.

4. Minocycline 100 mg once per day for 9 days.
5. Lymecycline 300 mg once per day for 10 days.

These drugs are also useful for the treatment of non-gonococcal, non-chlamydial urethritis, but about 30% of individuals have recurrence. Similar drug regimens are used in the treatment of women who are the known sexual partners of men with NGU. There is epidemiological evidence that the recurrence rate of non-chlamydial NGU is higher after resumption of sexual intercourse with a partner who has not been treated with antimicrobial agents.

When there is the possibility of early pregnancy, all tetracyclines are contraindicated and the following are recommended:

1. Erythromycin stearate 500 mg four times per day by mouth for 7 days.
2. Amoxycillin 500 mg three times per day for 7 days may also be used.

For the treatment of chlamydial PID, the following are recommended:

1. Doxycycline 100 mg twice per day for a minimum of 10 days plus metranidazole 200 mg three times per day for the first 7 days.
2. Ofloxacin 400 mg twice per day.
3. Clindamycin 450 mg four times per day as an alternative to metronidazole.

Tests of cure are not required for patients treated with the tetracyclines, treatment efficacy being > 95%. Consideration of a test of cure some 3 weeks after therapy should be considered in those treated with other regimens, but it should be noted that chlamydial antigen and DNA might still be detectable for up to 3 weeks after successful treatment. Cure is less certain with erythromycin or amoxycillin, given in the dosages noted above, and a test of cure should always be undertaken.

Partner notification is essential in all cases.

Bacterial vaginosis

This condition is being recognized with increasing frequency as a cause of increased vaginal discharge and results from the replacement of the normal lactobacilli with mixed organisms, including anaerobes, *Gardnerella vaginalis* and *Mycoplasma hominis*. In contrast to trichomoniasis and candidiasis, the vagina is not inflamed. The pathogenesis of bacterial vaginosis is uncertain and there is no clear evidence that it is a sexually transmitted infection.

Bacterial vaginosis may be associated with pelvic infection post-termination, and post operative wound infection, and there is increasing evidence that, in pregnant women, the condition may be associated with late miscarriage, premature rupture of the membranes, premature delivery, low birth weight, and postpartum infection.

Clinical features

1. Increased vaginal discharge, greyish-white in colour with a fishy odour, particularly after intercourse.
2. Pruritus vulvae is not a feature unless there is concurrent infection, e.g. with *Candida* spp.
3. Vaginitis is not a feature.

Diagnosis

Diagnosis is clinical, supplemented by a few simple microbiological tests.

1. A greyish discharge may be noted at the introitus, and on speculum examination the walls of the vagina may be coated with a discharge that is sometimes frothy.
2. The pH of the vaginal discharge is measured using narrow-range (pH 4–6) pH paper (Whatman) held in a pair of forceps, and avoiding the alkaline cervical secretions. The pH of vaginal secretions is normally less than 4.5 but in bacterial vaginosis it is greater than 5. However, the pH of vaginal fluid can be greater than 5 in women who do not have the condition.
3. A loopful of discharge is suspended in a drop of isotonic saline (8.6 g NaCl/L) on a microscope slide, covered, and examined microscopically using a × 40 objective. Polymorphonuclear leucocytes are few but 'clue cells' – epithelial cells that appear granular because of adherent bacteria – are usually obvious. The exceedingly mobile curved rods of *Mobiluncus* spp. may also be noted.
4. Although the 'sniff test' (performed by mixing some vaginal secretions with a drop of potassium hydroxide, 25% w/v, on a slide and immediately sniffing to detect the characteristic ammoniacal odour of volatile amines) is said to be a sensitive and specific test for bacterial vaginosis, it is subjective and requires some degree of practice.

Culture of vaginal discharge for *G. vaginalis* and anaerobes is not helpful diagnostically.

Treatment

Oral metronidazole (either 400 mg twice daily for 5 days or as a single dose of 2 g), or clindamycin cream 2% (a 5 g applicatorful inserted vaginally every night for 7 nights) are both effective. Recurrence, however, is common. There is no clear evidence that treatment of the sexual partner is indicated.

PROTOZOAL INFESTATION
Trichomoniasis

Trichomoniasis is caused by the protozoan flagellate *Trichomonas vaginalis* that colonizes but only rarely invades the mucosa of the lower urogenital tract. The organism is sexually transmitted. In recent years, the incidence of the disease has declined, perhaps because of the widespread use of metronidazole in a variety of conditions.

Clinical features

In women

1. A thin, yellow, offensive vaginal discharge, vulval soreness, dysuria and dyspareunia are the classic symptoms.
2. The vaginal wall is reddened and a frothy, yellow discharge pools in the posterior fornix; punctate red spots on the ectocervix ('strawberry cervix') may be noted. These features, however, are not always present and are not pathognomonic of trichomoniasis.
3. Up to 25% of infected women are symptomless.

In men

1. Most men who are infected with *T. vaginalis* are symptomless, but a few present with an NGU.
2. Trichomoniasis can occasionally be identified in urethral material or urine from men who are known sexual contacts of women with trichomoniasis.

Diagnosis

1. In women, saline mount preparation of material from the posterior fornix is examined microscopically at a magnification of ×400. Urethral smears or a centrifuged deposit of urine from men can be examined similarly. The protozoa are recognized by their size (10–30 μm in length), oval shape, rapidly-moving anterior flagella, undulating membrane and their jerky movement.
2. Material in Stuart's or Amies' medium can be sent to the laboratory for culture, a method considered more sensitive than microscopy.
3. The rapid detection in secretions of trichomonal antigen by latex agglutination is also a possible diagnostic test.
4. Sometimes, trichomonads may be found in Papanicolaou-stained smears, but this method is not recommended for routine diagnosis.

Treatment

1. Metronidazole (a single oral dose of 2 g or 200 mg by mouth every 8 hours for 7 days) is usually curative.
2. The regular sexual partners of women with trichomoniasis should be treated similarly, even when the protozoan cannot be detected in genital secretions.
3. Patients taking metronidazole should be advised to avoid alcohol (because of unpleasant side effects from their interaction) until treatment has been completed.

FUNGAL INFECTION

Candidiasis

Vulvovaginal candidiasis is caused by yeasts of the genus *Candida*, particularly *Candida albicans*. This yeast is saprophytic in humans, but certain conditions, including pregnancy, uncontrolled diabetes mellitus, use of broad-spectrum antimicrobial agents, use of immunosuppressive drugs, and HIV infection, favour its transition to a pathogen, and, these conditions should be considered when a woman presents with candidal vulvovaginitis. Candidal balanoposthitis may be the presenting feature of diabetes mellitus in men.

Clinical features

In women

1. Pruritus vulvae and burning of variable severity are the principal features; there may be associated superficial dyspareunia. However, these are non-specific symptoms and the diagnosis should be confirmed as below.
2. Erythema of the vulva that sometimes extends to the perineum, perianal region, genitocrural folds and the medial aspects of the thighs.
3. Oedema of the labia minora is common.
4. Vaginitis is less frequently found but there may be a curdy white vaginal discharge with white adherent plaques.
5. Primary cutaneous candidiasis affects the genitocrural folds and outer aspects of the labia majora. The lesions are initially papular with small satellite vesicles or pustules, but progress to superficial ulcers.

In men

1. Pain or itching of the penis and often a subpreputial discharge.
2. The prepuce may be oedematous and fissured, resulting in phimosis. Usually the glans is reddened with multiple maculopapules that may progress to superficial ulceration.

Diagnosis

Material from the posterior fornix of the vagina or from plaques can be examined microscopically for yeasts and mycelia after mounting in a drop of saline or potassium hydroxide solution (10% w/v); these structures may also be seen in Gram-stained smears. *Candida* spp. can be cultured, but the presence of yeasts does not imply that they are the cause of vulvo-vaginitis.

Treatment

1. The azoles are the treatment of choice for acute candidal vaginitis. Table 13.2 indicates the more commonly used preparations and their mode of administration. As there is little difference in efficacy between the available drugs, patient choice is important. If there is concurrent vulvitis, as there often is, clotrimazole, econazole or miconazole creams may also be used; nystatin cream can also be used but it stains underclothes. These antifungal creams and oral preparations are also useful for the treatment of candidal balanoposthitis.
2. Although persistence of symptoms may indicate infection with a *Candida* spp. that has reduced susceptibility to the azoles (e.g. *C. glabrata*), treatment failures are usually the result of misdiagnosis, and failure to respond should prompt re-assessment of the diagnosis.

Table 13.2 Treatment regimens for acute candidal vaginitis

Drug	Dose and route of administration	Comments
Polyenes		
Nystatin	100 000 unit pessaries; one or two inserted vaginally nightly for 14 nights	Can stain underwear; long course necessary
Imidazoles		
Clotrimazole	500 mg pessary inserted vaginally at night as single dose OR 200 mg pessary nightly for 3 nights OR 100 mg pessary nightly for 6 nights	
Econazole	150 mg pessary (Ecostatin 1 or Gyno-Pevaryl 1) inserted vaginally at night as single dose OR 150 mg pessary inserted nightly for 3 nights	
Miconazole	5 g intravaginal cream inserted vaginally once daily for 10 days OR 100 mg pessary inserted vaginally twice daily for 7 days OR 1.2 g vaginal capsule inserted vaginally once at night	
Triazoles		
Fluconazole	150 mg as single oral dose	Avoid in pregnancy
Itraconazole	200 mg twice daily for 1 day	Avoid in pregnancy

3. Symptomless candidiasis found, e.g., on a routine cervical smear does not require treatment.

Recurrent candidiasis. In women with proven recurrent candidiasis, antifungal therapy should be given until the patient is symptomless, and culture for *Candida* spp. is negative. Thereafter, the woman should be given suppressive therapy with either fluconazole 150 mg orally every month, or with a 500 mg clotrimazole pessary inserted vaginally every week. The duration of such suppressive treatment needs to be tailored to the individual patient, but these regimens usually require to be continued for at least 6 months. There is no evidence that treatment of the sexual partner reduces the frequency of recurrent candidiasis.

VIRAL INFECTIONS

Herpes simplex virus

The incidence of genital herpes simplex virus (HSV) infection has been increasing over the past 20 years. In most areas of the UK, HSV 2 has been the principal type that affects the genitalia. However, HSV 1 is the infecting type in about 50% of men and women with primary genital herpes. In most cases, this type of virus has been acquired from oro–genital contact. In developed countries, the prevalence of antibodies against HSV 1 in adolescents has been declining, and it has been suggested that the increasing incidence of genital herpes may reflect lack of protection against HSV 2 if there has been no prior exposure to type 1 virus.

Symptomless infections are common. More than 80% of those whose sera contain antibodies against HSV 2 have no history of infection. Transmission can occur when a symptomless individual excretes the virus in genital secretions.

After replicating in the skin or mucous membranes, the virus is transported via the axon to the neurones in the sacral ganglia. Further replication occurs and the virus then spreads via the sensory nerves to the skin or mucous surface, where clinical signs of infection may develop. After resolution of the primary disease, the virus becomes latent or hidden in the ganglia. Reactivation by unknown mechanisms is followed by transport of viral genomes to the skin surface where replication can occur. This occurrence may or may not be associated with the development of clinical signs.

Natural history

The long-term natural history of genital herpes is uncertain.

1. Within 1 year about 55% of individuals who have had symptomatic primary herpes associated with HSV 1 and 90% who have had primary HSV 2 infection will develop a recurrence.

2. In general, there is less frequent recurrence and a longer interval between the primary episode and recurrence in patients who have had HSV 1 infection compared with those who have had HSV 2.

Recent evidence suggests that in some patients, the frequency of recurrences declines over time.

Clinical features

Primary genital herpes develops after a variable latent period.

1. Systemic symptoms are common, particularly in women and include fever, headache, malaise and myalgia.
2. Pain, which can be severe, in the vulva or penis, dysuria and increased vaginal discharge.
3. Tender enlargement of the inguinal lymph nodes usually develops more than 1 week after the onset of the illness.
4. Lesions are initially papular but quickly become vesicular and ulcerate. They persist for up to 2 weeks until crusting.
5. In women, extensive ulceration of the labia majora, labia minora, adjacent skin, introitus, perineum, perianal region, vagina and cervix is found.
6. In men, ulceration of the coronal sulcus, glans penis, prepuce, shaft of the penis and perianal region may be noted; in the uncircumcised, phimosis with secondary bacterial infection may develop.
7. In both sexes, herpetic proctitis may be a feature.
8. New lesion formation is noted during the first 10 days. Sacral radiculitis, presenting as constipation, urinary retention and paraesthesiae in the distribution of the sacral nerve is an uncommon complication of primary HSV 2 infection.
9. Systemic features usually resolve within 7 to 10 days and genital lesions usually heal within about 21 days.
10. Clinical features in women tend to be more severe than those in men.
11. Clinical features of first-episode genital herpes in individuals who have been exposed previously to HSV appear to be less severe than those suffering a true primary genital infection.

Recurrent genital herpes. Clinical features in general tend to be less severe than those of primary disease.

1. Systemic symptoms are not a feature, but prodromal symptoms occur commonly and consist of a tingling sensation in the affected area or shooting pains in the distribution of the sciatic nerve.
2. Lesions are similar to those of the primary disease but are usually much less extensive and heal more quickly.

Diagnosis

It is good to make a definitive diagnosis so that proper counselling can be undertaken.

1. Material obtained by gently scraping the base of an ulcer using an applicator stick tipped with cotton wool should be sent in the appropriate transport medium (e.g. Hank's) for viral isolation in tissue culture.
2. The detection of HSV antigens by immunofluorescence or enzyme-linked immunoabsorbent assay (ELISA) may become a practical alternative to tissue culture in the non-pregnant woman.
3. Blood should be taken at the first clinical attendance, and again 10 to 14 days later, for serological studies, particularly using complement fixation test (CFT). Individuals with primary infection will develop antibodies in this interval.

The CFT cannot detect initial infection with HSV 2 in the presence of HSV 1 antibodies. Serological tests that are type specific have been developed but their place in clinical practice has yet to be defined.

Treatment

Primary or initial infections

1. Aciclovir (200 mg orally five times per day for 5 days), famciclovir (250 mg three times per day for 5 days), or valaciclovir (500 mg twice daily for 5 days) are the treatments of choice. Compared with placebo, the lesions heal more rapidly, pain is relieved more quickly, new lesion formation ceases, and systemic features resolve more speedily. Recurrences, however, are not abolished or reduced in frequency.
2. Patients should be warned about the possible risk of autoinoculation of other parts of the body, particularly the cornea, and about the need for strict hygiene.
3. Resumption of sexual intercourse should be delayed until the lesions have healed.

Recurrent disease. The use of the above antiviral agents is less certain. Although the clinical course of the disease is shortened somewhat, in general this is of marginal benefit to the patient. When given early, e.g. during the pro-dromal stage, they may reduce significantly the duration of the recurrence.

Suppressive treatment. Aciclovir (200 mg orally four times per day or 400 mg twice daily), or famciclovir (250 mg twice daily) reduces the frequency of recurrences and may be useful in the occasional patient with very fre-quent or disabling recurrences. When given for 1 year, the subsequent recurrence rate may be reduced.

Aciclovir has few side effects but its safety in pregnancy has not yet been established. Counselling plays an important part in the management of patients with genital herpes.

Genital herpes in pregnancy

Primary infection may be associated with spontaneous abortion, intrauterine growth retardation and preterm labour. Guidelines for the management of genital herpes in pregnancy are available (Smith et al 1998). Neonatal herpes infection may occur intra- or post-partum. Over one-half of infants born to mothers with primary HSV infection at term are likely to become infected and to develop overt disease with its high mortality rate. In these women, caesarean section reduces the risk of neonatal infection, and should also be considered if the woman presents with primary infection during the last 6 weeks of pregnancy. The risk to babies born vaginally to women who have recurrent HSV at term is low, but caesarean section should be undertaken if genital lesions are present at term. As 60% of women who deliver babies with HSV infection do not have any clinical features of the infection or a history of genital herpes, routine screening during pregnancy is not appropriate.

Human papilloma virus

Warts are caused by HPV of which there are over 70 types. Most hyperplastic genital warts (condylomata acuminata) are associated with types 6 and 11 but other types, including types 16, 18 and 31, are sometimes detected in tissues. The importance of the latter types is that DNA sequences that hybridize with HPV types 16 and 18 are identified frequently in biopsies from women with premalignant and malignant disease of the genital tract. Whether the association is causal remains uncertain as HPV DNA sequences homologous to those of HPV types 16 and 18 can be found in healthy tissues. The role of co-factors, such as cigarette smoking, in carcinogenesis, is also unclear. Vulval intraepithelial neoplasia (VIN) has also been associated with HPV infection, but progression to malignant disease appears to be uncommon in young women. Similarly, the significance of penile intraepithelial neoplasia found in male contacts of women with HPV infection and cervical intraepithelial neoplasia (CIN) is uncertain.

The virus is highly contagious through sexual contact, but the latent period is variable, being on average 3 months from exposure. Genital warts in prepubertal children should raise the possibility of sexual abuse.

Clinical features

1. The most common manifestation of genital HPV infection is the fleshy hyperplastic wart (condyloma acuminatum).

In women, these lesions are located at the introitus or at the labia majora and minora, perineum, perianal region, vagina, urethra and cervix.

In men, they are found most frequently in the coronal sulcus and frenum, but also on the prepuce, skin of the shaft of the penis, within the distal urethra, in the perianal region and on the scrotum.

Although condylomatous lesions of the cervix are noted in only about 6% of women with genital warts, cytological or colposcopic evidence of HPV infection is found in at least 25% of cases. There are often associated dysplastic-like changes of variable severity. Although spontaneous regression of the milder dysplastic changes has been described, the natural history of these lesions is uncertain.

2. At least 50% of women with VIN complain of pruritus vulvae, burning and pain. The lesions are single or multiple, macules or papules on the skin that may be white and lichenified; mucosal lesions are usually erythematous macules. Blanching is noted after the application of 5% acetic acid. Some lesions are pigmented. Biopsy is essential for diagnosis (Campion and Singer 1987).

3. Subclinical infection with HPV of the skin of the penis is now well documented.

Management

1. Every effort should be made to exclude a concurrent sexually transmitted infection (present in over 30% of patients) as treatment of this often facilitates the treatment of genital warts. In the absence of specific antiviral chemotherapy, treatment is largely symptomatic. Although the condylomata acuminata eventually undergo spontaneous regression, perhaps as a result of cell-mediated immunity, persistence for many months is common. As the lesions are psychologically disturbing and as they may become secondarily infected and bleed, some form of therapy is usually indicated.

2. At the first consultation, counselling about the infection and its protracted course should be undertaken. The sexual partner should be encouraged to attend for examination, counselling and treatment, if necessary.

3. The use of condoms to prevent the spread of infection should be encouraged.

4. Table 13.3 indicates some treatments that are available for condylomata acuminata. With every treatment, however, recurrence is common.

Cervical screening policy. Women who have had genital warts, or who are known sexual contacts of men with warts, must undergo regular cervical screening given the association between certain types of HPV and cervical

Table 13.3 Treatments available for condylomata acuminata

Treatment	Method of use	Comments
Antimitotic/antimetabolite		
Podophyllin resin	Suspension 20–25% w/v in ethanol or liquid paraffin applied topically once weekly. Protect surrounding surfaces with petroleum jelly. Wash off in 6 hours	Batch variation in potency. Avoid in pregnancy. Avoid use in vagina, on cervix, or in anal canal
Podophyllotoxin	0.5% solution or 0.15% cream applied twice daily for 3 days; further treatments at 7-day intervals	Generally more satisfactory than podophyllin. Avoid in pregnancy and above sites
Ablative methods		
Cryotherapy		If extensive, may need general anaesthesia
Electrocautery		
Laser ablation		
Scissor excision		
Trichloroethanoic acid	50% w/v applied carefully to surface of wart	May cause burns
Immunomodulatory agents		
Inosine pranobex	Given orally	Efficacy unproven
Interferons -α, -β, -γ	Given by subcutaneous injection or intralesionally	Efficacy unproven
Imiquimod	Applied topically	Place in therapy as yet uncertain

cancer. Local policies will usually dictate whether screening can be more frequent than the standard 3-yearly examination.

Human immunodeficiency virus

The human immunodeficiency viruses (HIV 1 and 2) selectively infect and destroy cells that bear the CD4 antigen – T4 (helper/inducer) lymphocytes and cells of the macrophage/monocyte system. After entry into the cell, the viral genomic RNA is transcribed into DNA by reverse transcriptase and some becomes circularized and integrated into the host cell genome. Throughout the course of HIV infection, there is constant replication of the virus, with progressive impairment of the immune system, as manifest by the decrease in CD4 cells in the peripheral blood. In addition, brain cells – microglia, astrocytes and possibly neurones – can be infected by HIV and, even in the absence of secondary infection, neuropsychiatric features may develop.

Epidemiology

HIV can be detected in blood, semen, cervicovaginal secretions, breast milk and saliva although there is little evidence that the last fluid is important in the transmission of infection. In developed countries, men who have had unprotected anal intercourse with an infected man constitute the group at greatest risk of HIV infection, but data show clearly the propensity for heterosexual spread. In central Africa, the majority of infected individuals, both men and women, have acquired the virus heterosexually. The presence of a concurrent sexually transmitted infection, particularly an ulcerative condition, such as genital herpes, facilitates infection with HIV.

As the duration of HIV increases, so does infectivity through sexual intercourse, whether homo- or heterosexual. Infection from artificial insemination with infected semen is rare.

Intravenous drug users who share contaminated syringes and needles are also at risk of HIV infection. Since the introduction of self-exclusion policies and screening of donated blood for anti-HIV, the risk of acquisition of the virus through blood transfusion in developed countries is now very low. Heat treatment of blood products such as Factors VIII and IX has reduced significantly the risk of infection to haemophiliacs.

Although there have been reports of probable infection of neonates by breast-feeding, most infants have acquired HIV from an infected mother before or during parturition. There is good evidence that infection can occur very early in pregnancy, but by no means every infected mother transmits the infection to the fetus. The risk of neonatal infection varies from 22% to 51% and it is likely that there is a direct relationship between duration of maternal infection and risk to the child. In women with symptomatic infection, pregnancy may influence adversely the outcome. Recent studies have suggested that treatment of the mother with zidovudine or nevirapine during pregnancy may reduce the risk of transmission to the fetus.

Clinical features

1. Many HIV-infected individuals are symptomless, the infection only being detected by serological testing.
2. Within a few weeks of infection, and before antibodies become detectable, some patients develop a mononucleosis-like illness with pyrexia, malaise, skin rash, sore throat, lymphadenopathy, diarrhoea, arthralgia and, sometimes, neurological features. These symptoms usually resolve within 3 weeks, but the lymphadenopathy may persist.
3. Persistent generalized lymphadenopathy is common, even in symptomless infected individuals. The lymph nodes are enlarged (> 1 cm in diameter) but discrete and usually not tender. The spleen may also be enlarged.
4. Dermatological abnormalities are common (and may occur in the absence of lymphadenopathy) and include seborrhoeic dermatitis of the face and scalp, facial warts, extensive tinea pedis and cruris, pityriasis

versicolor, multiple molluscum contagiosum, extensive folliculitis and purpura (resulting from thrombocytopenia).
5. Oral manifestations include candidiasis, hypertrophic gingivitis and oral hairy leukoplakia.
6. The development of herpes zoster, persistent weight loss and diarrhoea are associated with a deteriorating immune system.
7. The secondary neoplasms and infectious diseases that constitute the acquired immune deficiency syndrome (AIDS) are detailed in standard medical textbooks.
8. HIV infection may present as a dementing illness without evidence of other secondary infections.

Features of AIDS in children include failure to thrive, lymphadenopathy, disseminated candidiasis, *Pneumocystis carinii* pneumonia, disseminated mycobacterial infection, lymphocytic interstitial pneumonia and parotitis.

Course of infection

The natural history of HIV infection is still uncertain. Up to 50% of individuals who have been infected for 10 years have not developed serious infectious diseases or neoplasms. Within a few days of infection, there is a rapid increase in the number of copies of viral RNA that can be detected in the plasma. Within a few weeks, the viraemia is markedly reduced probably as the result of cellular immune responses, and a steady state is reached until the individual becomes symptomatic (Fig. 13.3). The plasma titre of

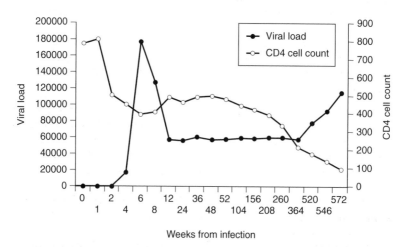

Figure 13.3 Plasma viral load and CD4 cell count in the peripheral blood of an untreated HIV-infected individual.

viral RNA (viral load) at this stage correlates well with disease progression, individuals with high viral loads developing symptomatic disease sooner than those with low viral loads. Shortly after infection, the CD4 cell count in the peripheral blood falls, but usually increases within the next 3 to 4 months to almost normal levels. There is then a progressive decline in the number of these cells. Serial estimations of the number of CD4 cells in the peripheral blood, and the viral load are essential in assessing prognosis and the need for treatment.

Diagnosis

In a family planning setting, it is generally the 'worried well' individual who seeks help and advice and, hopefully, reassurance. Careful, sympathetic, knowledgeable counselling, even before embarking on blood testing to establish the diagnosis, is essential. Pre-test counselling is time-consuming, and should be carried out with great sensitivity and should take into account:

1. The anxiety felt by individuals about themselves, particularly the possibility of having to face not only the stark reality of the diagnosis and ultimate prognosis but also the effect on their partner and their families.
2. Fear and embarrassment that secret hidden parts of their lives will be revealed.
3. Concern that their general practitioners will not keep them on their lists nor dentists be prepared to treat them.
4. Implications for future applications for mortgages, life insurance and even jobs.
5. Provision of up-to-date information about the disease, current tests and the relevance of false-negative results. Myths must be dispelled.
6. Advice on contraception, safer sex techniques and alteration of lifestyle as appropriate.

In most cases, the infection is detected by testing serum for antibodies against core antigens (e.g. by ELISA). There is, however, an incubation period before serum antibodies become detectable which may vary from a few weeks to 3 months, or, rarely, longer. In general, if blood obtained 3 and 6 months from exposure has yielded negative results, testing can be discontinued.

Where available, the detection of viral RNA by polymerase chain reaction has almost replaced testing for HIV p24 antigen in the diagnosis of the acute seroconversion illness.

A different type of virus (HIV 2) has been recognized in West Africa, but there is little evidence of its widespread distribution elsewhere.

As sera showing positive results in one test will always be checked by another system, a 'false-positive' report is most unlikely. Technical errors (e.g. a wrongly labelled blood tube) can and do occur, however, and it is good practice to obtain a second blood sample from a patient who has no clinical features of HIV infection before telling him or her the result.

Note. Blood is a source of contamination in a person who is HIV-positive. Gloves should be worn for venepuncture, and the thicker latex variety rather than the fine plastic gloves should be used for pelvic examination. As the virus is sensitive to chemical agents, sodium hypochlorite 2% can be used to decontaminate surfaces.

Management

Counselling. When an infected individual is identified, counselling is essential. Some issues that should be considered are indicated in Box 13.1.

The means of transmission of the virus should be explained and the appropriate steps taken to avoid the spread of infection to others. Partner notification should be considered so that the partner(s) can be counselled, tested if consent is obtained, and offered treatment if infected. Within a relationship, considerable anxiety is often encountered when one partner is seropositive for HIV and the other is apparently uninfected. Anal intercourse should be avoided, but if this is to occur, a more robust sheath, lubricated with a water-soluble lubricant, should be used.

In addition to the risk to the fetus, there has been some suggestion that pregnancy can affect adversely the course of the infection in women with late-stage disease. When pregnancy occurs in a seropositive individual, the risk should be explained to the patient in a sympathetic manner. Although termination should be discussed, taking into account the known predictors, it is the individual and her partner's decision whether to continue with

---

Box 13.1 Points to be considered in counselling* a symptomless HIV-infected individual

1. Means of transmission of the virus and the avoidance of spread of infection to others.
2. Lack of risk to others through social contact.
3. Natural history of infection and, with the advent of combination antiviral therapy, the better prognosis than previously.
4. Medical and dental. The individual should inform practitioners of his/her infection. Otherwise only trusted individuals should be informed. Attendance at self-help groups may be useful.
5. Regular attendance at a specialist clinic for counselling, and clinical assessment.

* Counselling is time-consuming and should be undertaken only by those familiar with HIV infection. Particularly in the months following diagnosis, frequent counselling sessions are often required. At each visit, the individual should be encouraged to discuss his/her feelings.

the pregnancy or not. If the pregnancy continues, the woman must receive optimal antenatal care including the offer of antiviral therapy (see below). Although in developed countries breast-feeding by seropositive women is not recommended, this advice may be different in countries where breast-milk may be the only safe source of infant nutrition.

Contraception. The knowledge that HIV is transmissible sexually has created the need for policies on contraceptive provision for affected individuals which not only prevent unwanted pregnancy but also protect the partners from infection. It must be remembered, however, that the most effective contraceptive is the one that they are prepared to use.

1. *Condoms* meeting BSI requirements should be recommended, either alone or in addition to other contraceptives, as protection against transmission of HIV and other STIs (p. **149**).
2. *Female barriers.* Diaphragms alone are not protective against HIV transmission but some benefit may accrue when they are used with spermicides containing nonoxynol-9. The female condom offers more protection.
3. *Spermicides.* Creams and pessaries containing nonoxynol-9 may provide an additional barrier to HIV infection, but the irritant effect of this agent in some individuals may be disadvantageous (p. **153**).
4. *Hormonal contraception.* The combined pill (COC) is known to depress the immune system but there is no evidence that it adversely affects the progression of HIV disease. Because of its effectiveness, it is particularly suitable, but women in high-risk groups should be encouraged to ask their partners to use a condom in addition.

   Progestogen-only contraception has less effect on immunity and liver function than COC. The progestogen-only pill (POP) and depot-medroxyprogesterone acetate are both appropriate methods for HIV-positive women but should be used with condoms.

   Liver function should be checked in all drug-users and ex-drug-users before hormonal contraception is prescribed.
5. *Intrauterine devices* are not recommended for HIV-positive women or for those at risk of infection. If such women already have an IUD in situ, they would be best advised to change to another effective method. The presence of an IUD increases the risk of PID in the HIV-positive woman who is already immunocompromised, and recurrent acute episodes might lead to more rapid disease progression. Insertion may cause transient inflammatory reaction with trauma to the endometrium, which may facilitate virus entry. IUDs increase the discharge of monocytes and lymphocytes into the vagina and are often associated with heavier, longer and irregular menstrual bleeding, all of which could increase the risk of transmission of the virus. It is not known if the hormone-releasing intrauterine system would offer less risk.

6. *Sterilization.* This is not contraindicated for either partner.
7. *Emergency contraception.* There is no contraindication to hormonal emergency contraception.

Initial assessment and follow-up

Table 13.4 outlines the assessment of a newly diagnosed HIV-infected individual. Individuals are generally assessed at 3-monthly intervals or more frequently immediately after initiation of therapy. At these consultations, it is important to discuss issues regarding lifestyle, general health, worries and fears, and to offer referral for appropriate counselling and psychological and social support.

A physical examination is undertaken and any new findings that may indicate progressive disease are sought.

Table 13.4 Assessment of a newly diagnosed symptomless HIV-infected individual

	Comments
1. Repeat anti-HIV test	Need to exclude technical error
2. History	Note sexual history, past history of sexual diseases, drug use, occupational risk, blood or blood product transfusion, residence abroad, BCG vaccination, menstrual cycle, obstetric history, social circumstances
3. Physical examination	Note particularly skin and mucosal abnormalities, lymphadenopathy, hepatic or splenic enlargement. Genital examination for warts or candidiasis
4. Haematological examination	May be anaemia, leucopaenia or thrombocytopaenia
5. Plasma enzyme tests of liver function	Often minor elevation of alanine aminotransferase
6. Immunological tests:	
a. CD4 cell count	Normally > 500/mm^3. Repeat in 1 month to establish baseline
b. serum immunoglobulins	Often elevated
c. β_2-microglobulin	Elevated in later stages of infection
7. Plasma HIV RNA estimation	Viral load correlates well with rate of progression of infection. Useful in determining need for therapy. Repeat at 1 month to establish baseline (note that intercurrent infection or vaccination can raise levels). Note high levels immediately after infection, falling within 3 months
8. Serological tests for:	
a. *Toxoplasma gondii*	In individuals with a CD4 cell count of <200/mm^3, consider prophylaxis
b. cytomegalovirus	Possible reactivation in late stage infection; avoid transfusion of CMV-positive blood to CMV-negative recipient
c. syphilis	Past infection
d. hepatitis B and C viruses	May cause chronic hepatitis/cirrhosis
9. Cervical cytology/colposcopy	Increased risk of HPV infection; annual screen
10. Chest X-ray	Baseline film

Blood is taken for:
1. Haematological tests – haemoglobin, white cell count, platelet count.
2. Clinical chemistry, particularly in those on antiviral treatment.
3. Immunological tests – CD4 cell count.
4. Plasma HIV viral RNA titres.

Treatment

A detailed discussion about HIV therapy is outwith the scope of this book. Combination therapy with at least three drugs is preferred practice and the British HIV Association issues guidelines on when to initiate treatment and on preferred drug regimens. The use of highly active antiretroviral therapy has been successful in prolonging life and increasing the individual's well-being, and the incidence of opportunistic infections and secondary neo-plasms has fallen in countries where the necessary drugs are available. A good response to treatment is shown by the rapid reduction in viral load and a progressive increase in the number of CD4 cells in the peripheral blood.

Giving a pregnant woman zidovudine orally during the last 6 weeks of her pregnancy, intravenously during parturition, and treating the neonate with oral zidovudine for 6 weeks, reduces significantly the risk of vertical transmission of the virus. Nevirapine may also be used to prevent neonatal infection. It has also been noted that elective caesarean section reduces the risks of transmission of HIV from mother to child, independently of the effects of treatment with zidovudine.

Hepatitis B virus

Although hepatitis B virus (HBV) infection is endemic in certain geographical areas (e.g. South-East Asia), in temperate climates most infections are acquired by the inoculation of infected blood (e.g. by sharing contaminated syringes and needles) or sexually, mostly through homosexual contact. Heterosexual transmission is also now considered important.

As the detection of e-antigen in serum is associated with active viral repli-cation, infected individuals who are e-antigenaemic are the most infectious and should be counselled about their infectivity to sexual contacts and, during parturition, to a child.

Hepatitis B vaccine is available and, at least in the short term, provides a high degree of protection against infection. The vaccine should be offered to men who have sex with other men and to female sex industry workers.

Hepatitis C virus

Hepatitis C virus is usually acquired parenterally, e.g. by sharing contamin-ated syringes and needles. Although the virus can be transmitted sexually, the degree of risk is still uncertain; the use of condoms should be encouraged. The virus can also be transmitted vertically, particularly when the plasma viral load is high. Chronic liver disease is a common sequela of infection.

Molluscum contagiosum virus

Molluscum contagiosum, caused by a poxvirus, presents as hemispherical, umbilicated, pearly, flesh-coloured skin nodules 2–5 mm in diameter. When acquired through sexual contact, they are found on the penis, vulva and inner aspects of the thighs. In the immunocompromised individual, including those with HIV infection, they may be extensive and recalcitrant to treatment. The diagnosis is clinical but can be confirmed by electron microscopy of the core of a lesion that has been removed using a needle and fine forceps. Treatment is by curettage, electrocautery or piercing with a sharpened orange stick, the tip of which has been dipped in iodine solution.

Cytomegalovirus

Cytomegalovirus (CMV) is another herpes virus that can be acquired by sexual contact and congenitally. CMV can be isolated from semen and cervicovaginal secretions, and there is direct evidence of sexual transmission. Young children, however, may also be the source of maternal infection. 30–40% of pregnant women with primary CMV infections transmit the virus to the fetus. In 10% of cases, congenital infection may result in neonatal death or abnormalities, particularly a sensorineural deafness.

There is, however, little information on whether termination should be offered to women who have had primary CMV infection in pregnancy. Permanent damage is more likely if infection occurs in the first half of pregnancy. Information to pregnant women on how long conception should be delayed after primary infection is not available. Viral shedding from the cervix certainly can continue for many months after clinical features resolve.

In severely immunocompromised patients with HIV infection, CMV can cause retinitis, colitis, and pneumonitis, and various neurological abnormalities, including painful sacral radiculopathy.

ARTHROPOD INFESTATIONS
Phthiriasis

Phthirus pubis (the crab louse) is 1.2–2 mm in length and infests the strong hairs of the pubic and perianal areas, abdomen, thighs, axillae and, rarely, the eyebrows, eyelashes and beard. The louse is transferred by sexual contact but can be acquired from clothing. Itch is the principal symptom.

Treatment. Treat with phenothrin (0.2%) or malathion (0.5%) lotions.

Scabies

Scabies is caused by the mite *Sarcoptes scabiei* var. *hominis*. Most infestations are acquired by non-sexual contact.

1. The principal symptom is itch which is particularly noticeable at night and develops up to 6 weeks after a first infection, but earlier in second or subsequent attacks.
2. Burrows may be found on the hands and wrists, extensor surfaces of the elbows, feet and ankles, penis and scrotum, buttocks, axillae and, less frequently, elsewhere. When hygiene is good, burrows may not be apparent.
3. An erythematous rash with urticarial papules, not associated directly with the presence of the mite, is also noted in infested patients; penile and scrotal lesions are common.
4. Indurated nodules are sometimes found on the genitals and elsewhere.

Treatment. Treat with malathion (0.5% in an aqueous base) or permethrin cream (5%).

REFERENCES

Campion MJ, Singer A 1987 Vulval intraepithelial neoplasia: clinical review. Genitourinary Medicine 63(3): 147–152
Central Audit Group in Genitourinary Medicine. Clinical guidelines and standards for genital chlamydial infection. 1998 Health Education Authority, London
Fitzgerald M, Bedford C 1996 National standards for the management of gonorrhoea. International Journal of STD & AIDS 7: 298–300
McMillan A 1986 Vaginal discharge. British Medical Journal 293: 1357–1360
Smith JR, Cowan FM, Munday PE, on behalf of pregnancy subgroup of the Herpes Simplex Advisory Panel 1998. Guidelines for the management of herpes simplex virus infection in pregnancy. British Journal of Obstetrics and Gynaecology 105: 255–260

FURTHER READING

Adler MW 1993 ABC of AIDS, 3rd edn. British Medical Association, London
Editorial 1999 Short course zidovudine for prevention of perinatal infection. Lancet 353: 766–767
Editorial 1999 Elective cesarean delivery to reduce the transmission of HIV. New England Journal of Medicine 340: 1032–1033
Holmes KK et al 1998 Sexually transmitted diseases, 3rd edn. McGraw–Hill, New York
McMillan A, Scott GR 2000 Colour aids in transmitted infections. Churchill Livingstone, Edinburgh

Appendix 13.1

Suggested routine for examination of women for sexually transmitted infections:

1. Examine woman in semi-lithotomy position in a warm, well-lit room.
2. Inspect mouth and, if indicated, take material from tonsils or tonsillar fossae for culture for *Neisseria gonorrhoeae*.
3. Inspect skin (note particularly lesions suggestive of scabies or secondary syphilis, icterus, needle marks, ectoparasites).
4. Collect blood for serological tests for syphilis and, if indicated, for hepatitis B virus and human immunodeficiency virus infection (in latter, only after counselling).
5. Inspect pubic area for *Phthirus pubis* infestation, warts or molluscum contagiosum.
6. Palpate inguinal lymph nodes (if enlarged, note whether uni- or bilaterally enlarged and whether tender or not).
7. Inspect labia majora, labia minora, urethral orifice, introitus, perineum and perianal region. Note swelling of Bartholin's gland.
8. With the right forefinger in the vagina, gently massage urethra and look for expression of mucopus. Using an applicator stick tipped with cotton wool, collect secretions and prepare slide for microscopy. Collect more secretions and send for culture for *N. gonorrhoeae*.
9. Palpate Bartholin's glands and inspect expressed secretions. If mucopus exudes, collect for microscopy and culture for *N. gonorrhoeae*.
10. Pass speculum and inspect vaginal walls. Note character of secretions.
11. Using applicator sticks tipped with cotton wool, collect material from posterior fornix for microbiological examination for *Trichomonas vaginalis* (saline mount), *Candida* spp. (Gram-stained smear) and bacterial vaginosis (saline mount and Gram-stained smear).
12. When indicated, a cervical smear must be taken before other tests are performed.
13. Gently wipe cervix with cotton wool held in sponge-holding forceps and note characteristics of cervical secretions (perfectly adequate specimens for microbiological examination can be obtained during menstruation).
14. Using an applicator stick tipped with cotton wool, collect material from the endocervical canal and smear on a slide for later microscopic examination. Send another swab in transport medium for culture for *N. gonorrhoeae*.
15. Collect material from the endocervical canal for microbiological examination for *Chlamydia trachomatis* (see p. 289).
16. Pass an applicator stick tipped with cotton wool about 3 cm into the anal canal and send in transport medium for culture for *N. gonorrhoeae*.
17. Undertake bimanual vaginal examination, unless contraindicated.

Transport medium for *N. gonorrhoeae*

Using charcoal-impregnated swabs for the collection of material, Stuart's medium has proved valuable. In Amies' modification, the charcoal is incorporated into the medium, thereby allowing the use of untreated swabs. The clinician must be guided by the local laboratory on which transport system to use.

14

Sexuality and family planning

John Bancroft

The functions of sex   314
  Fertility   314
  Pleasure   315
  Pair-bonding and fostering
    intimacy   315
  Asserting masculinity or
    femininity   316
  Bolstering self-esteem   316
  Achieving power or dominance in
    relationships   316
  Expressing hostility   317
  Reducing anxiety or tension   317
  Risk-taking   318
  Material gain   318
The unfolding of sexuality and the
  evolving of sexual
  relationships   318
  Adolescence   319
  The couple and early marriage   320
  Early parenthood   321

Middle age   322
Common forms of sexual
  difficulty   323
  Female problems   324
  Male problems   326
  Problems that involve both
    partners   328
Sexual effects of contraceptive
  methods   328
  Hormonal contraception   329
  Intrauterine devices   330
  Diaphragms   330
  Condoms   331
  Withdrawal (coitus interruptus)   331
  Natural methods of fertility
    regulation   331
  New methods of male
    contraception   332
  Sterilization   332
Helping with sexual difficulties   333

Family planning is only necessary because people engage in sexual behaviour. The implications of this statement are often overlooked or ignored, as is shown by the neglect of sexuality in contraceptive research, the lack of appropriate training in dealing with sexual issues for staff working in family planning clinics and primary care, and the shortage of provision of appropriate help when issues or problems relating to sexuality arise.

During a family planning consultation, issues of sexuality are or should be open for discussion. By seeking advice on contraception, individuals or couples are implicitly stating their involvement, current or intended, in a sexual relationship, and one in which, at least for the time being, they do not wish to bear children. This is important for two principal reasons. First, the impact of a particular contraceptive method on the individual or the sexual relationship needs to be considered; this reflects on the direct consequences as well as the psychological effects of the method. Second, the obvious sexual implications make talking to the family planning doctor or nurse an opportunity to express concerns or seek advice about broader aspects of sexual life. Increasingly, individuals or couples contact family planning clinics simply to seek such help, often reluctant to approach their general practitioner, either for reasons of confidentiality or uncertainty about how the enquiry will be received.

Doctors and nurses working in family planning therefore need to be informed about the impact of sexual attitudes on the acceptability and choice of different contraceptive methods, as well as the direct effects of contraceptive methods on sexual life and, above all, to feel comfortable enough to discuss broader issues of sexuality to allow patients to express their concerns.

In many cases, listening and empathizing will be helpful. In others, simple advice, requiring some general understanding of sexuality rather than special expertise, may be all that is required. Occasionally, referral to those with special training in the management of sexual problems will be appropriate.

In any case, the health professional should be able to respond in ways which make it easier, rather than more difficult, for patients to express their concerns. There are many in the medical profession who believe that it is intrusive to enquire about their patients' sexual lives. In some circumstances that is the case. But when discussing contraception it *is relevant*, and the important aim is that one's approach should allow patients to respond in the way that suits them best; to say little or nothing if that is their choice, or to respond feeling secure that one's comments will be listened to appropriately. There is little doubt that a key factor in determining whether a patient discusses sexual concerns with a doctor or nurse is the patient's expectation of whether or not the health professional's response would be sensitive and unembarrassed.

THE FUNCTIONS OF SEX

Although reproduction is the fundamental purpose of sex, the human species is one in which sexual behaviour has come to serve a variety of other functions. In understanding patients' sexual concerns, it is often helpful to have a clear idea of the range of these functions. Not infrequently, problems arise in a sexual relationship because the two participants are, at the time, using sex for different and conflicting purposes. Fertility remains an important and influential factor even for those seeking contraceptive advice.

Fertility

In general, in our society, the majority of men and women expect and want to have children at some stage in their lives, although many are happy to delay this stage until they have established themselves in a relationship and a career, and feel economically secure enough to start a family. Other pressures may play a part and reflect individual characteristics, cultural or religious influences.

In some cultures, a young woman may feel a powerful need to demonstrate her fertility even when she does not want a child at that point in her life. These are societies where traditionally a woman is only regarded as worthy of marriage when she has proved herself to be fertile. The relevance of such influences in European societies is complex but of considerable interest. Up to the end of the 19th century, there was a striking contrast in this respect between the north of Europe (e.g. Scandinavian countries, northern Germany) and the south or Mediterranean regions. In the north, the importance of proving fertility before marriage was evident; in the south, the emphasis was on proving virginity. There are signs that these contrasting patterns still apply with greater acceptance of single mother-hood in the north, more evidence of 'double standards' of sexual morality and the 'virginity ethic' in the south. But whatever the social context, some young women may approach contraception with an ambivalent attitude because of this underlying, quite possibly unconscious, need to prove their fertility. To embark on many years of contraception, *not knowing whether you will be fertile at the end of it*, can cause concern for some.

Religion can also be a powerful influence. In the Roman Catholic Church, women are encouraged to believe that sexual pleasure is acceptable only if it is associated with the possibility of conception. The majority of women in the Roman Catholic Church, and other religions with similar teaching, escape from this restraint on their sexual expression and come to terms with their need for effective contraception – but not all.

Pleasure

Perhaps the primary, or most basic, reinforcer of sexual behaviour is the pleasure that can be experienced, a combination of sensual pleasure and the uniquely sexual pleasure associated with orgasm. In some individuals, this becomes a powerful motivation for their behaviour; for others, it is of sec-ondary importance. In either case, it will reflect that individual's capacity for sexual responsiveness and orgasm, and this capacity can be affected by psychological factors – relationship problems, illness, including depression, drugs and sometimes contraception.

Pair-bonding and fostering intimacy

This becomes the most rewarding factor for many people, particularly after the excitement of a new relationship has subsided. In an exclusive sexual relationship, the couple do things together which they would not do with others. This is the essence of sexual intimacy. The effectiveness of sex in fos-tering such intimacy stems from the inherent psychological risks that are involved; in particular, the risks of being rejected, laughed at, found unat-tractive, or losing control in ways which one's partner finds off-putting. To express ourselves fully in a sexual relationship, we therefore need to lower our defences. To do so and to feel safe in the process provides a particularly powerful form of bonding between two people. Experiencing and giving pleasure no doubt contributes to this process, but may be less crucial to bonding than the experience of emotional security that is engendered. It is for this reason that the bonding effect of sexuality within a relationship is so readily threatened by sexual involvement outside the relationship.

Asserting masculinity or femininity

'Gender identity' is how we feel about ourselves as male or female. During childhood, sexuality is relatively unimportant to gender identity; at that stage, a sense of gender is established in terms of non-sexual interests, activities, and peer-group relationships. Following puberty, when secondary sexual characteristics develop and hormonal and social milieu change, sexuality becomes important. How attractive or effective we feel in sexual terms becomes an important reinforcer of how masculine or feminine we feel, amongst other things. Much of early adolescent sexuality can be understood in this way. Throughout our lives, particularly at times when gender identity is threatened in other ways (e.g. when facing redundancy or the effects of ageing), we may use our sexuality for this purpose.

Bolstering self-esteem

Feeling sexually attractive to others, or succeeding in one's sexual endeavours, may generally improve self-esteem (and conversely, in the face of sexual failure, lower it). For both these functions, reinforcing gender identity and bolstering self-esteem, there are differences as well as similarities in the ways in which men and women use sexuality, e.g. a man's capacity to 'perform' sexually may become central to his sense of manhood, particularly his ability to develop an erection. This is of considerable importance in understanding problems of erectile dysfunction.

Achieving power or dominance in relationships

The 'power' of sexuality tends to be regarded as an aspect of masculinity, with the male, for both social and physical reasons, typically being in a position of dominance. However, sex can be used to control relationships by both men and women and, as such, is often an important aspect of the dynamics of a relationship. Power may be exerted by controlling access to sexual interaction, determining the form that a sexual encounter takes, and whether the process has a positive or negative effect on the partner's self-esteem. While this can continue to be a factor within an established relationship, it is also an important and interesting aspect of early 'courtship' behaviour.

Whereas women have legitimate reasons for fearing the abuse of power by men in sexual interaction, the extent to which women control normal sexual exchanges is perhaps underestimated. Typically, during 'courtship', the man makes obvious approaches; the woman decides whether or not they should be allowed to progress to the next stage. This pattern, while tending to become obscured once sexual relationships are established, can nevertheless be influential in determining the response to 'rejection'; men get used to the idea that their requests for sex may be turned down, while women may feel particularly vulnerable if they invite sexual activity, and the invitation is rejected or ignored.

Expressing hostility

An important aspect of the 'dominance' issue of male–female sexual inter-action is the use of sexuality to express hostility. This is of most relevance to the problem of rape and sexual assault. Many instances of sexual assault or coercive sex can be seen as an extension of dominance or power, usually by the male over the female. There are also instances when the sexual assault can be understood as an expression of anger, either against the individual woman, or against the woman as a representative of other women, or against the man whose property the assaulted woman is seen to be. There is much controversy about the extent to which rape should be understood as either an act of aggression or a sexual act. To understand many cases of rape and sexual assault it is necessary to understand how aggression and sexual arousal can interact.

For many people, anger and sexual arousal seem incompatible; for them, sex becomes difficult if not impossible until anger subsides. For others, anger can enhance sexual arousal, and aggressive sex can become a means of expressing the anger. This is the basis of much of the sexual assault that occurs within established relationships although, mainly because of the physical dominance that is required, it is largely an expression of anger that men use towards women. A woman has other ways of expressing her anger through the sexual relationship; she may deny her partner sexual access; she may deny him the satisfaction of knowing that she enjoyed his love-making, and she may in a variety of subtle ways, make him feel sexually inadequate.

Reducing anxiety or tension

The reduction in arousal that typically follows orgasm may be used as a device to reduce anxiety or tension. Interestingly, for most people the presence of anxiety (or depression) reduces sexual interest and arousal. But in a minority the arousal associated with anxiety (or, as mentioned above, anger) can serve to augment sexual arousal. In such individuals, sexual arousal and orgasm are more likely to be used as a 'mood regulator', giving at least transient relief from the negative mood state. In more extreme cases, this pattern may become established as a form of compulsive sexual behaviour.

Risk-taking

Sexual interaction provides a variety of risks, ranging from the relatively benign, such as being found out, to the serious, such as pregnancy or sexually transmitted infections. Such risk-taking has taken on a special and more disturbing significance in relation to the HIV and AIDS epidemic. It remains an unanswered question why some individuals, in the face of obvious sexual risk, persist in exposing themselves to that risk. Explanations are likely to be complex, though a mechanism, similar to that discussed under 'anxiety and tension', may be playing a part. Thus, for most people, the awareness of risk may inhibit sexual response thereby making avoidance of the risk that much easier. For some individuals, on the other hand, the arousal associated with the perception of risk augments the sexual response. For some such individuals taking sexual risks becomes a form of excitement which they seek. (For a detailed discussion of this pattern, see Bancroft (2000).)

Material gain

Offering oneself as a sexual partner for payment or other material benefits is a well-established aspect of human sexuality. Prostitution, the institutionalized form of such sexual transaction, has long been established in most human societies. The social function of prostitution, i.e. the extent to which it serves the needs of a society, has been an issue of considerable debate at various times. A cynical view of marriage sees it as a barter between sex, provided by the woman, and material security, provided by the man. In some marriages, the woman may take this view, making it more difficult for her to realize her own sexual identity. If she feels that her partner is not keeping his side of the bargain, she may tend to withhold hers, denying herself as well her partner the potential benefits of a good sexual relationship.

THE UNFOLDING OF SEXUALITY AND THE EVOLVING OF SEXUAL RELATIONSHIPS

Following the sexual development of the individual and his or her subsequent sexual relationships, a temporal pattern evolves in which particular functions are more important at some stages of the lifespan than at others. Contraception and the choice of method have varying implications through these life stages.

Adolescence

In early adolescence, much of sexuality is to do with re-establishing gender identity and self-esteem. Most of us reach the end of childhood reasonably confident in our identities as children, whether boys or girls, and up till then sex is of limited relevance, if any, unless we have been unfortunate enough to have been abused or exploited sexually as a child. With the onset of puberty, bodily changes occur in an unpredictable fashion and hormonal changes have an impact on our emotional reactivity.

Capacity for sexual arousal is heightened, probably reaching its peak for males during the adolescent years, and society informs us in a variety of ways that we should now be evaluating ourselves as sexual beings. Much of early adolescent sexual behaviour, whether it be 'innocent' dating (i.e. with no expectations of sexual interaction), or more obviously sexual exploration, is principally motivated by the need to establish what sort of sexual person we are, whether or not we are successfully masculine or feminine in our sexuality and whether we are sexually attractive to others. Somewhat lower on the agenda is concern about sexual competence – do we know what to do, and can we effectively do it? While struggling with these new and complex issues, the young 'dating' couple will be starting to explore their ability to establish and cope with intimacy. The sense of vulnerability, of emotional risk, will be particularly acute for both boy and girl at this stage, and their earlier experiences at negotiating close relationships will prove important in determining their success.

Not surprisingly, considering the complexity of this new situation, there is much scope for 'dysfunction' of sexual response. The adolescent or young adult male, who is at the peak of his sexual responsiveness, may find it difficult to control his arousal, and rapid ejaculation may be a problem, further lowering his self-confidence. The young woman, until she has developed a sense of security and comfort with her emerging sexuality, may find it difficult to experience orgasm, at least in the presence of her partner.

In most such cases, one can justifiably take an optimistic approach and anticipate that with time these difficulties will be resolved. Those whose earlier experiences have made them particularly vulnerable (as a consequence of earlier emotional traumas or sexual abuse) may now start to establish more overt sexual difficulties.

At this stage, the implications of contraception are probably more complex as well as more important than at any other time. Clearly, the teenage girl needs to avoid an unwanted pregnancy which can have disastrous consequences. But her approach to avoiding conception will be inextricably caught up in how she sees herself as a sexual person. While 'going on the pill' may be a sensible way to deal with the issue, it might have other meanings to her. By taking the pill, is she declaring herself 'sexually available' and by doing so, will her suitability as a sexual partner be devalued? Would her self-esteem be better served by avoiding any such forward planning so that sexual activity when it does occur is in the 'heat of the moment'?

Several studies have shown that young women with negative feelings or guilt about their sexuality are less likely to use contraception, or to use it inconsistently, when they are sexually active (Fisher et al 1983, Gerrard et al 1993). A study of young female university students found that women using oral contraceptives were not only more sexually active than their fellow students using other methods of contraception, but were also more sexually interested and more comfortable with their sexual relationships (Bancroft et al 1991a). Their choice of this method of contraception may not simply have improved their sex lives, it may, in the first place, have reflected their greater comfort with their own sexuality.

In the last few years, the emphasis on safer sex and the importance of condoms have added a further complexity to the decision-making of adolescents and young adults. At the time in their lives when they are first exploring issues of intimacy and trust in their sexual relationships, they are advised to act on the assumption that no sexual partner should be trusted. In other words, they should use condoms as a protection against sexually transmitted infection, regardless of what their partner tells them about his or her previous experience. The difficulties of such a situation for an adolescent should not be underestimated, and it is noteworthy how little attention has been paid to helping adolescents learn how to cope with these sensitive negotiations in their early relationships.

The couple and early marriage

Once the relationship is established, particularly after marriage or cohabiting begins, the challenge is to develop the security of the established sexual relationship, which is also starting to lose the powerful impact of 'novelty'. It is at this stage that establishing good communication becomes crucially important to the continuing development of the sexual relationship. If the couple does not establish ways of letting each other know what they enjoy and what they find unpleasant, then problems, which otherwise would be sorted out and resolved, will become established.

A common type of problem for the young couple stems from an interesting difference between males and females. As already mentioned, the younger male has a tendency to ejaculate quickly when he is sexually aroused. His developmental task is to learn to control his sexual responses so that he can ejaculate when he wants to. The young female often has to overcome established, socially conditioned patterns of inhibition which tend to delay or prevent her experiencing orgasm; she has to learn to 'let herself go' sexually. Unfortunately, once anxiety enters the situation, as it may do when the couple feel they are facing a problem of adjusting sexually, the effect of the anxiety is to aggravate the man's rapid ejaculation and to further delay or inhibit the woman's response. In such circumstances, the young woman, after a few years in which she is frequently aroused but seldom satisfied sexually, finds that she is losing interest, preferring not to get involved so that she avoids further disappointment and frustration. Her male partner, aware of his poorly controlled ejaculation, fails to establish confidence in his sexual performance, making him vulnerable, sooner or later, to other problems such as erectile failure.

Approximately half of the young to middle-aged men who present at sexual problem clinics with erectile problems report lifelong lack of control over their ejaculation. Occasionally, in couples who have delayed sexual intercourse until after marriage or until they start cohabiting, the woman may be unable to tolerate vaginal intercourse; spasm of her perivaginal muscles makes penile insertion difficult or impossible. This condition is known as vaginismus. Usually it results from a tendency for a woman's pelvic floor muscles to go into spasm as soon as insertion of anything into the vagina is attempted (she may also find it difficult or impossible to use tampons). Such women may be responsive and able to enjoy love-making until vaginal entry is attempted. In other cases, the vaginismus is part of a more general aversion towards sexuality. This is a problem typically of the young woman and seldom develops as a secondary problem after a woman has experienced satisfactory sexual intercourse.

In the young couple, failure to fulfil the broader expectations of the relationship can also lead to withdrawal from the sexual relationship by one or other partner. Thus, for the young man or woman who finds their partner failing to give them the emotional and practical support they expected while continuing with their individual-oriented interests, it may become increasingly difficult to engage in sexual activity which will be sexually pleasurable for both.

Contraception at this stage is primarily concerned with avoiding unwanted pregnancy. But the choice of method can have various implications which we will consider in more detail below.

Early parenthood

Pregnancy, and the few months following childbirth, pose further needs for sexual adjustment. The woman is likely to experience a diminution of her sexual desire and capacity for sexual enjoyment towards the end of the pregnancy largely because of the major physical and mechanical changes. It may be as long as a year after childbirth before she regains her previous level of sexual interest and enjoyment.

Postnatally, a number of factors conspire to delay her return to sexual enjoyment. She is likely to be tired, and if she is feeding her infant through the night, this will be a major factor. Sexual intercourse may be painful for several weeks following a delivery, particularly if she had an episiotomy or perineal tear. Depressive mood changes are common, and these will serve to dampen her sexual interest. The dynamics of her relationship with her partner undergo major change with the arrival of a child and many couples find this disrupts their closeness and in particular their sense of sexual intimacy, at least temporarily.

Resentments may arise in either partner which may have sexual repercussions. How the couple negotiate the return to love-making can certainly test the man's sensitivity to his partner's needs. Breast-feeding, particularly when this is the only form of feeding, delays the return of ovarian cyclicity; the hormonal state of the fully breast-feeding woman is comparable to that after the menopause, with oestrogen deficiency which can impair normal vaginal response and cause discomfort during intercourse (Alder and Bancroft 1988).

The postnatal period, for these various reasons, is one of the commonest times for sexual difficulties to arise, which, if the couple have not developed the appropriate methods of resolving them, can become established long-term difficulties. The commonest of such long-term problems is the woman's loss of sexual desire.

Middle age

The sexuality of the long-established relationship typically encounters some different obstacles. By this stage, the novelty of the sexual relationship has long gone. For many that is not a problem; they have established a comfortable form of sexual intimacy which remains an integral part of their relationship. But for others, a routine quality to the sexual relationship takes its toll. In such circumstances, it is all too easy for stresses, at work for example, to distract causing tiredness and to dampen any spontaneous enthusiasm for sexual activity that might occur. Love-making becomes infrequent, and tensions may develop in the relationship as a consequence.

What does this infrequency mean? Does my partner no longer love me, or find me attractive? Is he or she sexually interested or involved with someone else? Not infrequently, such couples can be reassured to find that, when they escape from their normal day-to-day pressures, such as on holiday, they recapture some of their earlier sexual enthusiasm. All too often, the lessons of such a discovery are not learnt, and they return from holiday to their previous routines and pressures, and somewhat barren sexual existence.

Other factors impinging on sexual function become increasingly important with the ageing process. A gradual reduction in the speed and intensity of our sexual responses occurs and physical disease becomes increasingly common. Cardiovascular and neurological diseases are particularly important in men, impairing erectile function. Women experience gynaecological problems which can generally impair their well-being and hence their capacity for sexual interest and pleasure.

As women enter their 40s, menstruation frequently becomes more heavy, prolonged or frequent and directly interferes with their sexual lives. It is common for women passing through the transitional period of the peri-menopause to experience a decline in their sexual interest and responsiveness. To some extent, this is a direct result of hormonal changes; oestrogen deficiency will, in some menopausal women, result in impaired vaginal lubrication which makes sexual intercourse uncomfortable or even painful. However, the loss of sexual interest that commonly occurs can only be partially explained in such terms, and we remain uncertain of the causes of such mid-life sexual decline in many women. It may be relevant that the evidence of such decline is most apparent in women from lower socio-economic groups, amongst whom satisfaction with the premenopausal sexual relationship tends to be less (Garde and Lunde 1980, Cawood and Bancroft 1996).

By the time women are considering the relevance of the menopause, they are often encountering a variety of other new challenges. It is a time when many women are moving on from major commitments of mother-hood to consider new alternative roles, when men are contending with the consequences of their age in their career (e.g. threat of redundancy, being overtaken by younger colleagues), as well as the impact of faltering physical health.

Choice of contraception for this age group becomes confounded by other health issues and is considered elsewhere in the book (Ch. 17).

With yet older age groups, the sexual problems we see are mainly erectile problems in men and loss of sexual interest in women. The effects of ageing do have an impact on sexuality but not all negative by any means. These couples are less likely to seek help within a family planning or reproductive health context.

COMMON FORMS OF SEXUAL DIFFICULTY

There are interesting sex differences in the way that sexual problems are presented. Men tend to formulate their sexual problems mainly in terms of sexual function. In general, they are more comfortable with a physical rather than a psychological explanation, and consequently tend to seek more physical types of help. Women are more likely to see their difficulties in terms of the 'quality of the sexual experience' and its relevance to the relationship. They are more likely to feel comfortable with a psychological explanation as well as psychological types of help. In general, physical factors are more commonly implicated in male than in female sexual dysfunction, though the study of physical aetiology in women has been somewhat neglected. In both sexes, we remain very uncertain how psychological problems become translated into the physiological failure of sexual dysfunction, but we can recognize a variety of psychological problems that are commonly associated. (For a more detailed account, see Bancroft (1989).)

Female problems

Loss of enjoyment

This is probably the commonest sexual complaint of women. A woman may participate in love-making, but fail to experience the pleasure and excitement which she has been used to. If she does not become aroused, then normal vaginal lubrication and vulval tumescence may fail to occur and vaginal intercourse may become uncomfortable or even painful, further blocking her capacity for enjoyment.

Loss of sexual interest

Frequently this occurs together with the loss of enjoyment; such women have no desire to make love and do not enjoy it when it occurs. But in many cases the capacity for enjoyment, once love-making is underway, may remain; the woman simply does not experience any spontaneous sexual desire. As with men, factors leading to loss of sexual desire are varied and often difficult to identify. Mood change is particularly important in women, not only as chronic depressive illness but also as the variations in depressive mood around menstruation that some women experience. Many women are aware of feeling more sexually interested and arousable at certain stages of the menstrual cycle, though the timing of this varies from woman to woman. But those women who typically feel low premenstrually usually lose sexual interest at that time, and find the postmenstrual phase the best time for them sexually.

In some women with marked perimenstrual mood changes, their capacity for sexual desire becomes restricted to a few days postmenstrually, and not infrequently this is eventually lost as well. Unresolved conflicts or resentments in the relationship can underlie both loss of enjoyment and interest. In recent years, it has become much more common for women with such problems to reveal earlier sexual traumas or abuse.

Women contending with life-threatening forms of cancer, such as breast or gynaecological cancer, may react psychologically to both the stress of the illness and the impact of treatment (e.g. mastectomy). Physical factors may also play a more direct role. Loss of desire is to be expected in states of ill-health and may specifically be caused by abnormal hormonal states. Testosterone appears to be important for sexual desire in many, if not all women, as it is in men. Substantial reduction in testosterone, as occurs following ovariectomy or other forms of ovarian failure or suppression, may result in loss of desire.

Sexual aversion

In some cases, the thought of sexual activity causes so much fear or anxiety that a pattern of avoidance of sexual contact becomes established. Often in such cases the cause can be identified from earlier traumatic experiences, but sometimes the origins of the problem remain obscure.

Orgasmic dysfunction

Some women present specifically with difficulty in experiencing orgasm, either in the presence of their partner or in any situation. This may be part of a more generalized loss of sexual enjoyment, or be relatively specific, with sexual arousal and enjoyment still occurring but failing to culminate in orgasm. Although occasionally drugs may block orgasm in women, in most cases psychological factors are likely to be responsible.

Vaginismus

This tendency to spasm of the pelvic floor and perivaginal muscles whenever vaginal entry is attempted may result from some earlier traumatic experience of vaginal insertion (e.g. rape or a particularly clumsy pelvic examination by a doctor). More often there is no obvious antecedent cause and it appears to be a particular tendency for reflexive spasm of these muscles when challenged to relax. If the problem is simply one of vaginismus, there is a good likelihood that the condition can be treated relatively simply, with appropriate training in vaginal relaxation and use of vaginal dilators. If the vaginismus is associated with more deep-seated psychological problems, often presenting as a reluctance to accept the maturity of a full sexual relationship, the prognosis is much less certain, and such cases may be resistant to treatment.

Vaginismus is usually a primary sexual difficulty affecting women at the start of their sexual lives, often resulting in 'non-consummation' of the sexual relationship. It is unusual for it to arise later in a woman's life after a phase of normal sexual intercourse, particularly if she has experienced childbirth. When it does, it is important to look for local causes of pain or discomfort that might lead to the muscular spasm.

Dyspareunia

Pain when intercourse is attempted is a common and often treatable problem. If it is a recurring problem, then anticipation of pain can easily lead to inhibition of normal sexual response thus aggravating the problem by impairing normal vaginal lubrication. The pain or discomfort may occur at the vaginal introitus, resulting from spasm of the perivaginal muscles (as in vaginismus) or inflammation or soreness of the introitus that can follow episiotomy or perineal tear. A Bartholin's cyst or abscess may cause pain simply as a result of sexual arousal, because of the tendency of the Bartholin's gland to secrete in response to sexual stimulation.

Soreness of the vaginal wall is commonly associated with vaginal infections, and persistence of the soreness for some hours after intercourse is attempted is a common description.

Pain experienced when the partner thrusts deeply, or when certain positions are adopted during love-making, suggests some pelvic problem, such as endometriosis, a low-placed ovary or pelvic inflammatory disease.

Sometimes, pain or discomfort results from the vasocongestion that arises in the pelvic tissues supporting the uterus during sexual arousal, particularly if previous surgery or infection has resulted in adhesions.

Although dyspareunia can be the symptom of a psychological problem (e.g. a conversion symptom), this is relatively unusual, and a local explanation for the pain should be carefully sought. This should include a systematic and careful pelvic examination in which an attempt is made to elicit the pain that normally occurs. Some forms of superficial dyspareunia, usually referred to as vulvo-vestibulitis, are characterized by painful ultrasensitivity of the vulva to touch. The pain, therefore, is not confined to sexual activity. This condition is not well understood and it is often difficult to find either physical or psychological explanation (Meana et al 1997).

Male problems

Premature ejaculation

Difficulty in controlling ejaculation so that love-making can continue is typically a problem of younger men. It is seldom, if ever, the result of physical disease, though in some older men physical impairment of erection may need prolonged stimulation before an erection develops, by which time ejaculation is difficult to control. Premature ejaculation is made worse by anxiety. Sexual counselling can often help; the first task is to enable the couple to establish tension-free love-making, so that the anxiety which aggravates the ejaculatory problem is reduced. Then the man, with the co-operation of his partner, learns how to delay ejaculation, using such techniques as the 'stop–start' or 'squeeze'.

Occasionally the use of drugs, such as the new selective serotonin re-uptake inhibitors (SSRI) (e.g. fluoxetine), is justified to pharmacologically delay ejaculation. However, improvement seldom continues once the drug is stopped.

Erectile dysfunction

This is the commonest sexual complaint of men, affecting about 50% of the men who attend our sexual problem clinics, and being increasingly common in older age groups. The aetiology of this problem is varied and still not well understood. Ageing itself plays an important part, for reasons which are also not clear. It is possible, for example, that there may be an age-related loss of responsiveness to crucial neurotransmitters in the central nervous system which normally lead to sexual arousal. But there are a variety of physical diseases, many of them associated with age, which impair erectile response, cardiovascular and neurological disease being the most important.

Psychological factors are undoubtedly important and often combine with physical causes to make the problem substantially worse. In younger men with erectile dysfunction, psychological causes are more likely to predominate and a variety of psychological factors can often be identified in such cases. However, we still know very little about the mechanisms which link such psychological problems to erectile failure. In many cases, some form of direct neurophysiological inhibition of erectile response is involved, but research into such mechanisms is at a very early stage. (For a theoretical discussion of this issue, see Bancroft (1999).)

Many men, having experienced erectile difficulty, lose confidence in their capacity for sexual response, which in some way serves to maintain the problem. Fortunately, in many such cases confidence, and with it sexual function, returns or can be regained with help, either professional or from a sympathetic and supportive partner. An important breakthrough in the pharmacological treatment of erectile dysfunction has been the advent of sildenafil (Viagra), a phosphodiesterase V inhibitor which is effective in a substantial proportion of cases, though its precise indications and limitations remain to be elucidated.

Ejaculatory failure

Taking a long time to ejaculate or being unable to do so at all in the presence of the partner, or intravaginally, does arise, but less commonly than the above two problems. About 6% of men attending Edinburgh sexual problem clinics have this complaint. In many cases, it results from psychological problems, presumably involving inhibition. In some cases, this inhibitory tendency can be seen as part of a more general pattern of emotional inhibition. In other cases, it appears to be more specifically sexual. In a few cases, physical factors, such as testosterone deficiency, can be responsible.

A number of drugs can interfere with ejaculation. Just as SSRIs can be used to treat rapid ejaculation, so can delayed ejaculation (and orgasm in women) be a side effect of such drugs. With some adrenergic antagonists, ejaculation but not orgasm is blocked, resulting in a so-called 'dry run' orgasm. Neurological damage, as can occur in diabetes, and structural damage after transurethral resection of the prostate, may result in retrograde ejaculation into the bladder.

Loss of sexual desire

Spontaneous desire for sexual activity, or sexual appetite, is a difficult concept. For both men and women, it involves the capacity to become aroused by sexual thoughts or situations, leading to a state which motivates them to pursue further sexual stimulation, and ultimately orgasm. Some men seek help because they are aware that their sexual desire has markedly declined. In some cases, this is an understandable reaction to other types of sexual dysfunction and it is important to establish whether the loss of desire preceded or followed the onset of the dysfunction (e.g. erectile failure).

A variety of psychological factors appear to be associated with loss of sexual desire, including depression, unresolved tension or resentment in the relationship. Sexual desire is also likely to be blunted if general health is poor, or if the man is chronically tired or stressed. A specific physical cause is a deficiency of testosterone, the principal androgen, which can result from various forms of hypogonadism. Prolactin-secreting tumours of the pituitary may present as loss of sexual desire, the raised prolactin producing effects very similar to those of androgen deficiency.

Problems that involve both partners

It is often said by sex therapists that there is no such thing as an uninvolved partner. While that might be a slight exaggeration, it is certainly true that there are many ways in which one partner can contribute to the difficulties that are mainly presented or experienced by the other, e.g. the way in which premature ejaculation can eventually result in loss of interest on the part of the woman. Erectile problems can be aggravated by problems in the woman, such as dyspareunia. Not infrequently, vaginismus can obscure the fact that the man also has an erectile problem. There are also many ways in which problems in communication or subtle ways of causing anxiety or insecurity in one's partner may contribute to or serve to maintain a sexual difficulty.

SEXUAL EFFECTS OF CONTRACEPTIVE METHODS

Having considered the ways in which attitudes to contraception and its significance to the user vary at different stages during the reproductive span, it is appropriate to consider the effects of different contraceptive methods on sexuality.

Hormonal contraception

The contraceptive efficacy of such methods, together with their lack of intrusion into love-making, have probably enhanced the sexual lives of many women. Several large-scale studies have shown that frequency of coitus is higher in oral contraceptive users than in users of other contraceptive methods. However, a review of the literature (Bancroft and Sartorius 1990) concluded that a proportion of women react adversely to combined oral contraceptives (COCs), with depressive mood changes, or loss of sexual desire, or both, and that many such women probably discontinue COC use for that reason, and do not therefore feature in large cross-sectional studies of regular COC-users. However, the size of this proportion experiencing such adverse effects could not be estimated at that time because relevant studies had not been carried out. The sexual effects of the progestogen-only pill (POP) has, until recently, received no attention at all, which is surprising considering that progestogens are used to inhibit sexual desire in male sexual offenders.

The impact of oral contraceptives on sexuality will be compounded by the implications to the couple of using that type of method. Does the male partner simply leave contraceptive management to the woman, giving evidence of his reluctance to take a fair share of the responsibilities of the relationship? Does this cause any resentment in the woman and consequently affect the relationship? Some women dislike the idea of altering their 'body chemistry' by taking a form of medication every day. Others may dislike the direct contact with their partners' ejaculate, which previously had been contained in condoms. It is difficult to disentangle the psychological implications of hormonal contraception from any direct effects on sexuality or well-being.

One unique study (Graham et al 1995) has assessed the direct effects of the COC and POP independently from the psychological implications associated with their use as a method of contraception. Volunteers from Edinburgh and Manila (Philippines) who had been sterilized or whose partners had undergone vasectomy took either the COC or POP or a placebo for 4 months. Careful evaluation before starting on the treatment phase showed many differences between the two centres. In particular, the Edinburgh women reported more interest in sex, more enjoyment, arousal, closeness to their partners during love-making, and more preparedness to initiate. The Manila women reported a somewhat higher frequency of sexual activity. COC significantly reduced sexual interest in 50% of the Edinburgh women, whilst producing little change sexually in the Manila women. POP, on the other hand, had no apparent adverse effects on sexuality in either centre and some positive effects on mood. Its only negative effect was the expected disruption of the bleeding pattern.

The mechanism for this negative hormonal effect of the COC is not yet understood. It could be an effect of the progestogen. The COC and POP in this study contained the same progestogen, but it was in substantially larger amounts in the COC. Alternatively, it could result from a reduction in free testosterone. Further research is required to answer these questions. Whatever the explanation, this negative effect on sexual interest could result in some women discontinuing a COC early in its use, and in others could produce subtle negative effects on their sexuality which are not really noticed until the COC is stopped, and an improvement in sexuality occurs (Bancroft et al 1991b).

The relevance of such effects to the acceptability of oral contraceptives has recently been investigated in a study at the Kinsey Institute which has not yet been published. Ninety-six women were assessed in considerable detail before starting on a COC for contraceptive purposes. They were followed-up for 1 year or until discontinuation if earlier. 24% discontinued within the first 3 months. Not surprisingly, these discontinuers had substantially more negative side effects of the method. More surprising was that the side effects which most strongly distinguished continuers from discontinuers were decreased sexual interest and negative mood change. It thus appears that the adverse effects observed in the first placebo-controlled study are indeed relevant to acceptability of oral contraceptives.

Such adverse effects are, of course, only relevant for a proportion of women, and for many the advantages may result in net gains in the quality of their sexual lives. The possibility of a negative effect on sexuality, particularly sexual interest, and to some extent on mood, should be considered when helping women to decide on the method which suits them best. The rather positive message about the POP from Graham's study should also be borne in mind when weighing up the alternatives. Newer methods of hormonal contraception, such as Norplant, await assessment in this respect.

Intrauterine devices

There has been little research into the effects of intrauterine devices (IUDs) on sexuality. Any adverse effects that do occur are secondary to the effects of the IUD on menstruation. An important aspect of this method is that the fitting of the IUD is the responsibility of a doctor. For some women, this has psychological implications which make the method more acceptable.

Diaphragms

This method, while reasonably effective when used conscientiously, is unacceptable to many women. It interferes with the spontaneity of love-making;

either the woman has to disrupt the love-making to go and fit her diaphragm, or she has to anticipate when love-making is likely to occur, which can be particularly problematic for young couples. It also requires handling of the genitalia for fitting and removal, with which some women are uncomfortable. Some women find that a diaphragm interferes with their sexual enjoyment with loss of cervical and some vaginal sensation. Occasionally, the male partner is aware of its presence during intercourse.

Condoms

This barrier method has been extensively promoted as offering protection against transmission of HIV. It is disliked, however, by many men who find not only that putting on a condom disrupts the spontaneity of love-making, but also that their erotic sensitivity is noticeably reduced. If premature ejaculation is a problem, this effect can be an advantage. On the other hand, if a man is unsure of his ability to maintain his erection, the process of fitting a condom can pose quite a threat, as he is likely to fear loss of the erection in the process. Many of the disadvantages of condoms could probably be avoided, or at least reduced, if couples learned to use condoms properly.

Withdrawal (coitus interruptus)

Withdrawal of the penis from the vagina before ejaculation occurs has a very long history. For many couples, the level of awareness and focused attention necessary to use this method distracts from the enjoyment and 'abandonment' of the love-making. As the male produces urethral secretions before ejaculation which can contain sperm, this method is particularly unreliable. For some couples, however, this method works quite well, particularly when the women dislikes intravaginal ejaculation.

Natural methods of fertility regulation

The various methods for identifying the fertile period of the woman's cycle and avoiding sexual intercourse around that time are the only methods of fertility control acceptable to the Roman Catholic Church. They have a high failure rate, and require not only conscientious monitoring of the cycle by the woman but also the preparedness to abstain at the stage of the cycle when some women feel particularly interested sexually. An interesting aspect of the Church's approach to this method is the importance that is attached to the abstinence that is prescribed, the implication being that the self-control required is beneficial to the relationship. In fact, the method can be used with avoidance of vaginal intercourse without avoidance of love-making and mutual orgasm. It may well be true, however, that for some couples the pacing of their sexual activity and the periods of abstinence which result may enhance the enjoyment of their love-making when it does occur.

New methods of male contraception

Apart from the condom, the traditional male method, considerable effort is being made to develop alternative forms of reversible male contraception. The method most likely to succeed, which is currently being evaluated, is the suppression of testicular function (and hence spermatogenesis). This can be achieved in various ways, but unless testosterone levels are maintained, a predictable loss of sexual interest will result. High doses of exogenous testosterone serve the double purpose of suppressing spermatogenesis by means of negative feedback on the pituitary, whilst maintaining circulating testosterone levels.

As yet, such methods appear to work without adversely affecting the man's sexuality, although possible effects on his mood or aggression have not yet been satisfactorily excluded (Anderson et al 1992). It is an interesting fact that concern about possible effects of a male method on the man's sexuality has been in the forefront of researchers' minds, whereas female methods have been in use for decades with negligible concern about possible adverse sexual effects on the woman.

Sterilization

A number of studies have now followed up men and women who have been sterilized and the general impression is of either no effect or an enhancement of the couple's sexual life thereafter (Bancroft 1989). The selection of the method is an opportunity for the couple to demonstrate their sharing of responsibilities and their joint problem-solving. The sexual relationships of couples where the woman had been sterilized were found to be less positive than those where the man had undergone vasectomy (Alder et al 1981). Clearly, the reasons for the decision to choose sterilization are relevant to the consequences; sterilization carried out for medical reasons, often soon after childbirth, is more likely to be followed by an adverse reaction and feelings of regret. It is also important that the person being sterilized is not doing so because of pressure from the partner. Apart from these aspects, however, and providing there are no postoperative complications, there are no reasons why either method should adversely affect sexual response or enjoyment.

HELPING WITH SEXUAL DIFFICULTIES

The ability not only to facilitate the patient's expression of concern about his or her sexual difficulties, but also to listen empathetically, can be of considerable help. Not infrequently, this will be the first time the patient has actually talked about the problem, and being able to do so may make it much easier to get the problems and likely causes into perspective. In many cases, there will be a lack of relevant information about normal sexual response and what to expect. This can be readily rectified. Common examples are the assumption that couples should experience orgasm simultaneously, or that women should experience orgasm simply as a result of vaginal intercourse.

By talking with the couple, it is often possible to help them gain a better understanding of each other and what the sexual experience means to each of them. Enabling the couple to talk more openly and comfortably about their sexual feelings is often of crucial importance, paving the way for the couple to sort things out for themselves.

An important responsibility in the family planning setting is to identify cases of dyspareunia and establish whether any treatable condition, such as a vaginal infection, is present. The impact of other physical problems, such as cardiovascular or neurological disease, on sexual function may require more specialized diagnostic assessment. It certainly should not be assumed, e.g. that because a man has diabetes, his erectile problems are simply the result of the diabetes.

Simple advice can be helpful; not only suggesting particular things to do (e.g. involving masturbatory techniques or vibrators, using the 'stop–start' technique for rapid ejaculation), but also 'giving permission' to the couple to try something that they might previously have felt was 'not normal' or not acceptable. Encouraging them to see that 'normal sex' does not have to involve vaginal intercourse, and consequently the inevitable erection, can reduce the pressure on the couple and allow them to relax and enjoy their love-making in new ways.

Such simple counselling is unlikely to do any harm, and hence it is entirely reasonable for the non-expert to provide this type of help. What is required is a modest amount of knowledge, as covered in this chapter, and the ability to talk about it comfortably and without embarrassment. If such a simple approach fails to help, then referral to the specialist should be considered. Vaginismus probably warrants early referral, as do cases of ejaculatory failure, sexual aversion and loss of sexual desire, which are often difficult to assess as well as treat. However, it is important to establish clearly with the patient or couple whether such referral is really what they want at that time.

REFERENCES

Alder E, Bancroft J 1988 The relationship between breastfeeding persistence, sexuality and mood in the post-partum woman. Psychological Medicine 18: 389–396

Alder E, Cook A, Gray J, Tyrer G, Warner P, Bancroft J 1981 The effects of sterilization: a comparison of sterilized women with wives of vasectomized men. Contraception 23: 45–54

Anderson R A, Bancroft J, Wu F C W 1992 The effects of exogenous testosterone on sexuality and mood of normal men. Journal of Clinical Endocrinology and Metabolism 75: 1503–1507

Bancroft J 1989 Human sexuality and its problems, 2nd edn. Churchill Livingstone, Edinburgh

Bancroft J 1999 Central inhibition of male sexual response; a theoretical perspective. Neuroscience and Biobehavioral Reviews 23: 763–784

Bancroft J 2000 Individual differences in sexual risk taking; a psycho-socio-biological theoretical approach. In: Bancroft J (ed) The role of theory in sex research. Indiana University Press, Bloomington

Bancroft J, Sartorius N 1990 The effects of oral contraceptives on well-being and sexuality. Oxford Reviews of Reproductive Biology 12: 57–92

Bancroft J, Sherwin B B, Alexander G M, Davidson D W, Walker A 1991a Oral contraceptives, androgens, and the sexuality of young women: I. A comparison of sexual experience, sexual attitudes, and gender role in oral contraceptive users and nonusers. Archives of Sexual Behavior 20: 105–120

Bancroft J, Sherwin B B, Alexander G M, Davidson D W, Walker A 1991b Oral contraceptives, androgens, and the sexuality of young women: II. The role of androgens. Archives of Sexual Behavior 20: 121–135

Cawood EHH, Bancroft J 1996 Steroid hormones, the menopause, sexuality and well-being of women. Psychological Medicine 26: 925–936

Fisher WA, Byrne D, White LA 1983 Emotional barriers to contraception. In: Byrne D, Fisher WA (eds) Adolescents, sex and contraception. Erlbaum, Hillsdale, NJ, 207–239

Garde K, Lunde I 1980 Social background and social status; influence on female sexual behaviour. A random sample of 40-year-old Danish women. Maturitas 2: 241–246

Gerrard M, Gibbons FX, McCoy SB 1993 Emotional inhibition of effective contraception. Anxiety, Stress and Coping 6(2): 73–88

Graham CA, Ramos R, Bancroft J, Maglaya C, Farley TMM 1995 The effects of steroidal contraceptives on the well-being and sexuality of women: a double-blind, placebo-controlled, two centre study of combined and progestogen-only methods. Contraception 52: 363–369

Meana M, Binik YM, Khalife S, Cohen DR 1997 Biopsychosocial profile of women with dyspareunia. Obstetrics and Gynecology 90: 583–589

15

Gynaecological problems in the family planning consultation

Anna Glasier

Vulval, vaginal and cervical
  conditions 335
  Bartholin's cyst and abscess 335
  Lichen sclerosus 336
  Atrophic vaginitis 336
  Vaginal wall cysts 337
  Congenital malformations 337
  Cervical ectropion ('erosion') 337
  Cervical polyp 337
Pelvic masses 338
Endometriosis 338
  Treatment 339
Adenomyosis 340
Menstrual dysfunction 340
  Menorrhagia 340
  Menstrual irregularity 340
  Intermenstrual and postcoital
    bleeding 341
  Clinical management 341
  Treatment 341
Postmenopausal bleeding 342
  Clinical management 342
Oligomenorrhoea and
  amenorrhoea 343

Causes 343
Clinical management 343
Hirsutism 345
  Clinical management 345
Dysmenorrhoea 346
  Clinical management 346
Menstrual migraine 347
Pelvic pain 347
  Clinical management 347
Dyspareunia 347
Vaginal discharge 348
Urinary problems 348
  Urgency and frequency 348
  Stress incontinence 348
  Clinical management of urgency,
    frequency and stress
    incontinence 349
  Dysuria 349
Pre-pregnancy counselling 350
Bleeding in early pregnancy 351
  Management 351
Recurrent miscarriage 352
Infertility 352
  Clinical management 352

A wide range of gynaecological problems may become apparent during a family planning or well woman consultation. Not all are related to contraception and many can be dealt with without referral to a specialist. Increasingly a medical approach to gynaecological problems is reducing the need for surgical intervention. In large clinics, it may be helpful to have access to a standard gynaecological textbook (Shaw et al 1997, Edmonds 1999).

VULVAL, VAGINAL AND CERVICAL CONDITIONS

Bartholin's cyst and abscess

A Bartholin's cyst arises as the result of an obstruction to the duct of the Bartholin's gland. It presents as a cystic swelling in the labium majorum.

Cysts are usually less than 5 or 6 cm in diameter and are painless. Infection of a cyst can result in abscess formation presenting as a hot, red and very painful swelling. Recurrent infections may occur if the abscess bursts and drains spontaneously. Both cysts and abscesses are dealt with surgically and should be referred to a gynaecologist – the latter as an emergency.

Lichen sclerosus

Lichen sclerosus accounts for some 25% of referrals to specialist vulval clinics. Although commonest in postmenopausal women, lichen sclerosus can occur in young women and rarely in children and men. Lichen sclerosus most commonly occurs when endogenous oestrogen is low; however, neither systemic nor local oestrogen treatment is of benefit. An association with abnormalities of androgen metabolism in the skin has been suggested but treatment with testosterone is of limited benefit. Most women present with vulval itch (pruritus vulvae) or less commonly with vulval pain or dyspareunia. Asymptomatic lichen sclerosus may be noted during a well woman examination. The vulval skin looks white, thin and crinkly (because of loss of dermal support). There may be fusion of the labia minora with clitoral adhesions and shrinkage of the introitus. The changes may extend around the anus and on to the thighs. Women with lichen sclerosus may also have autoimmune disorders and atopy.

The condition may sometimes be found adjacent to vulvar carcinoma and will itself progress to invasive carcinoma in some 5% of cases. The recommended treatment is topical potent steroids (e.g. Dermovate). Since this requires expert supervision and as biopsy may be needed to exclude neoplasia, referral to a specialist is recommended. Symptomatic lichen sclerosus can be extremely debilitating and is often resistant to treatment. Support groups may be helpful for women who are severely affected.

Atrophic vaginitis

Oestrogen deficiency in postmenopausal women results in thinning of the vaginal epithelium. In atrophic vaginitis, the vaginal walls look reddened with occasional punctate bleeding points. Atrophic vaginitis is a common cause of postmenopausal bleeding. It responds rapidly to local oestrogen treatment. Most vaginal oestrogen preparations are absorbed systemically. Prolonged treatment may therefore have the same effect on the endometrium as oral unopposed oestrogen and should not usually be given for more than 3 months without additional cyclical progestogens. Very low dose preparations are probably safe to give for much longer without added progestogens; the low-dose vaginal oestrogen ring can be used for up to 2 years.

Vaginal wall cysts

Thin-walled cysts can arise anywhere in the vagina but are most common in the upper portion. They are remnants of the lower Wolffian duct. They are regular in outline and rather translucent in appearance. These cysts can usually be ignored although if they appear to be enlarging, the patient should be referred to a gynaecologist. Vaginal wall cysts should not be confused with *vaginal adenosis*, a rare condition in which multiple glandular cysts occur often accompanied by profuse mucus secretion. Vaginal adenosis may be premalignant and can occur in young women exposed to diethylstilboestrol (DES) in utero. Women with a history of DES exposure should have regular colposcopic examinations of the vagina and cervix.

Congenital malformations

Rarely congenital malformations such as vaginal agenesis or vaginal septum may be found on routine pelvic examination or present in patients with sexual difficulties. Referral to a gynaecologist is indicated.

Cervical ectropion ('erosion')

The vaginal surface of the cervix is covered with squamous epithelium and the skin is pale pink and smooth. The cervical canal is lined with columnar epithelium and has a red, glandular appearance. Eversion of the edges of the external cervical os (ectropion) thus exposes the columnar epithelium. The vaginal surface of the cervix may be covered by quite an extensive area of columnar epithelium which appears rough and red ('eroded').

This is usually a chance finding on routine vaginal examination and needs no treatment. It is more likely to occur at adolescence, during pregnancy and in women using the combined oral contraceptive (COC) pill.

Occasionally, the exposed columnar epithelium may bleed if touched and can cause postcoital bleeding. A large 'erosion' may be associated with a profuse vaginal discharge.

Cervical erosion causing symptoms may be cauterized provided a normal cervical smear has been obtained. Squamous epithelium grows back over the cauterized area restoring a healthy looking cervix. Cautery causes a profuse watery discharge and patients should be warned of this. It is better to avoid cauterizing the cervix if the patient is about to go away on holiday!

Cervical polyp

Single or multiple small, red, so-called 'mucus' polyps may sometimes be found at the external cervical os. Usually asymptomatic, they may sometimes cause intermenstrual or postcoital bleeding. Polyps arise from within the cervical canal and, if small, can be twisted off with polypectomy forceps. The polyp should be sent for histological examination. Larger polyps, particularly those with a thick stalk, may bleed profusely and should be left for the gynaecologist to remove.

PELVIC MASSES

A pelvic mass may sometimes be diagnosed on routine vaginal examination and, if large, may also be felt abdominally.

Premenopausal women. Pregnancy should always be excluded. The likely cause is either uterine fibroids or an ovarian cyst and these may often be distinguished on the basis of the history or examination. Small 'functional' ovarian cysts are not uncommon and usually disappear with menstruation. If a symptomless cyst is found on vaginal examination in a young woman – particularly if she is using low-dose progestogen-only contraception – it can be left and the examination repeated after the next menstrual period. It is not always possible to distinguish between a uterine mass and an ovarian swelling, even with an ultrasound scan. Women with symptomatic or persistent cysts should always be referred to a specialist.

Postmenopausal women. Ovarian cysts are present in 6% of asymptomatic postmenopausal women. Most are benign. The prevalence of ovarian cancer is 61 per 100 000 women aged 68. Vaginal ultrasonography is more than 95% accurate in predicting the benign nature of a tumour and CA125 is much more likely to be elevated if the cyst is malignant. While ultrasound appearance and CA125 concentrations may be reassuring, post-menopausal women with ovarian cysts should always be referred for further evaluation.

ENDOMETRIOSIS

Endometriosis is one of the commonest benign gynaecological conditions and is present in up to 25% of women consulting with gynaecological symptoms. It is probably inherited as a complex genetic trait since among first-degree relatives of affected women the prevalence of the disease is significantly increased. It is characterized by the presence of functional endometrial tissue outside the uterine cavity. The commonest sites are on the peritoneum and in the ovary where endometriotic cysts (often filled with debris from cyclical bleeding – chocolate cysts) may develop. Endometriotic deposits respond to endogenous and exogenous steroid hormones in a similar manner to uterine endometrium.

Although a variety of theories exist, the aetiology of endometriosis is not clear. Pelvic endometriosis is probably a consequence of transplantation, during retrograde menstruation, of viable endometrial cells into the peritoneal cavity. Deposits outside the pelvis, e.g. in the lung or skeletal muscle, are better explained by metaplasia of cells of the original coelomic membrane.

Endometriosis causes pain which may present as dysmenorrhoea, dyspareunia or pelvic pain unrelated to menstruation or intercourse. Endometriosis is also diagnosed in 20–40% of subfertile women. Severe endometriosis can cause structural damage to the tubes and ovaries but the mechanism by which mild endometriosis is associated with infertility remains unclear.

The only definitive way to diagnose endometriosis is by visualizing the deposits at laparoscopy. Magnetic resonance imaging (MRI) scan is being tested in some centres as a non-invasive screening tool. Infrequently, endometriotic cysts or nodules can be seen in the vagina or on the cervix. Pelvic examination may reveal thickening of the uterosacral ligaments, nodules in the pouch of Douglas, or fixation of the uterus as a result of adhesions. In most cases, however, pelvic examination is unremarkable. Women with severe endometriosis sometimes have elevated CA125 levels but this lacks both the sensitivity and specificity required for a screening test.

Treatment

Since the definitive diagnosis can only be made at laparoscopy, treatment is usually instigated by a specialist. In a woman presenting with symptoms suggestive of endometriosis, a trial of medical treatment often helps towards making a diagnosis. Laser ablation of endometriotic lesions at laparoscopy is of benefit in relieving pain, and surgical treatment is required for removing endometriomas. A medical approach to treatment involves drugs which suppress ovarian function or induce pseudopregnancy. The COC pill given continuously for three cycles at a time – danazol 400–800 mg daily and gestrinone 2.5–5 mg twice weekly – have all been shown to relieve symptoms with concomitant resolution of endometrial deposits. Gonadotrophin releasing hormone (GnRH) agonists give rapid and effective symptom relief but are associated with a 3–5% loss of vertebral trabecular bone density in the lumbar spine after 6 months of use and should be used only by specialists.

'Add-back' hormone replacement therapy (HRT) used with GnRH agonists may protect against bone loss without reversing the beneficial effects on the endometriosis. There is no evidence that the treatment of mild endometriosis increases the chance of conception and pregnancy is either prevented by the treatment itself or contraindicated during its use, thus effectively prolonging the duration of infertility.

ADENOMYOSIS

Adenomyosis, the presence of endometrial tissue deep within the myometrium, is probably a separate pathological entity from endometriosis with a different aetiology, and affecting a different population. It can present simply as an enlarged uterus on routine pelvic examination or may be associated with dysmenorrhoea or menorrhagia. It is usually diagnosed retrospectively by a pathologist after hysterectomy but can be diagnosed by MRI scan.

MENSTRUAL DYSFUNCTION

Disturbance of menstruation is a problem commonly raised during family planning or well woman consultations. A particular method of contraception may be the cause of the problem: menorrhagia caused by an IUD; intermenstrual bleeding associated with low dose combined oral contraception; irregular menses resulting from use of the progestogen-only pill – these problems and their management are covered in the relevant chapters. Disturbances of menstruation unassociated with a contraceptive method are often short-lived and bleeding patterns which are normal for that individual may resume within a few cycles. Many women do not require sophisticated investigation or treatment but simply reassurance that a particular pattern of menstruation is not sinister. The commonest cause of persistent disturbance is dysfunctional uterine bleeding, defined as excessive bleeding (heavy, prolonged or frequent), of uterine origin, that is not due to organic pelvic disease or to a generalized medical condition. It is obviously a diagnosis of exclusion. (For review, see Crosignani and Rubin (1990).)

A pelvic examination is essential in every case to exclude pathology. In any woman, risk factors for endometrial cancer include treatment with tamoxifen or unopposed oestrogen, obesity and polycystic ovarian syndrome, hypertension and obesity.

1. Menorrhagia

One in 20 women aged 30–49 will consult a general practitioner because of menorrhagia. One in 5 women in the UK have a hysterectomy before the age of 60, half of them for menorrhagia and at least half of these women will have no identifiable pathology.

2. Menstrual irregularity

Occurs commonly in adolescents and in the perimenopause and is usually associated with anovulation. It may sometimes be associated with an ovarian cyst.

3. Intermenstrual and postcoital bleeding

Bleeding between periods (IMB) or after intercourse (PCB) may be due to a local cervical problem including ectropion, malignancy (see above) or more rarely an intrauterine polyp. Some women bleed around midcycle in response to the fall in oestrogen following the luteinizing hormone (LH) surge.

Clinical management

1. Take a careful history.
2. Pelvic examination to exclude any obvious cause.
3. Cervical smear if due or if cervix looks suspicious.
4. Women under 40 years complaining of menorrhagia or irregular menses without pelvic pathology do not need dilatation and curettage (D&C) or endometrial biopsy since the chance of finding any abnormality is negligible. Exceptions to this general rule (RCOG Guidelines No. 3 1994) include:
   a. failure of uterine bleeding to respond to medical treatment
   b. persistent intermenstrual bleeding.
5. Vaginal ultrasound allows endometrial thickness to be measured and may reveal endometrial polyps or other pathology.
6. Endometrial biopsy may be considered in women over 40 and can be done in the clinic/surgery using a disposable sampler.
7. In the absence of any obvious pathology, an endometrial biopsy and/or colposcopy or hysteroscopy should be considered in women with IMB or PCB.

Treatment

1. Menstrual dysfunction often resolves spontaneously. Reassurance is sometimes all the patient is seeking, particularly if she is adolescent or approaching the menopause.
2. In most cases, and in the absence of contraindications, the COC pill will often restore acceptable cycles.
3. Menorrhagia is associated with a local overproduction of prostaglandins which cause increased blood loss and myometrial contractions. It is often improved by the oral administration of prostaglandin synthetase inhibitors (e.g. mefenamic acid 500 mg tds) or aspirin during menses. Women appreciate an explanation of the rationale for prescribing these drugs and should be encouraged to take them regularly (e.g. 6-hourly) during days of heavy bleeding. If this approach is effective, treatment can be prolonged indefinitely. More effective than prostaglandin synthetase inhibitors is the antifibrinolytic drug, tranexamic acid (1 g tds

during menses). In a randomized trial in which menstrual blood loss (MBL) was measured, mefanamic acid reduced MBL by 20% while tranexamic acid reduced it by 54%.

4. Irregular dysfunctional uterine bleeding responds to cyclical progestogens (norethisterone 10–15 mg/day in divided doses from the 12th day of each month or day 12 of the cycle for 14 days). Progestogens given in this way replace the progesterone which is missing because of anovulation and stimulate the development of a secretory endometrium which breaks down when the progestogen is withdrawn, thus restoring regular bleeding patterns. It is worth stopping treatment after 6 months or so, as the problem may have resolved. Treatment can be restarted if menorrhagia resumes.

    Cyclical progestogens are usually ineffective in women with heavy regular bleeding as they are almost certainly ovulating.

5. If menstrual dysfunction persists despite the above approaches, or if any pathology is found on pelvic examination, the patient should be referred to a specialist.

POSTMENOPAUSAL BLEEDING

Irregular and infrequent bleeding episodes are of course common during the perimenopause.

Vaginal bleeding which occurs in a postmenopausal woman more than 1 year after the last menstrual period should always be investigated.

Clinical management

History

A careful history should be taken paying attention to the following

1. Date of LMP.
2. Associated pain or discomfort – postmenopausal bleeding (PMB) may simply be the result of a small amount of oestrogen secretion from a surviving ovarian follicle (the ovary having a 'last fling') in which case the bleeding often resembles a normal period and may be accompanied by premenstrual symptoms and dysmenorrhoea.
3. PMB occurring after intercourse may be due to atrophic vaginitis.
4. A history of associated discharge may suggest a vaginal infection.
5. A history of weight loss, malaise or apparent weight gain associated with a growing pelvic mass may suggest ovarian or uterine malignancy.
6. It is worth taking a full medical history including a drug history – some patients forget to tell the doctor that they are taking HRT. The history should take account of homeopathic remedies such as ginseng which has

some oestrogenic properties. Abnormal bleeding in association with HRT is discussed in Chapter 16.

Examination

1. Pelvic examination may reveal a local vulval, vaginal or cervical cause or a pelvic mass. Local vulval lesions are easily missed and should be actively sought. Atrophic vaginitis (see above) is common in postmenopausal women and, although it may be the cause of the PMB, its presence should not preclude consideration of other causes which may co-exist.
2. A cervical smear should be taken if there is any suspicion of abnormality or if one is due.
3. Vaginal ultrasound, if it is available in the clinic, may reveal an endometrial thickening if there is a carcinoma but a negative scan does not exclude pathology.
4. Endometrial biopsy using a disposable sampler is thought to be almost as good as a formal D & C for excluding endometrial cancer (especially if used in conjunction with vaginal ultrasonography) but may not be possible in elderly women with a narrow cervical os.
5. Even if a benign cause such as atrophic vaginitis is suspected, it is probably advisable to refer women with PMB for specialist opinion.
6. Rarely, a forgotten IUD may be found.

OLIGOMENORRHOEA AND AMENORRHOEA

Infrequent or absent menstruation occurs commonly. Pregnancy should always be excluded. The problem is often short-lived and simple reassurance should suffice. Depending on the woman's age, need for contraception or desire to start a family, investigation may be delayed for 6 months.

Causes

Both may be a result of hypothalamic, pituitary or ovarian dysfunction. Intercurrent illness, particularly endocrinopathy, e.g. diabetes or thyroid disease, or diseases which affect nutritional status, e.g. Crohn's disease, may be present. Amenorrhoea may be primary or secondary.

Clinical management

Investigation

1. Take a careful history, including a history of menstrual patterns since menarche. Problems which appear to have arisen after stopping the pill

in fact often pre-date its use and have simply been masked by the pill-induced regular withdrawal bleeds. A history of weight loss, excess exercise, diet (vegetarians seem to be prone to amenorrhoea), galactorrhoea or stress should be specifically sought. Recent use of depot medroxyprogesterone acetate should be excluded.

2. Examination – in addition to pelvic examination, a general physical examination should pay attention to body mass index, signs of thyroid disease, hirsutism and the presence or absence of galactorrhoea.

3. Primary amenorrhoea – measure LH, follicle-stimulating hormone (FSH), prolactin and oestradiol. If FSH is elevated, an analysis of karyotype should be undertaken. If this is abnormal, refer to a specialist.

4. For secondary amenorrhoea or oligomenorrhoea, measure serum gonadotrophin and prolactin concentrations. Testosterone estimation is helpful in women with clinical signs of either polycystic ovarian syndrome (PCOS) such as obesity, acne and hirsutism, or virilization such as clitoromegaly. Measurement of thyroxine and thyroid stimulating hormone (TSH) may be useful. Skull X-ray or MRI of the pituitary fossa is indicated if there is hyperprolactinaemia.

4. If biochemical investigations are abnormal, if the problem persists or a pregnancy is desired, refer to a specialist.

5. If investigations are negative, normal cycles may resume spontaneously within a few months. Review in 6 months time.

6. If investigations and clinical signs (and ultrasound scan if available) suggest PCOS and fertility is not required, COC will give regular cycles. Dianette which contains cyproterone acetate (an anti-testosterone) as the progestogen is particularly useful for treating acne or hirsutism and can be used for as long as other COC pills.

7. Although women with amenorrhoea or oligomenorrhoea are less likely to conceive than women with regular cycles, ovulation may occur and they should be encouraged to use contraception if they wish to avoid pregnancy. Once the nature of the underlying hormonal disturbance has been established, hormonal contraception may be considered. It is perfectly appropriate to prescribe COC for women with hypogonadotrophic or normogonadotrophic amenorrhoea and indeed it will protect them from osteoporosis caused by oestrogen lack. Pill use does not compromise future fertility although regular withdrawal bleeds will of course continue to mask the underlying disorder. Women with PCOS are at risk of endometrial cancer in later life as a result of long periods of unopposed oestrogen stimulation of the endometrium; for these women, the pill will restore regular cycles and protect them from endometrial cancer. Although COC is not absolutely contraindicated for women with hyperprolactinaemia, the oestrogen component does stimulate prolactin secretion and is better avoided or discussed with a specialist.

HIRSUTISM

Hirsutism is defined as the presence of excess hair growth in women. It is not by itself a disease but most women find hirsutism extremely distressing. In most cases, hirsutism results from a combination of mildly increased androgen production and increased skin sensitivity to androgens.

Hirsutism usually starts around puberty when androgen secretion increases, or after a period of weight gain or when oral contraceptives are stopped. Rapidly worsening hirsutism at any other time should raise suspicions of neoplasia.

At least 25% of all young women have coarse pigmented (terminal) hairs on the face (usually the upper lip), areolar and lower abdomen. Women tend to develop more body hair until the menopause after which time only facial hair development increases. 95% of women who complain of hirsutism have either idiopathic hirsutism or PCOS. PCOS (p. **344**) can be diagnosed on the basis of an elevated concentration of LH in the presence of a normal circulating FSH and an elevated testosterone concentration, together with an ultrasound scan confirming the typical appearance of the ovaries.

Idiopathic hirsutism is common in women whose mothers are of Mediterranean or Asian origin. Rare causes of hirsutism include adrenal hyperplasia, Cushing's syndrome, androgen-secreting tumours of the ovary or adrenal glands and drug treatment (anabolic steroids).

Clinical management

1. History and examination to exclude PCOS and/or virilism. Hormone evaluation is not necessary in women with mild, gradually progressive hirsutism and regular menses. For women with irregular menses, measure serum testosterone and arrange ovarian ultrasound. If serum testosterone is higher than 6 nmol/L without evidence of PCOS or if there are signs of virilism (male pattern baldness, clitoromegaly, muscle development and deepening of the voice), refer to a specialist.
2. Reassurance.
3. Cosmetic advice – bleaching, electrolysis, depilatory creams, shaving.
4. Medical treatment:
   a. Cyproterone acetate (an anti-androgen), most easily given as Dianette or alternatively 25–100 mg given for the first 10 to 11 days of a 21-day course of oestrogen (so-called reversed sequential regimen), or during the first 10 days of an oral contraceptive pill cycle, or, for women without a uterus 25 mg daily continuously
   b. Spironolactone 25–100 mg twice daily orally (contraindicated in women with renal insufficiency or with drugs which increase serum potassium).

The response to medical treatment is slow and it is best combined with cosmetic approaches. The success of treatment can be judged by a fall in the frequency of the need to remove hair mechanically (e.g. shaving).

DYSMENORRHOEA

Dysmenorrhoea (period pain) can be primary or secondary. It is said to occur in 60–70% of women with some 15% complaining that their activity is limited by dysmenorrhoea. Primary dysmenorrhoea is often present from menarche, and is probably due to an imbalance of prostaglandins. Secondary dysmenorrhoea occurs in a woman who has not had painful periods previously and may be associated with endometriosis or an intracavity uterine fibroid or polyp.

Clinical management

Investigation

1. Take a careful history, including the precise timing of pain. Classical primary dysmenorrhoea is often accompanied by vomiting and diarrhoea.
2. Pelvic examination to exclude underlying pathology. A normal pelvic examination does not exclude endometriosis. Although dysmenorrhoea is common, endometriosis should be seriously considered. In the UK, the average time from the onset of pain until a surgical diagnosis is made is 8 years.

Treatment

1. An explanation of the cause of dysmenorrhoea and simple reassurance are often enough. It is true that most young women grow out of it.
2. Simple analgesics – aspirin is a potent prostaglandin synthetase inhibitor. Other non-steroidal anti-inflammatory drugs such as mefenamic acid may be helpful. As is the case with menorrhagia, patients should be advised that they will get more relief by taking the medication at regular intervals and not just in response to pain.
3. Dysmenorrhoea is often improved by the COC pill. If it persists, two or three packets can be taken without a break in order to reduce the frequency of the problem (p. **57**).
4. If there is no response to these simple measures, referral to a specialist (preferably one with an interest in dysmenorrhoea) may be indicated. Presacral neurectomy using intra-abdominal lasers is being evaluated in a few specialist centres

MENSTRUAL MIGRAINE

Some women complain of severe headaches at the onset of menses. They may result from the relatively abrupt fall in circulating oestrogens at the end of the cycle and seem to be more common among pill-users than among women having spontaneous cycles.

Taking two or three packets of the COC pill continuously before having a break may help and, if nothing else, reduces the frequency of the headaches. The application of an oestrogen patch on the last day of pill-taking has been reported to be of value but there are few data on this approach.

PELVIC PAIN

Chronic pelvic pain is a common problem in young women and is often attributed to a gynaecological cause. More often than not, no pelvic pathology such as endometriosis or chronic infection is found.

Clinical management

1. Take a history – include careful exploration of urinary and gastrointestinal tract symptoms. Irritable bowel syndrome is a common cause of lower abdominal pain in young women who may not be constipated but will often admit to a bowel motion 'like rabbit pellets'.
2. Abdominal and pelvic examination.
3. Pelvic ultrasound – for some women, a normal pelvis on ultrasound is 'proof' that there is nothing seriously wrong.
4. Exploration of social and psychological factors – a demanding job (especially mother/wifehood), tension at home or low self-esteem can turn a mild and occasional 'tummy ache' into chronic pelvic pain. Women who have suffered from sexual abuse or domestic violence may first seek help by presenting with pelvic pain.
5. There is a school of thought that pelvic pain is due to 'pelvic congestion' and some researchers have demonstrated varices in pelvic veins. Short-wave diathermy may be helpful.
6. Referral for diagnostic laparoscopy – although it often seems pretty certain that no pathology will be found, some women remain concerned until someone has actually 'had a look'.

DYSPAREUNIA

Many women assume that pain on intercourse is the result of an organic problem and the issue is not uncommonly raised during a family planning or well woman consultation. Dyspareunia is described as superficial if it is felt at the vaginal introitus and deep if the pain is felt within the pelvis. It may be primary (i.e. present since the first attempt at intercourse), or secondary. Very rarely is dyspareunia caused by an organic lesion such as a pelvic mass. A pelvic examination should be undertaken in order to be able to reassure the patient. Management thereafter is described in Chapter 14.

VAGINAL DISCHARGE

See Chapter 13.

URINARY PROBLEMS

Urinary problems are common in women of reproductive age as well as among postmenopausal women. It is estimated that at least 20% of women suffer from urinary frequency (the passage of urine more than seven times during waking hours and twice or more during the night) and 15% report urgency (a sudden strong desire to micturate, which if unrelieved, may lead to incontinence). Stress incontinence (involuntary leakage of urine on coughing or sneezing) is also common, particularly in multiparous women who may not admit to the problem because of the embarrassment it causes. Dysuria may also present quite commonly in the course of the family planning consultation.

Urgency and frequency

May arise from:

1. Disease outside the urinary tract, including pregnancy, pelvic mass, diabetes, diuretic therapy, neuromuscular disorders and psychiatric disorders.
2. Renal disease.
3. Disease of the bladder, including tuberculosis, interstitial cystitis, functionally small bladder and detrusor instability.
4. Urethral conditions including urethral syndrome and diverticulum.
5. Surgery (hysterectomy) and radiation.
6. Oestrogen deficiency (menopause).

Stress incontinence

May be associated with:

1. Congenital weakness of the bladder neck.
2. Childbirth.
3. Trauma, e.g. pelvic fracture.
4. Fibrosis following surgery.

Clinical management of urgency, frequency and stress incontinence

1. Take a careful and detailed history. It is important to define the problem exactly since stress incontinence is much more amenable to surgery than urge incontinence or frequency.
2. Examination to exclude pelvic mass, prolapse, cystocele or abdominal pathology, neurological abnormality and medical or surgical conditions likely to exacerbate incontinence.
3. Mid-stream specimen of urine to exclude urinary tract infection (UTI): dipstick to exclude glycosuria.
4. Fluid intake and output chart and urinary diary (which the patient can take to the specialist if referral is required) if frequency or urgency appears to be the problem.

Treatment

1. Any obvious predisposing factors such as UTI should be investigated and treated.
2. Menopausal women may benefit from local or systemic oestrogen therapy.
3. Women with stress incontinence who are undecided about surgery or who intend further childbearing may benefit from pelvic floor exercises, if they are properly taught (usually by a physiotherapist) and continued for long enough.
4. Urgency and frequency may be helped by bladder training. The patient reduces her fluid intake, if it is excessive, and uses timed voiding to overcome urgency, slowly increasing the interval between voids.
5. Anticholinergic drugs such as tolterodine may be of value but often have troublesome side effects.
6. When there is evidence of organic disease or if conservative measures fail, referral to a specialist is indicated.

Dysuria

May result from:

1. UTI.
2. Vaginal infection.
3. Frequency dysuria syndrome (FDS) – sometimes called urethral syndrome – describes a condition of frequency and/or urgency, dysuria, strangury and nocturia without an obvious cause.
4. Oestrogen deficiency. Urogenital atrophy is a late manifestation of the menopause which is associated with recurrent UTI (occurs in over 10%

of women over 60), dyspareunia, urinary frequency, dysuria and incontinence.
5. Urethral prolapse or caruncle – the urethral mucosa may occasionally prolapse in elderly women. The everted portion becomes red and inflamed and is sometimes called a caruncle. Often symptomless, it can cause dyspareunia and dysuria.

Management

1. Take a careful history.
2. Examination is indicated if anything other than a simple UTI is suspected.
3. Urinalysis and bacteriological investigation of a mid-stream specimen of urine. *Chlamydia* should be excluded if FDS is suspected. Appropriate antibiotic therapy should be given.
4. Symptoms due/related to postmenopausal oestrogen deficiency respond well to local oestrogens. The improvement is very gradual and it may be some months before a benefit is obvious.
5. Referral to a gynaecologist/urologist for cautery or excision of a urethral prolapse.
6. Recurrent UTI or FDS can sometimes be prevented by simple education. Personal hygiene is important and patients should be instructed to wipe the perineum from front to back to avoid contamination of the urethra. Vaginal deodorants (of dubious value for anyone) and irritant bath additives should be avoided. Fluid intake should be encouraged particularly when symptoms occur. Alkalinizing agents (e.g. potassium citrate) may be of some help. Regular and complete bladder emptying is essential. Postcoital UTI may be associated with use of a barrier method and a change of method may help.

PRE-PREGNANCY COUNSELLING

Many women attending a family planning consultation intend to embark upon a pregnancy at some time in the future. If that time is imminent, the nurse or doctor has an opportunity to give some pre-pregnancy advice or counselling. For many women, general advice is sufficient; a few may need specialist help.

1. Stopping contraception. It is a myth that women should stop using the COC pill and change to a barrier method some months before embarking on a pregnancy. Recent use of the pill has no effect on the fetus and, as ultrasound scans are now widely available, conceptions which occur immediately after stopping the pill do not present problems with dating.

2. Diet. There are plenty of leaflets available. Pregnant women should be advised to have a healthy diet and to avoid foods such as unpasteurized cheese or substances which are known to carry organisms such as *Listeria* or *Salmonella*.

3. Folate supplements. Neural tube defects have been linked with folate deficiency. Women planning a pregnancy are advised to take folate supplements in addition to having a balanced diet. 400 µg/day should be taken orally until 12 weeks gestation.

4. Alcohol and smoking. Smoking has been associated with an increased risk of miscarriage, prematurity and intrauterine growth retardation. Pregnancy may offer a good incentive to stop. Alcohol, in small amounts, is not contraindicated but a regular moderate or heavy intake should be discouraged.

5. Antenatal screening/genetic counselling. Women over the age of 35 or those with a family history of genetically transmitted disease may need specialist counselling. The doctor involved in a family planning consultation should be aware of how and to whom in the area couples may be referred.

6. Rubella status should be checked particularly in nulliparous women in their early 40s who were not vaccinated at school (Ch. 12).

BLEEDING IN EARLY PREGNANCY

Women sometimes present to the family planning clinic with bleeding in early pregnancy. They may already know or suspect that they are pregnant, or pregnancy may be diagnosed at the consultation. Bleeding may be due to local causes such as cervical erosion or polyp or may be a sign of miscarriage or ectopic pregnancy.

Management

History. Take a careful history, including detailed menstrual history and history of accompanying abdominal pain. Unilateral iliac fossa pain rather than period-type pain should raise the suspicion of ectopic pregnancy. Other suspicious symptoms include feelings of faintness and shoulder tip pain. A history of pelvic infection, subfertility or IUD use should be sought specifically.

Examination. The patient's general condition should be assessed. Spontaneous abortion and ectopic pregnancy can both cause heavy bleeding and shock. If the patient is shocked, she should be transferred immediately to hospital preferably with an intravenous line in place. Products of conception distending the cervical os can cause shock in incomplete abortion. If the products are removed digitally from the os, the patient usually recovers immediately. In the absence of shock, abdominal and pelvic examination may distinguish between threatened, incomplete and missed abortion and ectopic pregnancy. Speculum examination may reveal a local cervical cause of the bleeding and the degree of dilatation of the cervical os can be determined. Products of conception may be seen. Pain on cervical excitation, unilateral forniceal pain and a mass may suggest ectopic pregnancy.

Pregnancy test may be helpful but a negative result does not exclude ectopic pregnancy, missed or complete abortion. Measurement of serum β-hCG is more sensitive than urinary pregnancy tests if it is available.

Referral. The patient should be referred to hospital as an emergency if ectopic pregnancy is suspected. Threatened abortion can be managed at home but a scan confirming an ongoing pregnancy is reassuring to the mother. Ultrasound scan is used to distinguish missed and complete abortion and where either is suspected or, if the abortion is incomplete, the patient should be seen by a specialist.

RECURRENT MISCARRIAGE

Some 20–25% of pregnancies end in spontaneous abortion. Some women who miscarry recurrently may ask for advice during a family planning consultation. Most gynaecologists do not investigate couples until three or more pregnancies have miscarried. Women should be reassured that one and even two miscarriages are not uncommon and that their chance of carrying a pregnancy to term next time is high. The only practical advice that can be given is that smoking appears to be associated with miscarriage. Women with recurrent miscarriage should be referred for investigation by a specialist. Useful investigations prior to referral include:

1. Karyotyping of both partners.
2. Full blood count of the mother.
3. Measure serum LH and FSH in the mother.
3. Lupus anticoagulant level from the mother.

INFERTILITY

Between 1 in 8 and 1 in 10 couples experience difficulty in conceiving. Some initial advice may be given and, if appropriate, investigations started in the family planning clinic. Depending on the woman's age, investigations should not usually be started until a couple have been trying to conceive for at least 1 year, as 90% will succeed within that time. The RCOG guidelines on The Initial Investigation and Management of the Infertile Couple (1998) provide a useful flow diagram (Fig. 15.1).

Clinical management

Take a history. The common causes of infertility are:

a. failure of ovulation
b. tubal disease
c. male infertility.

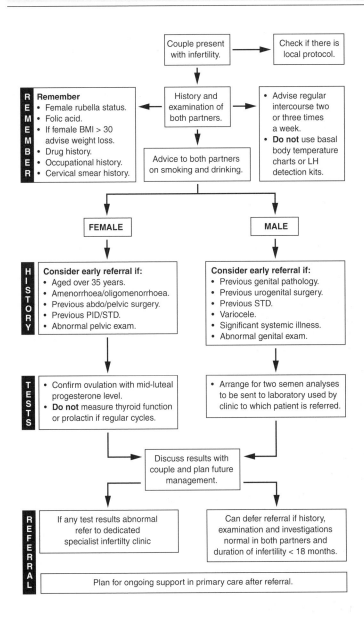

Figure 15.1   Flow chart for investigation and management of infertility in primary care. BMI, body mass index; LH, luteinizing hormone; PID, pelvic inflammatory disease; STD, sexually transmitted disease. (Reproduced with permission from Royal College of Obstetricians & Gynaecologists (RCOG) 1998. The initial investigation and management of the infertile couple. Evidence-based clinical guidelines no. 2. Guidence summary. RCOG, London.)

The history should explore these three areas. Women with regular cycles are almost certainly ovulating. Previous abdominal or gynaecological surgery or a history of pelvic inflammatory disease might suggest tubal disease. In the male, a history of undescended testes; hernia repair; mumps; intercurrent disease such as ulcerative colitis treated with drugs that are potentially toxic to sperm; heavy drinking or smoking might suggest male infertility.

Do not forget to ask about the frequency of intercourse, it may be very infrequent.

Give advice about the fertile time of the cycle.

With regular cycles, intercourse every other night during the fertile period is adequate. Basal body temperature measurement only defines the end of the fertile period. Patients who are keen to do so may be instructed in fertility awareness techniques and use them to achieve a pregnancy.

Commercial kits for identifying the LH surge are available to help define the fertile period. They are expensive and many couples find the strain of timing intercourse with such precision somewhat inhibiting. An ovulation monitor (similar to Persona) can be used to give an indication of days of high fertility.

Initial investigations which may be useful while a couple waits for an appointment for the infertility clinic include:

- Serum progesterone in the mid-luteal phase of the cycle (e.g. day 21 in a 28-day cycle; day 28 in a 35-day cycle). This confirms that ovulation is occurring.
- In a woman with oligomenorrhoea or amenorrhoea, it is worth measuring serum gonadotrophins, prolactin and testosterone concentrations.
- Semen analysis.

Referral to a specialist.   If a woman is over 35 years of age, it is probably better to refer after 6 months rather than waiting 1 year. Remember that there may be 2 or 3 months' wait for an appointment. If you identify a possible cause in the history or examination, it may be sensible to refer earlier.

REFERENCES

Crosignani PG, Rubin B 1990 Dysfunctional uterine bleeding. Human Reproduction 5: 637–638
Edmonds DK (ed.) 1999 Dewhurst's Textbook of Obstetrics and Gynaecology for Postgraduates, 6th edn. Blackwell, Oxford
Royal College of Obstetricians & Gynaecologists (RCOG) 1994 In-patient treatment – D&C in women age 40 or less. RCOG guidelines no. 3. RCOG, London
Royal College of Obstetricians & Gynaecologists (RCOG) 1998 The initial investigation and management of the infertile couple. Evidence-based clinical guidelines no. 2. Guideline summary. RCOG, London
Shaw RW, Soutter WP, Stanton SL (eds) 1997 Gynaecology. Churchill Livingstone, Edinburgh

RECOMMENDED READING

Powell JJ, Wojnarowska F 1999 Lichen sclerosus. Lancet 353: 1777–1783
Royal College of Obstetricians & Gynaecologists (RCOG) 1999 The management of
    menorrhagia in secondary care. Evidence-based clinical guidelines no 5. Guideline
    summary. RCOG, London

16

Premenstrual syndrome

P.M.S. O'Brien

Definitions   357
Symptoms   358
  Character   358
  Timing   358
Prevalence   359
Consequences   359
Quantifying symptoms and
  diagnosis   359
Aetiology and hypotheses   361
Management   362
  Range of proposed treatment
    regimens   362
Evidence-based approach   362
Non-hormonal therapy   362
Hormonal therapy   363
Surgical approach   364
Clinical management   365
Guide to treatment   366
Premenstrual syndrome in the context
  of family planning   366
Hormone replacement
  therapy-induced premenstrual
  syndrome   367
The future   368

DEFINITIONS

It is very important to be clear what is meant by the term premenstrual syndrome (PMS) as much confusion has been presented in the literature. The terms used in relation to PMS include premenstrual tension (PMT), premenstrual tension syndromes (PMTS), menstrual distress, late luteal phase dysphoric disorder (LLPDD) and premenstrual dysphoric disorder (PMDD). PMS is the term most often used in the UK but this may change.

There has been a reluctance, until relatively recently, to accept PMS as a serious condition. This has arisen because of a failure to distinguish true PMS from the milder physiological premenstrual symptoms, which occur in the normal menstrual cycle of 80–90% of women in their reproductive years. Both have a diverse range of symptoms that occur in the luteal phase of the cycle and resolve by the end of menstruation. Psychological research studies often attempt to deny the existence of PMS because of no or minimal changes in relatively asymptomatic volunteers (e.g. university undergraduates). These data are wrongly extrapolated to women with PMS.

What distinguishes PMS is that the symptoms are so severe that they disrupt the woman's normal functioning and her interpersonal relationships (work and family particularly). There are also women who have an underlying psychological disorder, which co-exists with PMS, and there can be premenstrual exacerbation of a pre-existing psychological disorder.

Finally, there are women who self-diagnose PMS but who actually have depression unrelated to the cycle; these are characterized by the fact that their symptoms fail to resolve after menstruation.

Box 16.1   Patients who may present at the premenstrual syndrome clinic

Physiological premenstrual symptoms
Occur only in the luteal phase.
Resolve completely with menstruation so that there is a symptom-free week between
menstruation and ovulation.
Are *not* severe and do not disrupt normal functioning.

Premenstrual syndrome
Occurs only in the luteal phase of the cycle.
Resolves completely with menstruation so that there is a symptom-free week between
the end of menstruation and ovulation.
Symptoms are severe and have a major effect on normal functioning and interpersonal
relationships.

Premenstrual exacerbation of medical disorder

Premenstrual exacerbation of psychological disease

Co-existing PMS and underlying psychological disorder
Either symptoms of an underlying disorder increase premenstrually or there is PMS
superimposed on an underlying problem. These are difficult to distinguish.
Symptoms resolve with menstruation but only to the level of the background disorder.

Non-cyclical psychological disorder
Patients complain of symptoms which typify PMS but they do not resolve by the end of
menstruation. Alternative diagnoses such as depression, personality disorder,
drug/alcohol abuse and other psychological/psychiatric diagnoses must be
considered.

SYMPTOMS

Character

An enormous range of symptoms has been described: they may be psychological and behavioural, or somatic. As many as 200 have been described in the literature. Typical psychological symptoms include irritability, aggression, tension, depression, mood swings and feeling out of control.

Commonly reported physical symptoms include bloatedness and breast swelling and pain.

It is usually the psychological symptoms that cause the most distress and bring women to seek medical attention.

Timing

The character of symptoms is less important than the timing and severity. For a diagnosis of PMS, the symptoms must occur in the luteal phase of the cycle and resolve by the end of menstruation.

The severity must be sufficient to have a major impact on normal functioning. Women may experience symptoms for any portion of the luteal phase; some in the few days immediately prior to the period, whereas others have symptoms from ovulation right through the luteal phase to the end of menstruation.

PREVALENCE

Accurate prevalence figures cannot be given.

Various papers quote 80–95% of women as having physiological symptoms, which are mild and normal.

Only 5% of women in their reproductive years appear to have absolutely no symptoms before the period.

Estimates for the prevalence of true PMS are around 5%.

CONSEQUENCES

Numerous consequences have been claimed to result from PMS. Though they are based on anecdotal reports, it does seem likely that many serious problems are due to the disorder. These include psychosocial events such as poor work performance, marital problems (perhaps leading to divorce), suicide, murder, arson and child battering.

Certain medical problems also appear to result from PMS, or at least occur in the luteal phase of the cycle; these include behavioural problems, migraine, epilepsy and asthma.

QUANTIFYING SYMPTOMS AND DIAGNOSIS

There seem to be as many methods to measure PMS as there are researchers! Research methods include specific charts, which may be Likert or visual analogue scales, and questionnaires such as the Moos' Menstrual Distress Questionnaire. Recently, a hand-held computer-based technique has been developed to record this information and it is currently under validation (Fig. 16.1). This can be contrasted with a PMS diary from an asymptomatic woman (Fig. 16.2).

For clinical purposes, a prospective symptom-rating diary is most appropriate but in reality most clinicians rely on the history at initial consultation.

The three essential clinical criteria for the diagnosis are that the symptoms:

a. occur in the luteal phase
b. have a major impact on normal functioning
c. disappear by the end of the period.

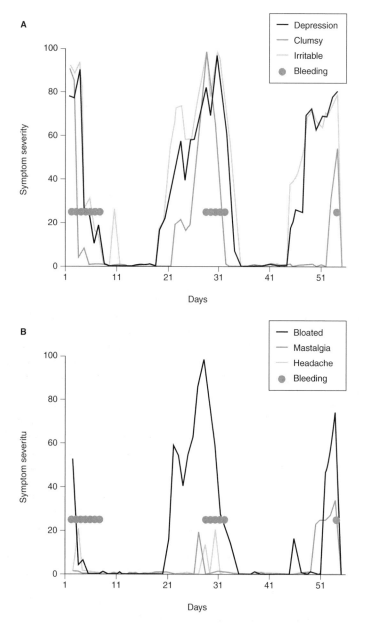

Figure 16.1 PC-screen data from hand-held computer-generated data of a severely affected woman with menorrhagia, dysmenorrhoea and severe psychological and somatic symptoms of PMS. (**A**) Typical psychological symptoms. (**B**) Typical somatic symptoms.

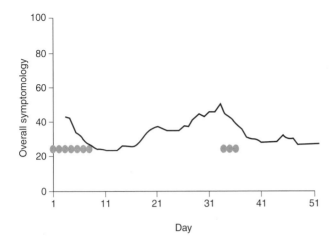

Figure 16.2   Asymptomatic woman with minimal physiological premenstrual changes.

AETIOLOGY AND HYPOTHESES

The underlying cause of PMS has not yet been elucidated but some recent theories are quite convincing and an understanding of them should enable the clinician to comprehend the thinking behind treatment methods currently recommended. Although the concept of a hormone imbalance has been popular, e.g. of progesterone deficiency, no evidence exists to support such theories. Indeed, the current consensus is that PMS sufferers and asymptomatic women do not differ regarding their hormone status. Women with PMS are thought to be *more susceptible to the effects of their normal ovarian hormone cycle* than are asymptomatic women. The reason for the increased sensitivity is thought to be related to neurotransmitter function. Candidates for this include abnormal function of beta-endorphins, GABA, dopamine, acetylcholine and serotonin.

All of the evidence in favour of these theories is indirect, e.g. the evidence for serotonin deficiency relies on research showing (a) that peripheral blood levels of serotonin are reduced and (b) that selective serotonin re-uptake inhibitors (SSRIs) improve symptoms.

If the broad philosophy of these theories is correct, then it appears that the *normal* ovulatory cycle provides the trigger for events in women who have an abnormal response to progesterone (or related steroids) which could result from a deficiency of serotonin function (or other neuropeptides). It is thus a psychoneuroendocrine disorder responding to an ovarian steroid trigger and so approaches to treatment fall into two broad strategies:

1. Correction of the neuroendocrine anomaly.
2. Suppression (or modulation) of the ovarian trigger.

MANAGEMENT

Range of proposed treatment regimens

Until recently, management has not been considered along the lines described above. There have been randomized controlled trials (RCTs) but, in general, most treatment approaches have been based on anecdote. The wide range of therapies claimed probably reflects the high placebo response where almost any therapy produces an apparently favourable initial response. As a result, claims have been made for ovarian irradiation, vitamin B6, progesterone, oestrogen, testosterone, dietary change, magnesium, endometrial resection, hysterectomy, oophorectomy, lithium, antidepressants, psychotherapy, hypnosis, yoga, diuretics and many other logical and illogical approaches.

Evidence-based approach

If we employ only methods that have adequate RCT evidence of accepted quality, then we risk missing some effective therapies; but this is where we should correctly start. In research into PMS therapy, symptoms must be quantified precisely and prospectively. Diagnostic inclusion and exclusion criteria must be strict. The studies must be randomized, double blind, placebo-controlled and include sufficient numbers of patients to demonstrate clinically and statistically significant differences in efficacy between active therapy and control. Clinicians must be aware of these requirements in order to avoid accepting the claims of poor quality treatment studies.

Few studies merit inclusion in good meta-analyses because they fail to meet the above standards. For this reason, few adequate meta-analyses have been published.

Non-hormonal therapy

Diet. All published dietary advice for PMS is not specific and is based on good dietary advice for health. This cannot be criticised but there are no controlled studies demonstrating a specific role for dietary modification in PMS.

The advice to take frequent carbohydrate meals is not supported by trials.

Vitamin B6. A recent meta-analysis by Wyatt et al (1999) has demonstrated the inadequacy of all studies but the trends demonstrated in favour of vitamin B6 provide the justification for large multicentre studies.

Prolonged overdosing with vitamin B6 can produce peripheral neuropathy.

Evening primrose oil. This contains a dietary source of gammalinolenic acid. One systematic literature review demonstrated possible beneficial effects but, at present, adequate evidence exists only for the positive treatment effect in premenstrual breast symptoms (Budieri et al 1996).

Minerals. *Calcium and magnesium.* Research studies are of insufficient quality to recommend magnesium or calcium treatment though limited studies suggest a possible benefit for both.

Alternative therapies. Many alternative therapies have been suggested but they have not been subject to appropriate trials. St John's Wort is the fashionable non-medical remedy and has many effects including serotonergic activity. It may therefore be acting as a weak SSRI.

There are controlled studies to suggest a benefit of exercise and relaxation therapy.

Psychotherapy. Cognitive behavioural therapy has gained widespread acceptance, particularly amongst clinical psychologists. There are some well-controlled studies which demonstrate efficacy over and above that of control therapy though others do not.

Psychotropic drugs. Benzodiazepines, lithium, monoamine oxidase inhibitors and tricyclic antidepressants have been used and assessed in a limited number of trials. SSRIs appear the most effective and there are many well-conducted studies of fluoxetine (at least seven) and sertraline (at least three) which fulfil criteria for meta-analysis (Steiner et al 1995). Dimmock et al (1998) have produced a meta-analysis of all RCTs of the SSRIs; this includes some of the best conducted trials with the most convincing results in PMS research. Somatic as well as psychological symptoms appear to improve with these drugs.

Diuretics. There is convincing evidence that fluid retention is *not* an essential prerequisite of PMS even where bloatedness is a major symptom. Thus there is little logic in giving diuretics. Despite this, diuretics have been prescribed for many years. In trials, only spironolactone demonstrates efficacy in PMS, particularly for somatic symptoms.

Prostaglandin inhibitors. Mefenamic acid and naproxen sodium have been assessed in five RCTs. All reported significant improvement in symptoms. Many PMS sufferers report co-existing menstrual dysfunction and therefore treatment of the latter may well improve general well-being.

Hormonal therapy

Progesterone/progestogens. Despite the popularity of progesterone and progestogens (and the fact that they are currently licensed in the UK for treating PMS) there are surprisingly few supportive data to justify this. There are no systematic reviews of progesterone treatment and of the 12 RCTs available, two of micronized progesterone and two using progesterone suppositories suggest benefit, whilst eight (seven with suppositories and one with an intramuscular injection) show no benefit over placebo (Freeman et al 1990). Three studies of dydrogesterone show benefit whereas four do not. Two of oral medroxyprogesterone acetate showed benefit whilst a third did not. There are no studies of the depot preparations. There are no trials of sufficient quality to assess the value of norethisterone.

Paradoxically, it should be remembered that all progestogens are capable of *causing* PMS when given with oestrogen in hormone replacement therapy (HRT) for the menopause.

The evidence is conflicting.

Oestrogen. Suppression of ovulation with oestradiol patches and implants has been shown to be effective. When given orally (one trial of conjugated oestrogens), there appears to be no benefit over placebo. Trials of oestradiol implants and oestradiol patches (100 μg and 200 μg) demonstrate significant benefit (Watson et al 1989). Oestrogen must be given with progesterone to prevent endometrial hyperplasia, which can result in the return of symptoms. Strategies to prevent this are outlined below.

Danazol. Danazol is no longer licensed for PMS because of concerns of potential masculinizing and lipid-altering side effects; danazol is now used less often. It is, however, very effective as evidenced by five good RCTs.

When given only in the luteal phase of the cycle, it is effective for premenstrual breast symptoms with no more side effects than placebo.

It is thus an effective drug but with the long-term risks of masculinization.

Gonadotrophin releasing hormone (GnRH) agonist analogues. GnRH alone has been demonstrated to be highly effective in seven separate trials. Menopausal side effects, including loss of bone mineral density, limit its use in the long term. These can be countered by administering add-back oestrogen/progesterone or possibly tibolone (Mortola et al 1991).

Bromocriptine. There are many trials which provide good evidence that bromocriptine is *not* effective for PMS except in the management of premenstrual breast symptoms.

Oral contraceptive pill. Four trials have failed to demonstrate superiority over placebo. In theory, continuous pill therapy should be effective but this has not yet been researched.

As many younger women will request the pill for contraception, it may seem worthwhile trying this empirically.

Surgical approach

Hysterectomy and bilateral oophorectomy should be and is, as shown in good studies, curative (Casson et al 1990). Hysterectomy alone reduces but does not eliminate symptoms.

Trials are limited because of the difficulty in providing true controls.

Bilateral oophorectomy alone (e.g. laparoscopically) should be effective, but the need for oestrogen (and thus progesterone) limits its potential.

There is no logical reason why endometrial ablation should be effective, as no 'menotoxin' has been demonstrated. There are no adequate trials in PMS except as an incidental finding in patients who have been randomized to treat menorrhagia.

CLINICAL MANAGEMENT

This evidence points to a large number of inadequately controlled trials on a large number of treatment regimens. It helps only a little with management.

Broadly, treatment aims either to suppress the ovarian cycle trigger by suppressing ovulation, or to correct factors that render women hypersensitive to their hormones by correcting neurotransmitter function.

The SSRIs have been shown to be extremely effective. There are recognized side effects but dependence is not a problem.

The most effective (and possibly permanent) approach is to eliminate ovarian function. However, the more effectively this is achieved, the more serious the unwanted side effects, e.g. hysterectomy with bilateral oophorectomy is the method nearest to achieving a cure for true PMS. The consequences of major surgery, surgical menopause and the need for long-term oestrogen virtually preclude this approach for all but a few severely affected patients and usually those who are to undergo hysterectomy for another indication.

When assessing the treatment for an individual patient, it is necessary to take into account several important factors:

A. The age of the patient and desire for pregnancy in the near or distant future. This will influence whether approaches that are also contraceptive or that require contraception can be used, or if hysterectomy would ever be acceptable.
B. Severity of the symptoms; impact on the quality of her life and that of her family. This will allow the clinician to use a hierarchical approach to therapy and determine if the more invasive means of treatment are justifiable.
C. A woman's preconceptions of the potential method available. She may be convinced that a certain approach is the only acceptable method.
    She may only accept non-hormonal methods, will not accept psychotropics and only wish to use non-medical techniques.
    The patient must always be involved in the decision-making process.
D. The nature of the symptoms:
    a. SSRIs are highly effective for psychological symptoms (but also somatic)
    b. breast symptoms respond to evening primrose oil, luteal phase danazol and bromocriptine
    c. pain responds to non-steroidal anti-inflammatory drugs
    d. somatic symptoms (particularly bloatedness) respond to spironolactone.

GUIDE TO TREATMENT

1. Patients will almost always have explored the simpler approaches including diet, evening primrose oil and vitamin B6. The next stage will involve both doctor and patient.
2. Early resort to the use of SSRIs is increasingly considered acceptable and when there is co-morbid depression, this is a particularly justifiable approach. Experience in the management of depression is required.
3. The use of danazol and GnRH analogues is usually limited by the inadvisability of long-term therapy; this can be prolonged by means of add-back HRT.
4. Oestrogen is an important approach, as it can suppress ovulation without inducing the risks of the menopause; it is effective as both implants and patches. If it proves ineffective in a particular patient, it is possible that a higher dose will be required to achieve suppression of ovulation. If PMS symptoms return in the progestogen phase, then a change of progestogen, reduced dose, reduced duration or intrauterine progestogen should be tried.
5. A symptom-directed approach (as in D above) can be very useful.
6. COC and depot medroxyprogesterone acetate (DMPA) may be useful if contraception is required.

    The levonorgestrel-releasing intrauterine system (LNG-IUS) will give contraception and treat co-existing menstrual problems. It can be used as an adjunct to oestrogen therapy.
7. Progesterone and progestogens are probably not effective but will be required to protect the endometrium when oestrogen is used. We have seen that these are associated, in many cases, with the recurrence of PMS symptoms. Alternative progestogens may then be tried resorting at an early or late stage to the LNG-IUS.

PREMENSTRUAL SYNDROME IN THE CONTEXT OF FAMILY PLANNING

No single medical speciality has ever accepted the responsibility for managing PMS. General gynaecologists rarely have sufficient expertise in the use of psychological interventions and psychotropic drugs.

Psychiatrists have very limited knowledge of endocrinology, gynaecology and family planning.

General practitioners' breadth of knowledge makes them ideally placed to manage most aspects of the problem.

Family planning or community gynaecology doctors will have much of this broad expertise and are in an ideal position to run a specialist PMS service.

As PMS appears in only fertile women, it will inevitably mean that PMS will, on many occasions, influence the choice of contraception:

Barrier methods will not affect PMS symptoms but will be required with several treatment regimens such as danazol, GnRH and oestrogen. There is good evidence to suggest that fluoxetine is safe in pregnancy but advice to use contraception may avoid potential legal difficulties.

Intrauterine device use will not affect symptoms. The LNG-IUS may suppress ovulation in the initial months of use and this is thought to explain a temporary improvement in symptoms. When used in conjunction with oestrogen for ovulation suppression, it appears to be potentially highly effective.

Combined oral contraception (COC) has not been shown to be effective but some patients do improve and in theory the continuous pill use (i.e. the tricycle regimen) should be effective and there is anecdotal experience to support this. An empirical approach is suggested, particularly for young women.

Progestogen-only pills. There is no evidence or rationale for an effect on symptoms.

DMPA. Ovulation is often suppressed and there is anecdotal evidence to suggest a beneficial effect.

Natural family planning, coitus interruptus. These will presumably have no effect on a woman's PMS.

Sterilization should have no influence on symptoms. It may, however, be difficult to convince a woman that, having been sterilized, she should then take hormones or indeed receive an LNG-IUS.

A large multicentre study is required, probably in a family planning setting, to determine the effects of continuous COC compared with DMPA compared with oestrogen plus LNG-IUS.

HORMONE REPLACEMENT THERAPY-INDUCED PREMENSTRUAL SYNDROME

As women with PMS do not have an ovarian hormone imbalance but an inappropriate response to the normal cycle, they also appear to have an inappropriate response when given conventional HRT. This is due to the progestogenic phase of therapy that is essential to protect the endometrium from endometrial hyperplasia or adenocarcinoma. Typically, they complain of mood disorders, irritability, aggression, bloatedness and breast tenderness during the 12 days of progestogen; this mimics PMS.

There are many possible strategies that may avoid this. Women vary enormously in their response. The approach must be empirical. There are no substantial trials to support the suggestions. The potential techniques are:

1. Change the progestogen – women appear to have individual responses to the different progestogens; this is often a disappointing venture.
2. Less frequent progestogen such as 3-monthly – bleeding problems are common when this regimen is used in perimenopausal women.
3. Shorter duration or a lower dose of progestogen in each cycle – this has to be balanced against the potential higher risk of endometrial hyperplasia.
4. Give unopposed oestrogen and no progestogen with regular endometrial assessment (by outpatient Pipelle biopsy) – a calculated risk requiring careful discussion.
5. LNG-IUS – good evidence of avoiding endometrial hyperplasia without significantly causing systemic side effects; irregular bleeding a common initial problem and the LNG-IUS is currently unlicensed for this indication in the UK.
6. Removal of the endometrium by hysterectomy. Hysterectomy is usually considered excessively invasive but may occasionally be the only acceptable treatment for a particular patient.
7. Continuous combined HRT regimens – some evidence that continuous progestogen is tolerated better than sequential preparations.
8. Tibolone – limited evidence though one study reported an improvement in PMS.
9. Selective oestrogen receptor modulators (SERMs) – they do not relieve menopausal symptoms but probably avoid PMS symptoms. Raloxifene could be a useful approach as an alternative to HRT if prevention of osteoporosis is the only indication.
10. Conventional HRT with SSRI – this is theoretical, although there appears to be a proven synergistic effect on mood.

As with the treatment of true PMS, the choice of regimen will depend on many factors including the severity of symptoms, previous PMS, the presence of co-morbid depression, time since menopause and whatever previous therapy the woman has received.

THE FUTURE

1. Education of general practitioners, practice nurses and community psychiatric nurses will provide them with the tools and expertise to diagnose and manage PMS within primary care groups. Healthcare professionals must be educated to distinguish the disorder of PMS from the mild premenstrual symptoms that are experienced by most women.
2. Refinement of cheap, hand-held, patient-friendly computers and programs to collect the large amount of data required to make an accurate diagnosis. The data can be down loaded to a conventional PC for a visual presentation of symptoms to patients and health professionals. This technique makes a very abstract concept highly visual.

3. The availability of an SSRI, which is capable of having an effect when taken intermittently, will increase the acceptability of these drugs, eliminate the stigma and reduce symptomatic side effects.
4. The development of a SERM which will have all of the desirable effects of raloxifene, treat menopausal symptoms, provide contraception and also suppress ovulation in premenopausal women.
5. The future of the management of severe PMS lies in the acceptance by the political and research bodies that this is a serious disorder and future developments in PMS should not be left solely in the hands of the pharmaceutical industry. Large multicentre studies should be established which will have the statistical power to demonstrate if there is evidence of efficacy over and above the high placebo response.

Acknowledgement

Figures 16.1 and 16.2 are reproduced by kind permission of Wyatt KS, Dimmock PW and O'Brien PMS 1999 Unpublished data.

REFERENCES

Budieri D, Li WP, Dornan JC 1996 Is evening primrose oil of value in the treatment of premenstrual syndrome? Controlled Clinical Trials 17: 60–68

Casson P, Hahn PM, Van Vugt DA, Reid RL 1990 Lasting response to ovariectomy in severe intractable premenstrual syndrome. American Journal of Obstetrics and Gynecology 162: 99–105

Dimmock PW, Wyatt KM, O'Brien PMS 1998 Selective serotonin re-uptake inhibitors: An interim systematic review of efficacy in treatment of premenstrual syndrome. British Journal of Obstetrics and Gynaecology 105: 104

Freeman E, Rickells K, Sondheimer SJ, Polansky M 1990 Ineffectiveness of progesterone suppository treatment for premenstrual syndrome. Journal of the American Medical Association 264: 349–353

Mortola JF, Girton L, Fischer U 1991 Successful treatment of severe premenstrual syndrome by combined use of gonadotrophin releasing hormone agonist and estrogen/progestin. Journal of Clinical Endocrinology 72: 252A–252F

Steiner M, Steinberg S, Stewart D, et al 1995 Fluoxetine in the treatment of premenstrual dysphoria. New England Journal of Medicine 332: 1529–1534

Watson NR, Studd JWW, Savvas M, Garnett T, Baber RJ 1989 Treatment of severe premenstrual syndrome with oestradiol patches and cyclical oral norethisterone. Lancet 2: 730–732

Wyatt KM, Dimmock PW, Jones PW, O'Brien PMS 1999 Efficacy of vitamin B6 in the treatment of premenstrual syndrome: systematic review. British Medical Journal 318: 1375–1381

FURTHER READING

Wyatt K, Dimmock P, O'Brien PMS 1999 Premenstrual syndrome, Clinical Evidence 2. BMJ Publishing Group 748–759

17

The menopause

Ailsa Gebbie

Endocrine changes at the
  menopause   372
  Changes in the
    perimenopause   372
Diagnosis of the menopause   372
Consequences of ovarian
  failure   373
  Short-term symptoms   373
  Intermediate symptoms   375
  Long-term symptoms   375
Treatment   378
  Non-hormonal treatment   379
  Oestrogen therapy   379
  Combined oestrogen–progestogen
    therapy   382
  'No period' hormone replacement
    therapy   383
  Contraindications to hormone
    replacement therapy   384

Complications of hormone
  replacement therapy   385
Special considerations   386
  Breast cancer   386
  Venous thromboembolism   387
  Adherence to therapy   388
Clinical management   388
  Assessment of a woman prior to
    hormone replacement
    therapy   388
  Monitoring   389
Contraception for older
  women   390
  Fertility in older women   390
  Pregnancy in older women   390
  Stopping contraception   391
  Contraceptive methods   391
  Hormone replacement therapy
    and contraception   393

The menopause is, by definition, a woman's last spontaneous menstrual period and is a diagnosis made in retrospect following amenorrhoea for 12 months. It occurs on average at the age of 51 years and historical texts reveal that this has remained unchanged for centuries. The majority of women in the UK can anticipate spending at least one-third of their lives in a post-menopausal state as the last century saw a striking increase in the average life expectancy of women to around 80 years.

The transitional phase of fluctuating ovarian function around the time of a woman's last menstrual bleed is known as the 'perimenopause' or 'climacteric'. For most women, this phase of menstrual irregularity lasts around 2 to 3 years although some women date the onset of symptoms attributable to the menopause considerably earlier than this. Women universally refer to the climacteric phase as 'going through the menopause'.

The last two decades have seen considerable scientific interest and research in the area of the menopause. Widespread media coverage has made hormone replacement therapy (HRT) a household name and, increasingly, doctors are offering HRT to women both for relief of acute menopausal symptoms and for prophylaxis against long-term sequelae of oestrogen deficiency. HRT is not a panacea for every ailment of middle-aged women and cannot be universally recommended for all. Although there is criticism of the medical profession by some who believe that the menopause is being over-medicalized, most women benefit from an individual assessment of their menopausal problems and how the risks and benefits of HRT relate to them.

ENDOCRINE CHANGES AT THE MENOPAUSE

The menopause signals the end of reproductive potential with the onset of irreversible ovarian failure. The exhaustion of the ovaries' store of oocytes leads to the cessation of follicular development and ovulation. This results in:

1. A gradual fall in circulating oestradiol and very low levels of circulating oestrogen once ovarian activity has ceased. The predominant oestrogen after the menopause is oestrone which originates from the peripheral conversion of adrenal androgens.
2. A rise in circulating gonadotrophins, follicle stimulating hormone (FSH) and luteinizing hormone (LH), as a result of the removal of the negative feedback effects of oestrogen.
3. Amenorrhoea resulting from the lack of endometrial stimulation by ovarian steroid hormones.

Changes in the perimenopause

The menstrual pattern shows great individual variation, and shortening of the cycle may be the earliest feature. The ovaries become progressively unresponsive to gonadotrophin stimulation with a rise in FSH concentration detectable in the follicular phase of the cycle. Months of amenorrhoea are often interspersed with spells of regular menstruation although there is generally a lengthening of the cycles as the last period approaches. Long cycles usually indicate lack of ovulation and the following menstrual bleed may be particularly heavy owing to prolonged stimulation of the endometrium by unopposed oestrogen.

DIAGNOSIS OF THE MENOPAUSE

Measurement of FSH concentration can be made for diagnostic purposes (> 30 IU/L indicating menopausal levels). A detectable rise of FSH may be found in the first 7 days of cycles early in the perimenopause. In practice, the diagnosis of the menopause is made clinically and it is only occasionally necessary to resort to biochemical investigation. FSH measurement may be helpful if:

1. A premature menopause is suspected, i.e. in a woman less than 45 years.
2. A woman has had a hysterectomy.
3. An older woman is taking the progestogen-only pill (POP) and is amenorrhoeic.

Measurement of oestrogen concentrations, despite being frequently recommended by women's magazines, is not a valid assessment of menopausal status as postmenopausal levels can be similar to those found in the early follicular phase of premenopausal women. Measurement of serum oestradiol levels may be used to monitor therapy in women receiving oestrogen implant therapy.

CONSEQUENCES OF OVARIAN FAILURE

Oestrogen deficiency is responsible for the symptoms experienced by women around the time of their last period. Acute, short-term symptoms, although very unpleasant, are generally self-limiting and are not life-threatening. The long-term consequences of ovarian failure have very important implications for future health and represent a large burden on healthcare resources in the UK.

Short-term symptoms

These symptoms are common, distressing, and cause many previously healthy women to seek medical advice. They are often insidious in onset and frequently misdiagnosed. Quality of life may be severely compromised in some women with menopausal symptoms and should not be ignored in any discussion on the risks and benefits of HRT.

Vasomotor symptoms

1. Hot flushes.
2. Palpitations.
3. Dizziness.
4. Weakness and faintness.

Hot flushes are the commonest menopausal symptom affecting around 80% of women. They tend to begin before the cessation of menstruation, persist on average for 2 to 5 years and are universally perceived as unpleasant and embarrassing.

The flush is felt as a sensation of heat, affecting the upper chest, neck and face, lasting only a few seconds or persisting for several minutes.

Reddening of the face may occur and intense flushes will often be followed by sweating although some women sweat without an initial flush.

Night sweats with disruption of the normal sleep pattern are often particularly troublesome, causing chronic sleep deprivation to both the woman and her partner. Subsequent lethargy and irritability are common.

Flushes can be triggered by stress, hot weather, alcohol and spicy food although most occur without an obvious precipitating factor.

The aetiology and exact physiological mechanism remain unclear. In response to fluctuating declines in oestradiol concentrations, the thermoregulatory centre within the hypothalamus triggers cutaneous vasodilatation and sweating with a rise in skin temperature of up to 5 °C.

Psychological symptoms

Many women report psychological symptoms as a problem in the climacteric years but there is little evidence to support an association between the menopause and frank psychiatric disease. Minor psychological disturbances, not dissimilar to those of the premenstrual syndrome, are common and often correlate with the phase of fluctuating hormone profiles prior to the actual menopause. They are listed in Box 17.1. For perimenopausal women with stressful jobs or in positions of responsibility, many of the symptoms are potentially very disabling. Chronic sleep disturbance from hot flushes and night sweats exacerbate many of these symptoms.

Social stresses can also affect the well-being of a woman around the time of the menopause and may be associated with events such as:

1. Death or illness of an elderly parent.
2. Marital separation or disharmony.
3. Poor job satisfaction.
4. Weight gain and obesity.
5. Difficult teenage children. The 'empty nest syndrome' is frequently quoted in this context but grown-up children who remain in the family home are often more of a problem than those who have 'flown the nest'.

Personality, cultural factors and attitudes to the menopause undoubtedly affect the incidence of psychological symptoms in the climacteric. In a society obsessed with youth and sexual attractiveness, feelings of low self-esteem and poor body image as women approach the end of their reproductive lives are hardly surprising.

Box 17.1   Psychological symptoms of the menopause

Depressed mood
Anxiety
Irritability and mood swings
Emotional lability
Inability to cope
Poor memory
Poor concentration
Indecision
Feeling of worthlessness

Intermediate symptoms

Urogenital atrophy

The tissues of the lower urogenital tract are highly oestrogen-dependent and undergo atrophy as a result of oestrogen deficiency. Older women frequently suffer these symptoms in silence through ignorance and embarrassment.

1. Dryness of the vagina causes dyspareunia, which in turn may result in loss of libido.
2. The vaginal pH increases and the vagina becomes prone to infection with bacterial organisms, as there is loss of the normal colonization with lactobacilli.
3. Dysuria, frequency, urgency and urge incontinence all increase in incidence with advancing age, and arise from atrophic change and loss of collagen support around the bladder neck.

Skin changes

1. There is a generalized loss of collagen from the dermal layer of skin postmenopausally.
2. Women frequently complain of thin, dry skin accompanied by hair loss and brittle nails.
3. Widespread joint and muscle aches are common symptoms and may also be explained by collagen loss.

Long-term symptoms

Osteoporosis

Osteoporosis is defined by the World Health Organization as a 'progressive systemic skeletal disease characterised by low bone mass and micro-architectural deterioration of bone tissue'. It is a silent condition and its clinical significance lies in the fractures that arise. The annual cost of osteoporosis to the UK National Health Service is currently over £940 million and osteoporotic fractures cause severe pain and disability to individual sufferers. Prevention of osteoporosis represents a major public health challenge and unless changes are made in present practice, there will be a doubling of the number of osteoporotic fractures over the next 50 years.

Bone density peaks in women in their mid-30s and, thereafter, declines slowly until a rapid acceleration in loss of bone mass occurs following the menopause. Whether or not a woman develops osteoporosis is determined by her peak bone mass and her rate of bone loss. Women are naturally endowed with a much less dense skeleton than men and their lifetime risk of osteoporotic fractures is more than double that of men.

376 HANDBOOK OF FAMILY PLANNING

Postmenopausal osteoporotic fractures classically affect three main sites:

1. Proximal femur.
2. Distal radius – the Colles' fracture.
3. Thoracic vertebrae – compression fractures cause the typical 'dowager's hump'.

The estimated risks of osteoporotic fractures faced by a 50-year-old woman in her remaining lifetime are:

16% risk of fractured hip.
1–3% risk of dying from complications of hip fracture.
15% risk of fractured wrist.
32% risk of fractured vertebra.
An overall 50% risk of sustaining some fracture.
(Cummings et al 1989).

Risk factors for osteoporosis (Box 17.2) are only, at best, a crude guide to a woman's risk of sustaining osteoporotic fractures. The two major risk factors are being female and postmenopausal! Bone mineral density is an important determinant of fracture risk but other factors such as liability to falls and type of fall also contribute.

Bone mineral density measurement. Assessment of bone mineral density (BMD) can be performed by highly accurate machines, e.g. dual X-ray absorptiometry (DXA). Measurement of BMD is recommended as a case-finding strategy, rather than for population screening, and to assess response to treatment. Quantitative ultrasound techniques can also be used to measure BMD much more cheaply with smaller, portable machines but abnormal results should be confirmed by DXA.

Role of oestrogen. The role of oestrogen in the prevention and treatment of osteoporosis:

1. Oestrogen has an anti-resorptive effect on bone, by suppressing osteoclast activity, and decreases bone turnover.
2. Oestrogen is of proven value and is the treatment of choice for preventing bone loss in perimenopausal women and, more importantly, reducing the incidence of fractures.

Box 17.2 Risk factors for osteoporosis

Premature menopause
Small, slim build
Caucasian racial origin
Steroid therapy
Immobilization
Inactive lifestyle
Cigarette smoking
Diabetes
Chronic liver disease

3. To prevent osteoporotic fractures occurring in women in very old age, treatment with HRT would have to be maintained almost indefinitely. Long-term adherence with HRT is currently poor as most women are only prepared to take it in the short term.
4. Oestrogen can also be used to treat women with established osteoporosis, by preventing further bone loss, and it decreases risk of subsequent fracture.
5. There is no upper age limit for commencing HRT for bone protection. However, elderly women are often intolerant of the hormonal side effects of HRT.

Alternative therapies. Alternative therapies in the prevention and treatment of osteoporosis:

1. Population-based strategies include increasing levels of physical activity, reducing the prevalence of smoking and increasing dietary calcium and vitamin D intake. A poor calcium intake in childhood can affect the peak bone density reached. Calcium supplements with vitamin D reduce risk of fracture in very elderly institutionalized women although there is no good evidence that supplements are of value in perimenopausal women.
2. Bisphosphonates such as etidronate and alendronate are being used primarily in the treatment of established osteoporosis in older age groups.
3. Calcitonin, sodium fluoride and various other agents have been claimed to prevent postmenopausal bone loss but oestrogen treatment is more effective.
4. The selective oestrogen receptor modulators (SERMs), raloxifene and tamoxifen, exert an oestrogen-like effect on bone and appear to decrease risk of breast cancer (p. 383).
5. Prevention of falls in elderly individuals is clearly important and use of hip protectors decreases risk of fracture.

Cardiovascular disease

Cardiovascular disease is the single most important cause of death in both men and women in the western world. Prior to the menopause, deaths in women from cardiovascular disease are uncommon, particularly when compared to men of similar age. There is a marked increase in the incidence of cardiovascular disease and coronary heart disease following the menopause and in women who have had a premature menopause. Loss of ovarian function at the menopause is associated with adverse changes in lipids, glucose and insulin metabolism, body fat distribution, coagulation and arterial function.

There is consistent epidemiological evidence that women using oestrogen replacement have a substantially lower risk of morbidity or death from cardiovascular disease (Grodstein et al 1996). The reduction in risk has been estimated to be about 40–50%. However, a criticism of these population studies is that women who opt to take HRT are a self-selected healthier group, generally at lower risk of cardiovascular disease in the first place. Moreover, most of the women involved in studies reporting a reduction in risk took oestrogen without additional progestogens. The findings of these epidemiological studies have yet to be confirmed by randomized controlled trials (RCTs). A primary prevention trial with large numbers of volunteers is now underway in North America although it is unlikely to report results for many years yet.

Oestrogen is thought to exert a protective effect by two main mechanisms:

1. *Beneficial effects on lipid profile.* Oestrogen appears to induce favourable changes in lipid metabolism but this varies with oestrogen type and delivery system, and can also be affected by choice of progestogen in combined HRT.
2. *A direct effect on the vascular system.* Oestrogen has vasoactive properties and increases blood flow by relaxation of arterioles through a number of synergistic pathways.

Epidemiological studies in the past have also suggested a major beneficial role for oestrogen in the prevention of cardiovascular disease in women with established ischaemic heart disease. However a large, randomized, trial from North America comparing HRT with a placebo in women with ischaemic cardiac disease showed an overall null effect after 4 years (Hulley et al 1998). In fact, in this study the HRT group actually had an excess risk of cardiac death in the first year of use compared with the placebo group.

At the present time, therefore, there is insufficient evidence to recommend universal treatment with HRT for all women for cardiovascular protection.

Other potential benefits

Recent epidemiological data suggest that HRT may offer significant protection against Alzheimer's disease, macular degeneration and colon cancer. These protective effects have yet to be proven by RCTs and at the present time there is insufficient evidence to offer HRT to individual women for the prevention of these conditions alone.

TREATMENT

Treatment of menopausal symptoms with agents other than oestrogen is frequently recommended but gives largely disappointing results. Most studies on alternative therapies for menopausal symptoms demonstrate a marked placebo response.

Non-hormonal treatment

1. The anti-hypertensive agent clonidine (50 µg b.d.) is effective in the short-term management of vasomotor symptoms but most women find that the beneficial effect wears off rapidly.
2. The use of tranquillizers and antidepressants in women with climacteric problems is widespread but, in the absence of frank psychiatric disease, these drugs are probably best withheld until HRT has been tried.
3. An enormous range of over-the-counter preparations is now available. Any benefit probably reflects a placebo response. The phyto-oestrogens, which are derived from plant sources, may exert a weak oestrogenic effect and can be taken by women with contraindications to oestrogen.
4. Progestogen-only therapy has been shown to have a mildly beneficial effect on hot flushes but side effects are frequently troublesome.
5. Some women find techniques such as relaxation, exercise regimens or aromatherapy helpful and self-help groups or nurse-counselling sessions may assist women to cope better with their symptoms.

Oestrogen therapy

As the symptoms of the menopause are caused by oestrogen deficiency, the logical treatment is oestrogen replacement. Progestogen is added to oestrogen in combined HRT preparations for women with an intact uterus to prevent the development of endometrial disease (p. 382).

The oestrogens used in conventional HRT are described as 'natural' because they give rise to plasma oestrogens identical to those produced by the premenopausal ovary. Their pharmacological effect is achieved with plasma levels of oestradiol well within the physiological range. Natural oestrogens are less potent in the dosages within HRT than synthetic oestrogens contained in combined oral contraceptive pills (COCs).

Oestrogen therapy is effective when administered by a variety of routes (Box 17.3) and generally causes few side effects. Choice of how to take systemic HRT is largely a matter of patient preference, although for the majority of women, the cheaper, oral preparations will be acceptable.

A very large number of HRT preparations is now available and in many different combinations of oestrogens and progestogens. A detailed list is available in the British National Formulary and is outwith the scope of this chapter.

Conjugated equine oestrogens (CEE) are widely prescribed for oral oestrogen replacement. Most of the long-term epidemiological HRT data is based on women who took CEE although some women may have ethical

---

Box 17.3   Oestrogen delivery systems

Oral
Transdermal: patches and gels
Subcutaneous: implants
Vaginal: creams, pessaries, tablets and rings
Sublingual or intranasal

---

objections to taking a preparation derived from animal sources. Oestradiol preparations can be prescribed as an alternative.

Oral oestrogens

Advantages

1. Cheap.
2. Convenient.
3. Well tolerated.
4. Easy to stop or change.

Disadvantages

1. 'First pass' through the liver – when oestrogen is taken orally, it passes through the portal circulation to the liver before reaching the systemic circulation and achieving the desired effect. During this 'first pass' through the liver, at least one-third is immediately metabolized to the weak oestrogen, oestrone, which is rapidly excreted. A higher dose of oral oestrogen has to be given compared to transdermal oestrogens to achieve the same therapeutic effect.
2. Occasional nausea and gastrointestinal upset.

Transdermal oestrogens

Transdermal delivery systems allow low-dose oestrogen therapy to be absorbed directly into the systemic circulation. Patches are designed to be changed once or twice weekly and are placed on smooth, dry skin anywhere below the waist. Oestrogen gels are administered once per day and, although widely used on the continent, do not have a large market share in the UK.

Advantages

1. Highly acceptable to women.
2. Convenient to use.
3. Avoid 'first-pass' effect through the liver; therefore, more 'physiological' and can be given in lower dosage. Less effect on hepatic synthesis of other products, e.g. clotting factors and lipoproteins.
4. Combination patches with progestogen are also available.

Disadvantages

1. Expensive.
2. Allergic reactions occasionally occur with patches but are much less common with the newer, single-layered matrix patches than with the older reservoir patches.

Subcutaneous oestrogen implants

These consist of crystalline pellets of oestrogen, which are inserted subcutaneously under local anaesthesia as a minor surgical procedure. The most common sites of insertion are the anterior abdominal wall or buttocks. The standard dose of implant is 50 mg, which is effective for around 6 months. Implants are now less widely used because of the increasing popularity of transdermal patches.

Advantages

1. Compliance is guaranteed.
2. Relatively higher serum oestradiol concentrations can be achieved with implants compared to other methods and this can be particularly beneficial in the treatment of established osteoporosis or severe vasomotor symptoms not relieved by standard dosages of oestrogen.
3. Can be given simultaneously with testosterone implants when loss of libido is a particular problem.

Disadvantages

1. Insertion involves a surgical procedure and a very small risk of bruising and infection.
2. Some women experience the return of many of their menopausal symptoms while their circulating concentrations of oestradiol are very high (tachyphylaxis). These women have to be 'weaned off' oestrogen implants in order to try to reduce their serum oestradiol levels and are a very difficult group to manage.

Vaginal oestrogen delivery systems

Local vaginal treatment with oestrogen is an effective way of improving atrophic change within the lower female genital tract and is prescribed as creams, pessaries, tablets or rings. Lower dose oestrogen preparations are preferable to the older, more potent, creams.

Advantages

1. Can be used by women who do not wish to take systemic HRT or where contraindications exist to its use.
2. Can be used in conjunction with systemic HRT if local symptoms persist despite standard doses of the latter being used.

Disadvantages

1. Elderly women often find difficulty in using creams and for some women they are unacceptably messy.
2. Most vaginal oestrogen preparations are only licensed for use over periods of 3 to 6 months because of the theoretical risk of endometrial cancer thereafter. If treatment is required for longer, the addition of cyclical oral progestogen is recommended for endometrial protection.

Other routes of oestrogen administration

Oestrogen is also rapidly absorbed by the intranasal and sublingual route and a nasal spray oestrogen product is available.

Combined oestrogen–progestogen therapy

Use of unopposed oestrogen replacement substantially increases risk of endometrial cancer. The addition of progestogen to oestrogen-replacement regimens removes excess risk of endometrial cancer. In sequential regimens, progestogen brings about a regular withdrawal bleed and must be given:

1. In adequate dosage.
2. For an adequate number of days each cycle.

In the standard sequential regimens, progestogens are added sequentially for around 12 to 14 days each month. The recommended daily dosages of different progestogens to oppose the effects of oestrogen are listed in Table 17.1. Calendar packs of combined oestrogen and progestogen regimens assist the woman to keep to the correct sequence. Separate prescriptions for oestrogen and progestogen can also be given if a particular combination is not marketed. A 'long cyclic preparation', with a larger dose of progestogen but only administered every 3 months, is also available and will give four withdrawal bleeds per year.

Women who have had a hysterectomy (with a few exceptions such as those with severe endometriosis) do not need to add additional progestogen.

Table 17.1 Progestogens licensed for use in standard, sequential HRT and dosages required

Progestogen*	Dosage
Norethisterone acetate	1 mg
Levonorgestrel	150 µg
Medroxyprogesterone acetate	5–10 mg
Dydrogesterone	10–20 mg

* Each to be administered for 12 to 14 days every month.

'No period' hormone replacement therapy

Continuous combined hormone replacement therapy

Continuous daily administration of both oestrogen and progestogen causes endometrial atrophy and thereby amenorrhoea. This regimen is suitable for women who are at least 1 year postmenopausal. Combined calendar packs are available commercially although separate prescriptions of oestrogen and progestogen can also be given.

1. Spotting in the early months is very common before complete amenorrhoea is achieved.
2. Women get the same beneficial effects on menopausal symptoms and prevention of osteoporosis as with sequential HRT.
3. When given to pre- or perimenopausal women, erratic bleeding frequently occurs because of endogenous ovarian activity.
4. As there is no cyclical effect with this regimen, women appear to tolerate the progestogen better with fewer PMS-type side effects.
5. Long-term adherence with HRT is improved as most women prefer to avoid the return of menstrual bleeding following the menopause.

Tibolone

The synthetic steroid tibolone (Livial) is a C-19 nortestosterone derivative which has weak oestrogenic, progestogenic and androgenic effects. As with other 'no period' preparations, its use should be restricted to women who are at least 1 year postmenopausal. As it has a weak androgen effect, it may have a beneficial effect in women with loss of libido and low mood. It is at present significantly more expensive than conventional HRT preparations.

Selective oestrogen receptor modulators

Several oestrogen-like compounds exist which exhibit differential effects on oestrogen receptors in the body.

Raloxifene is licensed for the prevention of vertebral osteoporosis and appears to exert a beneficial effect on lipid profile (Delmas et al 1997). It does not stimulate the endometrium and preliminary data suggest that it substantially reduces risk of breast cancer.

Tamoxifen is widely prescribed to prevent recurrence of breast cancer and is also protective to bone. In contrast to raloxifene, it causes endometrial stimulation and increases risk of endometrial cancer.

Neither raloxifene nor tamoxifen helps vasomotor symptoms which may be particularly troublesome with tamoxifen.

Contraindications to hormone replacement therapy

Absolute

The very few absolute contraindications to oestrogen therapy are listed in Box 17.4. Unfortunately, over the years, many contraindications to the COC pill have been extrapolated to HRT use and are inappropriately listed on the data sheets of HRT preparations.

Relative

Among those commonly encountered are:

1. Hypertension – women with controlled hypertension can be prescribed HRT but must be monitored carefully. If a woman is found to be hypertensive, an appropriate antihypertensive agent should be prescribed before HRT is commenced.
2. Previous episode of deep vein thrombosis or pulmonary embolism – this will require full evaluation and most women should be referred for a pretreatment thrombophilia screen and specialist advice.
3. Gallbladder disease – oestrogen can alter the composition of bile in a way that may predispose to gallstone formation. The non-oral routes of oestrogen delivery are probably preferable.
4. Fibroids – these may enlarge with HRT and cause bleeding problems. Withdrawal of treatment or even hysterectomy may have to be considered.
5. Endometriosis – this may be reactivated by oestrogen replacement but depends on the amount of residual disease present. Use of additional progestogen can reduce the risk of recurrence.
6. Previous myocardial infarction (MI) or cerebrovascular accident (CVA) – HRT can be given with careful monitoring after 3 to 6 months have elapsed.
7. Cancer – HRT has no effect on the majority of cancers.
   Endometrial cancer was previously considered an absolute contraindication. Women who have early stage disease and appear disease-free after treatment may take low-dose HRT following specialist advice.
   Breast cancer is still considered a complete contraindication for most women. Each woman should, however, be assessed individually and, for

Box 17.4   Absolute contraindications to HRT
Unexplained vaginal bleeding Pregnancy Breast cancer (see p. **385**) Severe, active liver disease Active thromboembolic disease

some with severe menopausal symptoms, improving quality of life with HRT may outweigh a theoretical risk of reactivation of breast cancer. Several small studies have in fact shown no increased risk of recurrence or death when HRT is prescribed for women with breast cancer.

Neither previous cervical nor ovarian cancer represents a contraindication.

Malignant melanoma is not a contraindication.

Complications of hormone replacement therapy

Oestrogen causes few side effects. Unfortunately, the addition of progestogen may cause troublesome side effects. These are common and lead to many women discontinuing HRT after only a few months of therapy.

Side effects of oestrogen

1. Nausea.
2. Breast tenderness and bloatedness.
3. Leg cramps.
4. Migraine.

Management

1. Reduce dose of oestrogen.
2. Change route of administration.
3. Try alternative oestrogen.

Side effects of progestogen

1. Regular monthly withdrawal bleeds which may be heavy, prolonged or painful.
2. Premenstrual syndrome-type symptoms of irritability, depression, breast pain, fluid retention and bloating.

Management

1. Reduce dose and duration of progestogen to minimum recommended for endometrial protection.
2. Change progestogen to C-21 progestogen derivatives (dydrogesterone or medroxyprogesterone acetate) which are less androgenic and generally tolerated better.
3. Change from oral progestogen to a vaginal progestogen gel or a progestogen-releasing intrauterine system.
4. Stopping progestogen completely is not recommended, but some women opt to do this. Regular endometrial biopsies and transvaginal scans are mandatory. The increased risk of endometrial cancer persists for many years after oestrogen treatment has been stopped.

5. Use of the continuous–combined regimen or tibolone (p. **383**).
6. Endometrial resection or ablation.
7. Hysterectomy.

SPECIAL CONSIDERATIONS

Breast cancer

Currently 1 in 12 women in the UK will develop breast cancer. Although it is still a much less common cause of death than arterial disease, it is a disease that affects relatively younger women and is universally feared.

A large re-analysis of 90% of the epidemiological data on the relationship between use of HRT and breast cancer has been undertaken (Collaborative Group on Hormonal Factors in Breast Cancer 1997).

Their findings are that:

1. Amongst current users of HRT, there is a small increase in the risk of breast cancer which rises with increasing duration of usage (Fig. 17.1 and Table 17.2).
2. The effect of HRT on risk of breast cancer is comparable to the effect of delaying the menopause.
3. Five years after stopping HRT, the excess risk of breast cancer disappears.
4. Women who develop breast cancer while taking HRT appear to have less risk of spread beyond the breast.

It is not known if the risk of HRT is increased in those with a strong family history of breast cancer or a past history of benign breast disease. There is no current consensus as to whether addition of progestogen confers any advantage or adds any additional risk in terms of development of breast cancer.

Table 17.2 Absolute risks of developing breast cancer whilst taking HRT. For women aged 50 not using HRT, about 45 in every 1000 will have breast cancer diagnosed over the next 20 years, i.e. up to age 70. For those who use HRT for long periods of time, the estimated number of extra cancers is shown below. (Reproduced with permission from Collaborative Group on Hormonal Factors in Breast Cancer 1997 Breast cancer and hormone replacement therapy: collaborative reanalysis of data from 51 studies of 52 705 women with breast cancer and 108 411 women without breast cancer. Lancet 350:1047–1059.)

Length of time on HRT	Extra breast cancers in HRT users, above the 45 occurring in non-users, over 20 years
5 years use	2 per 1000
10 years use	6 per 1000
15 years use	12 per 1000

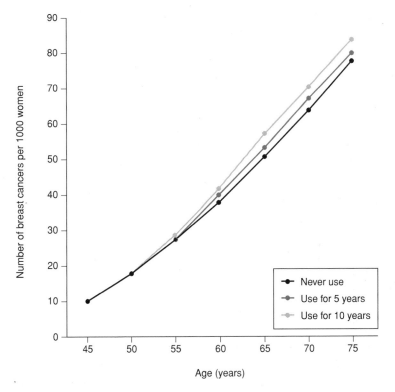

Figure 17.1 Estimated cumulative number of breast cancers diagnosed in 1000 never-users of HRT, 1000 users of HRT for 5 years, and 1000 users of HRT for 10 years (with assumption that HRT use began at age 50 years). (Reproduced with permission from Collaborative Group on Hormonal Factors in Breast Cancer 1997 Breast cancer and hormone replacement therapy: collaborative reanalysis of data from 51 studies of 52 705 women with breast cancer and 108 411 women without breast cancer. Lancet 350:1047–1059.)

Venous thromboembolism

Although it was originally thought that the natural oestrogens contained within HRT did not increase risk of venous thromboembolism (VTE), several epidemiological studies have now confirmed that there is a two- to four-fold increase in risk of VTE in women taking HRT. Women with risk factors for VTE such as obesity, varicose veins or previous superficial thrombophlebitis should be carefully counselled prior to commencing HRT. There is no indication to stop HRT routinely prior to surgery provided appropriate thromboprophylaxis, such as heparin, is used (RCOG Guideline 1999).

Adherence to therapy

Despite publicity of the well-established benefits, adherence to long-term therapy is relatively poor. Less than 60% of women who start HRT are still taking it after 1 year. Fear of breast cancer tends to discourage women from starting treatment and the withdrawal bleeds and cyclical progestogenic side effects often cause women to stop treatment after only a brief trial. Tolerance of 'no period' preparations is generally better than of those that cause withdrawal bleeding. Women also need to be given realistic expectations of what HRT will and will not help. Many women are disappointed when they try HRT and find that it is not the 'elixir of life'. Women taking HRT need good back-up support from healthcare advisers and may have to try several different preparations before they find one that suits them.

CLINICAL MANAGEMENT

Assessment of a woman prior to hormone replacement therapy

The initial consultation is an opportunity to discuss how the pros and cons of HRT relate to that individual woman. Use of menopause clinic proforma sheets can be helpful and a trained menopause nurse can do much of the basic information-giving.

History

1. Current symptoms attributable to the menopause; use of a symptom-rating questionnaire is often helpful.
2. Menstrual and gynaecological history.
3. Past medical history, noting any contraindication to HRT use.
4. Family history, particularly breast cancer, ischaemic heart disease and stroke at a young age, and osteoporosis.
5. Social history: employment, smoking, current relationship and any sexual problems.

Examination

1. BP.
2. Weight.
3. Teach breast awareness and self-examination.
4. Routine breast and pelvic examinations are not mandatory, but they should always be performed if there are any symptoms or significant past medical history. Women seeking HRT are generally in the peak age

group for breast and ovarian cancer and it may be wise to consider undertaking breast and pelvic examinations for medicolegal reasons.

Investigations

In practice, investigations are usually not necessary but may be indicated by the history or examination (Box 17.5).

In some younger women, particularly those who are still menstruating, it may not be clear whether symptoms are attributable to the menopause or not. A therapeutic trial of HRT for 3 months is often worthwhile and if there is no clear benefit in that time, an alternative diagnosis, such as premenstrual syndrome or depression, should be sought.

Monitoring

There is no absolute agreement as to how often women should be followed-up or what exactly should be monitored. By convention, however, the first follow-up visit is usually after 3 months and, thereafter, visits can be 6 monthly or more frequently if problems arise.

History

1. Assess degree of symptom relief; oestrogen dose can be increased if necessary.
2. Note bleeding pattern.
3. Assess any side effects.

Examination

1. BP.
2. Weight. Weight gain is a major issue with almost all women and is frequently attributed to HRT use. Excess weight gain is a feature of increasing age and studies show HRT-users put on less weight overall

---

Box 17.5   Investigations which may be indicated prior to prescribing HRT

Full blood count
Thyroid function tests
Hormone profile
Thrombophilia screen
Pelvic ultrasound scan
Endometrial biopsy and hysteroscopy
Bone density scan
Mammography
Lipid screen

than non-HRT-users. Advice and support on dieting and exercise should always be offered.
3. Confirm that women are 'breast aware'. Routine breast examination may be falsely reassuring and over 90% of breast cancers are detected by women themselves.
4. Routine 3-yearly cervical smear and mammogram if within the age limits for screening. Breast and pelvic examination should always be performed in the presence of any abnormal symptoms but are not mandatory at follow-up visits.

Duration of use

There is no hard and fast rule as to how long HRT can be continued. For relief of acute menopausal symptoms, most women will require therapy for 3 to 5 years. To prevent osteoporosis in very elderly women, treatment would have to be continued almost indefinitely and this has to be weighted against the small increase in breast cancer with prolonged duration of usage. The decision is an individual one and many women discontinue HRT without recourse to medical advice while others are extremely reluctant ever to stop.

CONTRACEPTION FOR OLDER WOMEN

Fertility in older women

The oldest mother on record in the UK to give birth following a natural conception was 54 years old although advances in assisted conception techniques using donor eggs have made pregnancy possible far beyond this age. Prior to the menopause, fertility decreases with age and conception rates begin to decline from mid-30s onwards. The quality of oocytes produced is generally poorer in older women and this is almost certainly the major factor which reduces conception rates. Ovulation usually continues to occur up to the perimenopause.

In stable relationships, frequency of intercourse declines with age. Married women aged 40 years have intercourse on average half as often as married women of 20 years do. However, as divorce rates rise, coital frequency inevitably increases as new relationships begin in relatively older age groups.

Pregnancy in older women

Pregnancy above the age of 40 years increases the risks to both mother and fetus although with optimum care, obstetric outcome should be good.

1. Maternal and perinatal mortality rates increase.

2. Miscarriages and chromosomal abnormalities, particularly Down's syndrome, increase in incidence. While screening and termination of pregnancy are an option, this presents moral and ethical dilemmas many older women could well do without.
3. Around 50% of all pregnancies in women over 40 years end in therapeutic abortion. This is a higher rate than in teenage populations.
4. Unwanted or unplanned pregnancies in this age group are often accompanied by a sense of shame or frustration and may well be psychologically and socially catastrophic.

Stopping contraception

As a rule of thumb, women are advised to continue contraception for 1 year after the last spontaneous period if aged 50 years or over, and for 2 further years following the last spontaneous period if less than 50. As fertility declines with age, most methods become almost 100% effective.

Contraceptive methods

Combined oral contraception

Selected, healthy, non-smoking women without risk factors can be prescribed low-dose combined preparations up to the age of 50 years provided they are carefully monitored.

Substantial benefits from taking COC in the later reproductive years include:

1. High contraceptive efficacy.
2. Excellent cycle control.
3. Reduced incidence of menorrhagia, dysmenorrhoea and premenstrual syndrome. Older women taking COC are much less likely to be admitted to hospital for minor and major gynaecological operations.
4. Probable added protection against osteoporotic fractures in later life.
5. Relief of early menopausal symptoms.
6. Protection against both endometrial and ovarian carcinoma.

However, these advantages have to be balanced against the possible disadvantages:

1. Very small risk of serious arterial thrombosis.
2. Very slightly increased risk of breast cancer with current COC usage (p. **68**).

Although overall the data on COC use and breast cancer are reassuring, the slight increase in relative risk of developing breast cancer is of more concern to older women because the background incidence of breast cancer is higher in their age group (Collaborative Group on Hormonal Factors and Breast Cancer 1996).

Women with risk factors, particularly those who smoke cigarettes, should still discontinue COC at the age of 35 years because of increased risk of serious arterial disease.

Stopping combined oral contraception. COC will stimulate withdrawal bleeds and mask any menopausal symptoms even though a woman may be menopausal. When a COC-user reaches the age of 50 years, the POP or a barrier method can be substituted. This will then allow assessment of the menstrual cycle and any menopausal symptoms. In the absence of subsequent menstruation, an FSH concentration can be measured. If this is within the menopausal range, the barrier method or POP should be continued for 1 further year. If FSH concentration is within the premenopausal range, the woman should continue the barrier method or POP and follow the general rules for stopping contraception.

Progestogen-only contraception

The progestogen-only pill. This is an excellent and safe form of contraception for older women with almost no contraindications. It is virtually 100% effective in this age group with failure rates equivalent to that of COC use in women in their 20s. Poor cycle control is its main drawback. Many older women become amenorrhoeic with POP use which causes them anxiety regarding possible pregnancy, although amenorrhoea is actually an indicator of high efficacy. Others experience excessive or irregular menstrual loss, which can lead to unnecessary gynaecological intervention.

Women who are amenorrhoeic on POP may be uncertain as to their menopausal status. Measurement of FSH concentration is a valid way of assessing this, as the POP does not exert a suppressive effect on gonadotrophins. It may be helpful to measure FSH concentrations annually in women over 45 years taking the POP who are amenorrhoeic.

Depot medroxyprogesterone acetate (DMPA). This is a highly effective method of contraception at all ages and amenorrhoea is a common feature. Some women who are amenorrhoeic with DMPA become relatively hypo-oestrogenic and this has led to concern regarding development of low BMD and increased risk of osteoporotic fracture (p. **93**). Although there is no absolute consensus on this issue, it may be wise to consider stopping DMPA at 45 years of age if treatment has been prolonged, in order to allow time for any recovery of bone loss before the menopause is reached.

Intrauterine devices

Failure, expulsion, infection, perforation and ectopic pregnancy rates are all reduced in older IUD-users. The criteria for insertion remain as for younger women, although careful account should be taken of the menstrual pattern prior to insertion in older women who may already have menorrhagia or dysfunctional bleeding. In this age group, copper devices remain effective far longer than the manufacturers' arbitrary 3 or 5 years, and any device inserted after a woman's 40th birthday can remain in situ, unchanged, until a year following the last menstrual period. IUDs should always be removed from postmenopausal women.

The levonorgestrel-releasing intrauterine system (LNG-IUS) is a particularly useful method of contraception for older women with excessive menstrual loss (p. 111). Although currently only licensed for contraception, it can be used in conjunction with systemic oestrogen as HRT in perimenopausal women, avoiding the need for systemic progestogen to be given.

Barrier methods

Condoms. Condoms should be recommended for personal protection against infection in new relationships at all ages although older couples may find it awkward to start using them for the first time. They may exacerbate erectile problems in older men although some men find they help them to maintain an erection. Some oil-based lubricants and antifungal vaginal preparations can affect the tensile strength of condoms and increase the chance of them bursting.

Diaphragms. These are relatively more popular in the older age group and for some the additional lubrication provided by spermicide is advantageous in the presence of vaginal dryness. Uterovaginal prolapse in a parous older woman may make secure retention of a diaphragm difficult.

Natural family planning

As this relies on the ability to recognize signs of ovulation, it is often difficult to use when cycles are irregular or anovulatory in the perimenopause. It can be appropriate if there are religious or ethical objections to all other methods.

Hormone replacement therapy and contraception

Conventional HRT is not reliably contraceptive and if it is given to a woman who is still menstruating, contraception should be recommended as well. Barrier methods, an IUD and POP can all be used in conjunction with HRT. For simplicity, the POP should be added to a sequential HRT preparation as a separate prescription. This appears to be effective and is being quite widely prescribed although no scientific data exist on the efficacy of this combination.

Once HRT has been started, it becomes impossible to give an accurate indication of when contraception can safely be discontinued. Two possible strategies exist:

1. Contraception can arbitrarily be continued until the age of 55 which is assumed to be the upper limit of fertility. For example, an IUD which is not causing any problems can remain in situ until this time.
2. HRT can be stopped briefly for around 2 months. If the woman is amenorrhoeic and has vasomotor symptoms, an FSH concentration can be measured. If this is raised, then contraception can be discontinued after 1 further year. If there is spontaneous menstruation or a low FSH concentration, then contraception should be continued and the exercise repeated 1 year later.

REFERENCES

Collaborative Group on Hormonal Factors in Breast Cancer 1996 Breast cancer and hormonal contraceptives: collaborative reanalysis of individual data on 53 297 women with breast cancer and 100 139 women without breast cancer from 54 epidemiological studies. Lancet 347:1713–1727
Collaborative Group on Hormonal Factors in Breast cancer 1997 Breast cancer and hormone replacement therapy: collaborative reanalysis of data from 51 studies of 52 705 women with breast cancer and 108 411 women without breast cancer. Lancet 350:1047–1059
Cummings SR, Black D, Rubin SM 1989 Lifetime risk of hip, Colles' or vertebral fracture and coronary heart disease among white postmenopausal women. Archives of Internal Medicine 149:2445–2448
Delmas PD, Bjarnason NH, Mitlak BH et al 1997 Effects of raloxifene on bone mineral density, serum cholesterol concentrations, and uterine endometrium in postmenopausal women. New England Journal of Medicine 337:1641–1647
Grodstein F, Stampfer MJ, Manson JE et al 1996 Postmenopausal estrogen and progestin use and the risk of cardiovascular disease. New England Journal of Medicine 335: 453–461
Hulley SB, Grady D, Bush T et al for the HERS Research Group 1998 Randomized trial of estrogen plus progestin for secondary prevention of coronary heart disease in postmenopausal women. Journal of the American Medical Association 230: 605–613
Royal College of Obstetricians and Gynaecologists (RCOG) 1999 Hormone replacement therapy and venous thromboembolism. Guideline No. 19. RCOG, London

18

Contraceptives of the future

Paul F. A. Van Look

The need for new contraceptives   395
Improving existing methods   398
  Male sterilization   398
  Female sterilization   399
  Combined oral
    contraceptives   400
  Progestogen-only pills   400
  Implants   401
  Injectable contraceptives   401
  Intrauterine devices   403
  Male condoms   403

Vaginal barrier methods   404
Natural family planning   405
The search for new methods   407
  Contraception for men   407
  Gonadotrophin releasing hormone
    analogues   409
  Steroid hormone receptor
    antagonists   409
  New delivery systems for steroid
    hormones   412
  Antifertility vaccines   413

THE NEED FOR NEW CONTRACEPTIVES

The 20th century witnessed extraordinary population growth. During the last century, world population increased from 1.65 billion to 6 billion, and experienced both the highest rate of population growth (averaging 2.04% per year) during the late 1960s, and the largest annual increment (86 million persons each year) in the late 1980s. According to United Nations population estimates, the 6 billion mark was reached on 12 October 1999 – an historic milestone. This was the shortest period of time in world history for a billion people to be added (Table 18.1). World population will continue to increase substantially during the 21st century; current projections indicate that it will stabilize at just above 10 billion persons after 2200. Thus, the 21st century is expected to be one of slower population growth than the previous century, and to be characterized by declining fertility and the ageing of populations. Demographic changes during the coming century, however, will be influenced markedly by the rate of decline in fertility which, in turn, depends strongly on the level of contraceptive use.

Over the last three to four decades, there has been an impressive rise in the use of contraceptives all over the world. It has been estimated that, in 1998, up to 58% of all married women of reproductive age or their partners were using a method of contraception (Table 18.2). At that time, the prevalence of use of modern methods in both developed and developing regions was about the same, 51% and 50%, respectively. However, significant differences exist between the more developed and the less developed parts of the world in the types of fertility-regulating methods used. In the less developed regions, some 45% of women practising contraception

Table 18.1 World population milestones

World population reached:
  1 billion in 1804
  2 billion in 1927 (123 years later)
  3 billion in 1960 (33 years later)
  4 billion in 1974 (14 years later)
  5 billion in 1987 (13 years later)
  6 billion in 1999 (12 years later)

World population may reach:
  7 billion in 2013 (14 years later)
  8 billion in 2028 (15 years later)
  9 billion in 2054 (26 years later)
  10 billion in 2183 (129 years later)

Source: UN Population Division, 1999a.

Table 18.2 Percentage of couples with woman at reproductive age using a contraceptive method

	World			More developed regions			Less developed regions		
	1983	1987	1998	1983	1987	1998	1983	1987	1998
All methods	51	53	58	70	71	70	45	48	55
Modern methods	42	44	50	46	47	51	40	44	50

Sources: Khanna et al 1994; UN Population Division 1999b.
Modern methods in this table include: female and male sterilization, oral pills, injectable methods, intrauterine devices, vaginal barrier methods (cervical cap, diaphragm, spermicides) and the condom.

rely on female or male sterilization and another 25% use an intrauterine device (IUD) (Table 18.3). In contrast, in the more developed regions, use is more evenly spread amongst the different methods and a substantial proportion of users relies on the more traditional methods of withdrawal and periodic abstinence (rhythm or natural family planning methods). Of interest to note is the nearly five-fold difference between the more developed and less developed regions in the use of the condom, and the apparent absence of any rise in condom use in the less developed regions in spite of the major condom promotion efforts made during the last decade by HIV/AIDS prevention programmes.

It has been estimated that there are some 120 million women in developing countries who are not practising family planning despite wishing to avoid pregnancy. This applies particularly in Africa where the needs of less than one third of all potential users are being met. But the most telling statistic by far of our inability to provide safe, effective, accessible, acceptable and affordable methods of family planning is the fact that, worldwide, some 46 million unwanted pregnancies are terminated each year. About 20 million

Table 18.3 Percentage distribution of current contraceptive users by type of method and year

	World		More developed regions		Less developed regions	
	1987	1998	1987	1998	1987	1998
Female sterilization	29	33	11	12	37	39
Male sterilization	8	7	6	7	9	8
Pill	14	14	20	24	11	11
Injectable	2	3	–	<1	2	4
Intrauterine device	20	22	8	9	25	26
Condom	9	8	18	19	5	4
Vaginal barrier	1	1	3	3	1	<1
Rhythm	7	5	13	9	4	4
Withdrawal	8	7	19	17	4	4
Others	2	1	2	1	2	1

Sources: Khanna et al 1994; UN Population Division 1999b.

of these abortions are induced under unsafe conditions and about 78 000 women each year die as a result (Division of Reproductive Health 1998). The yearly number of unplanned pregnancies caused by contraceptive failure has been estimated at between 8 and 30 million.

Until the 1970s, contraceptive research was for the most part carried out in the private sector by large pharmaceutical companies, but at the present time only a few major contraceptive manufacturers remain involved.

The reasons for this reduced involvement are cited as:

1. Product liability, coupled with the high cost of insurance to cover contraceptive development and introduction, particularly in the USA.
2. Stringent regulatory requirements for product approval, resulting in a long and expensive registration process and a concomitant decrease in patent protection.
3. A dearth of ideas for fundamentally new products.
4. A hostile political climate, particularly in the USA.
5. Competition from the public sector through the provision of free or low-priced contraceptives in developing countries.

More recently it has been suggested that there are two main reasons for the reduced involvement of industry in contraceptive research.

1. Pharmaceutical companies make most of their profit in developed countries where contraceptive use is already very high.
2. It is extremely expensive to develop new products – US$200–300 million over 10 to 15 years to bring a new drug on to the market, compared to US$25–50 million over 3 to 7 years to adapt existing drugs to new delivery systems.

Fortunately, a number of not-for-profit, public sector agencies such as the UNDP/UNFPA/WHO/World Bank Special Programme of Research,

Development and Research Training in Human Reproduction, the Population Council, and the Contraceptive Research and Development (CONRAD) Program, to name but three, continue their efforts to improve existing methods and develop new ones.

The main research leads currently being pursued and which may ultimately result in new contraceptive products are, first, work aimed at improving existing methods and, second, development of new methods.

IMPROVING EXISTING METHODS

In recent years, the improvements in several of the present methods of family planning include the introduction of new approaches to emergency contraception, once-a-month injectables and the development of new progestogen-only implants. Further advances can be expected for some of these methods in the near future.

The worldwide increase in the incidence of sexually transmitted infections (STIs), particularly HIV infection, has stimulated renewed interest in barrier methods for both men and women and has increased investment in the search for vaginal agents that have microbicidal as well as spermicidal activity (i.e. methods offering dual protection against pregnancy and infection).

Attempts are being made to develop simpler procedures for male and female sterilization in recognition of the fact that sterilization is the method of contraception used by the largest number of people in the world and that this is likely to remain so for the foreseeable future.

Male sterilization

Vasectomy is easier to perform and associated with fewer complications than female sterilization yet, worldwide, the number of couples with a woman of reproductive age who were relying on vasectomy was estimated in 1995 to be about 39 million whereas there were estimated to be more than 185 million couples relying on female sterilization. Behavioural research suggests that the necessity for a skin incision and lack of certain reversibility limit acceptability of male sterilization. Two major technical improvements, *no-scalpel method of vasectomy* and the *percutaneous, non-surgical vas occlusion technique*, have been developed to overcome these limitations (Ch. 7). A recent approach to non-surgical vas occlusion being studied in early clinical trials involves a single injection, into the vas deferens, of a preparation of styrene maleic anhydride dissolved in dimethyl sulphoxide (Guha et al 1998). In monkeys, this approach to intravasal sterilization has been shown to be reversible.

Valves and plugs

Various devices that are surgically inserted into the vas deferens to block sperm transport have also been tested but it has proved difficult to anchor them, and there have been problems with vas erosion and inflammatory reactions.

Female sterilization

Despite the large demand for female sterilization, there have been surprisingly few technological developments during the last few decades in methods either of approach to the fallopian tube or of tubal occlusion. Attempts to overcome the disadvantages of transabdominal approaches to the tubes initially focused, during the 1970s, on procedures carried out through the anterior or posterior vaginal fornix, but these procedures have gradually been abandoned. Subsequent research has been directed at occluding the cornual portion of the tubes via the uterine cavity either under direct hysteroscopic visualization of the tubal ostia or through blind instillation of occluding substances, but so far these attempts at transcervical sterilization have for the most part been unsuccessful. Procedures that have been investigated include those outlined below.

Cautery of the uterotubal junction and the interstitial portion of the tube

Failure rates are high and several interstitial or cornual ectopic pregnancies as well as thermal injury to bowel have been reported.

More recent attempts to use laser coagulation of the tubal ostia have also proved to be unsuccessful.

Occlusive plugs

Materials that may be either pre-formed or formed-in-place are used.

1. *The hydrogel plug or P-block.* This is a pre-formed plug that is inserted through the hysteroscope into the lumen of the tube where it hydrates and swells to occlude the tube.
2. *The Ovabloc.* A formed-in-place occlusive plug made of silicone. As in the male, it was hoped that these plugs would provide an effective and readily reversible method of tubal occlusion. However, rates of tubal occlusion and reversal are poor and insertion can be difficult.
3. *The Hamou tubal plug* blocks the tubes with a nylon or plastic thread. As with the other approaches, there have been problems with plugs migrating or breaking, resulting in high pregnancy rates.

4. *STOP*. This is a screw-like metal coil device that springs open upon release in the fallopian tube. It is in early clinical trials in Australia, Belgium and the USA and, if proven effective, could be available widely in 2 to 3 years according to its developers.

Chemical occlusion

This is the method that holds the greatest promise but the ideal chemical, i.e. one without toxic properties that will rapidly sclerose and occlude the tubal lumen and can be delivered in a reliable and simple manner to a defined segment of the tube, has yet to be found.

The most often used tubal sclerosant has been quinacrine hydrochloride (Ch. 7). Recently, the long-term safety of quinacrine has been questioned and this has led to the initiation of animal carcinogenicity studies. Another compound under study in animal models is streptomycin.

Combined oral contraceptives

Much of the research aimed at producing new types of oral contraceptive pills has resulted in lower dose, multiphasic and combiphasic preparations, and the development of new progestogens such as etonogestrel, gestodene and norgestimate and, more recently, trimegestone and drospirenone. This last compound also has antimineralocorticoid and anti-androgenic activities. The antimineralocorticoid (natriuretic) action counteracts the fluid-retaining effects of ethinyloestradiol, whereas the anti-androgenic activity has beneficial effects on acne and related skin conditions. Some work has been done to find new oestrogens such as oestrogen sulfamates to replace ethinyloestradiol in combined oral contraceptives (COCs), but these new compounds have not yet reached the stage of clinical trials.

In an attempt to reduce the incidence of side effects associated with oral pill use, a trial of vaginal insertion of the standard combined pills (50 μg ethinyloestradiol plus 250 μg levonorgestrel, marketed in Brazil as Lovelle) showed that there were no benefits and indeed there was an increased incidence of vaginal discharge (Coutinho et al 1993). The adverse metabolic effects on lipids and lipoproteins appeared to be reduced, but this requires confirmation.

For women who are comfortable with the vaginal route of administration, vaginal rings that release both an oestrogen and a progestogen may provide a better alternative (see below).

Progestogen-only pills

No major research is in progress in this area although it can be anticipated that progestogen-only pills (POP) containing the newer progestogens will be introduced in the next few years.

Implants

The basic concept behind implants is that by maintaining a continuous sustained release of steroid hormone, the contraceptive effect can be achieved with a much smaller daily dose than when the same steroid is given by the oral or intramuscular route. In addition, metabolic side effects are reduced by avoiding the first pass through the liver.

To date, all implants used in female contraception release a progestogen and their main side effects are menstrual disturbances and amenorrhoea, similar to other progestogen-only methods.

Research on second-generation implants is focusing on reducing the number of capsules and on using steroids with better pharmacological profiles.

Development of biodegradable implants that would not need to be removed was also being pursued in the 1980s and early 1990s. This work has been abandoned, however, because of concern about the long washout period that would exist after the physical integrity of the device was weakened to the point where it could no longer be removed. Contraceptive implants for men are also being investigated (p **408–409**).

Non-biodegradable implants

Norplant, Norplant II (Jadelle), Uniplant and Implanon – see Chapter 3

Sino-plant. This is a two-rod levonorgestrel-releasing system with each rod containing 75 mg of the progestogen. No data have yet been published outside China on the performance of this implant which is gaining increasing popularity in China with more than 300 000 users in 1999.

Nestorone. A single-implant system that releases the progestogen ST 1435 (16-methylene-17-acetoxy-19 norprogesterone) designed to be effective for 2 years with an effectiveness margin of about 6 additional months. This implant could be important for use in lactating women because, although small amounts of ST 1435 are secreted into breastmilk and thus reach the breast-fed infant, the progestogen is inactive by the oral route and would therefore have no biological effect.

The Nestorone implant is unlikely to become available for routine use within the next 5 years. A variant containing 50 mg of ST 1435 (also referred to as elcometrine) is approved in Brazil as a 6-month contraceptive implant for lactating women.

Injectable contraceptives

Injectable contraceptives have the advantage over subdermal implants in that they are easier to administer and do not require special training of providers. However, if the woman experiences side effects, she cannot discontinue use until the drug is depleted. To overcome the problem of poor cycle control, research has been carried out to develop combined oestrogen–progestogen formulations (which are injected once a month) and other progestogens with better pharmacokinetic profiles.

Combined oestrogen–progestogen preparations

These are currently being used by approximately 2 million women (Table 18.4).

The Chinese Injectable No. 1. This is used almost exclusively in China and neighbouring countries. The first injection is given on day 1 to 5 of the cycle with an additional injection 8 to 10 days later. Subsequent injections are given on day 10 to 12 after the onset of withdrawal bleeding, or 28 days after the previous injection if no bleeding occurs. In a World Health Organization (WHO) study, the 12-month life-table contraceptive failure rate of this regimen was found to be 0.8%, whereas the failure rate was 6% when the preparation was used on a strict once-a-month schedule.

The second preparation (Perlutal and various other proprietary names) is still used in Latin America even though the progestogen it contains was shown to cause breast abnormalities in beagle bitches.

Cyclofem (Cycloprovera, Lunelle) and Mesigyna. These two newer preparations are becoming available in an increasing number of countries. The 1-year life-table pregnancy rates with these preparations are less than 0.5% and discontinuation rates because of menstrual irregularity or amenorrhoea are generally less than half those seen with progestogen-only injectables such as depot medroxyprogesterone acetate (DMPA) or norethisterone enanthate (NET-EN).

Natural steroids. Research on aqueous suspensions of steroids has shown that, by controlling the range of crystal size, the release of the steroid from the injection site can be influenced. This approach using natural steroids could represent a new alternative in once-a-month injectable contraception and exploratory studies with a combination of 200 mg of progesterone plus 5 mg of 17β-oestradiol delivered as injectable microspheres are in progress.

Table 18.4 Once-a-month combined injectable preparations

Name	Progestogen	Dose	Oestrogen	Dose
Chinese Injectable No. 1	17 α-hydroxyprogesterone caproate	250 mg	Oestradiol valerate	5 mg
Topasel/Patector/ Perlutal (and various others)	Dihydroxyprogesterone acetophenide	150 mg	Oestradiol enanthate	10 mg
Cyclofem	Medroxyprogesterone acetate	25 mg	Oestradiol cypionate	5 mg
Mesigyna	Norethisterone enanthate	50 mg	Oestradiol valerate	5 mg

Progestogen-only preparations

With the objective of developing compounds that would provide contraception at low doses for long periods, some 230 derivatives of levonorgestrel and norethisterone have been synthesized. One of these, levonorgestrel butanoate, is currently being developed further as a microcrystalline suspension with a duration of action of 3 to 4 months and possibly longer.

A microsphere preparation of norethisterone, expected to provide efficacy for 90 days with less than half the dose of the standard injectable formulation, and one of natural progesterone for breast-feeding mothers, are at an early stage of clinical development.

Intrauterine devices

The most important reasons for discontinuing IUD use are pain, bleeding and expulsion. These side effects are thought to be related to the relative size of the frame or shape of the device. A 'frameless' IUD should, in theory, minimize the problems, and results from clinical trials are encouraging (GyneFix – see Ch. 4). Initial results with GyneFix 200, a 200 mm^2 copper-releasing IUD, show similar effectiveness to the regular 330 mm^2 device. Early clinical trials are also ongoing with FibroPlant-LNG, an intrauterine system consisting of fibres releasing levonorgestrel at a daily rate of about 14 μg.

Male condoms

Male latex condoms currently offer the best protection against STIs and HIV infection of any contraceptive. Unfortunately, they have a rather high contraceptive failure rate, probably owing more to user failure than to failure from condom rupture. However, latex does deteriorate if exposed to excessive heat, light or humidity, and it is rapidly destroyed by oil-based lubricants such as Vaseline. Furthermore, men in many areas of the world, including regions such as sub-Saharan Africa where the prevalence of STIs and HIV is highest, dislike condoms mainly because of loss of penile sensitivity and interference with the spontaneity of intercourse.

A range of plastic condoms currently under development could overcome many of these problems (Ch. 5). The main advantages of plastic condoms are that they are loose-fitting apart from the region of attachment at the base of the penis, are stronger than latex condoms in vitro and do not deteriorate on storage. Clinical testing of Tactylon, another version of a non-latex male condom, is scheduled to start in 2000 with the support of CONRAD.

Vaginal barrier methods

The worldwide increase in STIs, including HIV/AIDS, and the growing awareness of the need to expand the contraceptive method mix, have led to a re-examination of the role of barrier methods for women. Greater resources are being devoted to finding new methods as well as to improving existing vaginal barrier methods.

Diaphragms

Research is being directed towards improving acceptability and effectiveness.

Diaphragm used continuously without spermicide. The need to apply spermicide to the diaphragm and to insert it before intercourse and remove it later are all deterrents to its use (Ch. 5). In a retrospective study in Brazil, women who used the diaphragm with spermicide in the usual way had a significantly higher failure rate (9.8 pregnancies per 100 women at 12 months) than women who used it continuously without spermicide (2.8 per 100 women). Women in the latter group removed the diaphragm once a day for cleaning and during menses. Furthermore, there were significantly more discontinuations because of vaginal discharge and other medical reasons in the women using spermicide. Prospective randomized trials are required to confirm these findings.

Lea's shield. Made of flexible silicone rubber, this combines features of the diaphragm and of the cervical cap (see Ch. 5).

Cervical caps

Some modifications have been made in the design of the cervical cap, and in the materials used, to try to reduce the failure rate.

Contracap. A 'personalized' device made from a mould of the woman's cervix, this had an unacceptably high failure rate and trials were stopped. A modified device (KoCap) has been developed but not yet tested clinically.

FemCap. This is made of silicone and shaped like an American sailor's cap. It is claimed to fit the cervix better and to adapt more easily to changes in cervical shape and size during the menstrual cycle. Clinical experience is still limited.

Female condoms

Current research on the female condom is focusing on acceptability and contraceptive efficacy when used with or without spermicide (Ch. 5).

Vaginal sponges

The sponge has a lower efficacy and higher incidence of problems than other vaginal barriers.

Today sponge (see Ch. 5). Improvements in the sponge's performance will probably require a different material and a better spermicide as well as alterations in design to achieve better retention and coverage of the cervix. Little, if any, research towards attaining these goals appears to be in progress, and the company which produced the sponge has withdrawn it from the market.

Chemical agents

Currently marketed spermicidal agents – foam, jelly, cream, suppository, film – inactivate spermatozoa by immobilizing them. The large doses of these substances required for contraceptive efficacy in vivo compared to in vitro, particularly if used repeatedly over prolonged periods, are thought to contribute to problems of vaginal irritation. Long-term use disturbs the normal vaginal flora and enhances the risk of vaginal infection and irritation.

A variety of new chemical agents has been tested in recent years that immobilize sperm, interfere with sperm function through mechanisms other than spermicidal ones or harden cervical mucus so that sperm penetration is prevented. These compounds generally have antibacterial properties which could be considered an advantage in preventing STIs. Some of these compounds are not irritating to the vagina and do not disturb the normal flora. Several have recently entered clinical trials.

A variety of other, sometimes ill-defined agents, including several plant products such as gossypol have been tried with little success.

As far as vaginal chemical contraception is concerned, we have made some progress since the days when women were advised to smear tar in the vagina or insert the pulp of pomegranates or elephant's dung, but a greater research effort is needed in this area if we are to control the spread of STIs.

Natural family planning

Successful use of a natural family planning method depends on correct identification of the fertile days of the cycle and, equally important, consistent abstinence from sexual intercourse on those days (Ch. 6). Better ways of identifying the beginning and the end of the fertile period should improve the performance of currently available methods and may widen the appeal not only of periodic abstinence by attracting the new, more 'technology-oriented' users but also users of barrier methods by limiting the need to use the barrier method to only a few days in each cycle.

Electronic devices

Devices such as the BabyComp, Cyclotest-D, Rite Time, Fertil-A-Chron and Bioself 110 have been developed for predicting the fertile and infertile days based on the basal body temperature (BBT) changes and on information, stored in the device, about previous cycle lengths. Among these devices, Bioself is probably the most sophisticated and user-friendly; it uses BBT measurements for up to 12 preceding cycles to predict the beginning and end of the fertile period. Although marketed in several countries, few of these devices have been rigorously tested for their accuracy in defining the fertile period and their effectiveness as a family planning aid. They are also expensive.

In future, skin patches containing heat sensors may eliminate the need for thermometers.

Simple assay methods

Easy-to-use home tests for the measurement of hormones in urine are now available over the counter. They delineate the end of the fertile period through identification, in urine, of the luteinizing hormone (LH) peak (which is assumed to occur 3 days before the fertile period ends) or of the rise in pregnanediol glucuronide, the major metabolite of progesterone. Examples of such home kits are Ovutest, Clearplan-One Step (for LH) and the ProgestURINE RAMP test (for pregnanediol glucuronide).

Identification of the beginning of the fertile period, which requires detection of the pre-ovulatory rise in oestrogen, has been much more difficult to achieve. Persona, the 'Personal Contraceptive System', uses the pre-ovulatory rise in oestrogen and the ovulatory LH peak for delineating the fertile period. It is easy to use but requires a sophisticated reader with built-in programme to interpret the hormone changes. Only limited information is available about the effectiveness of this system as a family planning aid and its cost is a rather prohibitive factor.

Mucus-measuring devices

It is well established that the water content of the cervical mucus increases significantly beginning approximately 4 to 5 days before ovulation and decreases sharply shortly after ovulation occurs. A device to measure cervical mucus hydration, with a degree of sensitivity and specificity appropriate for alerting the woman to her impending and completed ovulation, is in the final stages of development. Other attempts to develop devices to characterize objectively mucus with respect to either amount or chemistry have been less successful.

Disposable calibrated syringes have been developed to allow women to aspirate cervicovaginal fluid and record daily volumes. A miniature magnifying device designed to detect 'ferning' in saliva and tests to measure the content of various enzymes and proteins in saliva or mucus have been investigated with generally poor results.

Low technology approaches

Recognizing that a significant number of women who would choose a natural method are deterred by the complexity of observations and calculations required by currently available methods, two very simple methods are being developed. One, the 'Standard Days method', is based on the determination of the 'fertile window' by a fixed calculation. This method, which is now being tested in several countries, identifies the woman's fertile days as days 8 to 19 of her cycle. It is most effective for women whose cycle lengths fall between 26 and 32 days. Another method, the 'TwoDay method', is based on the presence or absence of cervical secretions on the current or immediately-previous day. It also is undergoing field trials. These methods have the potential for increasing interest in and access to natural methods, since they require substantially less time to learn and are easier to use.

THE SEARCH FOR NEW METHODS
Contraception for men

The development of safe, reliable and reversible methods of contraception for oral or systemic use has proved to be much more difficult for men than for women. The process of spermatogenesis is still not fully understood and suppressing the production of some 1000 spermatozoa per second is a much more formidable task than preventing the release of a single egg once a month.

In spite of inherent difficulties, a contraceptive 'pill' for men, based on systemically administered steroid hormones, which acts through inhibiting the secretion of LH and follicle-stimulating hormone (FSH) by the pituitary gland, could be ready for more widespread testing within the next 5 years.

Hormonal methods

The ideal hormonal method of contraception for men should suppress sperm production while leaving testosterone secretion intact, thus rendering the man infertile but not impotent. To date, no hormonal approach has achieved this. It is also proving difficult to find a method which will completely inhibit sperm production (azoospermia) in the majority of men, which is cheap, effective within a short time of starting treatment and rapidly reversible.

A trial of weekly injections of 200 mg testosterone enanthate (WHO 1990) resulted in azoospermia in 65% of 271 men after 6 months of treatment. After 12 months of relying on the method for contraception, only 1 pregnancy occurred (0.8 conceptions per 100 person-years) among the azoospermic men.

A second trial in which men who did not achieve azoospermia but whose sperm count fell to less than 3 million/mL (nearly 99% of subjects) resulted in a failure rate of 1.5 per 100 person-years.

Research efforts are now concentrated on the development of long-acting methods, and regimens combining more potent androgens with either a progestogen (such as intramuscular DMPA or oral etonogestrel), a progestogen with anti-androgenic properties (cyproterone acetate), or a gonadotrophin releasing hormone (GnRH) antagonist.

Non-hormonal agents acting on sperm

Affecting sperm production. A wide variety of chemical agents have been shown to suppress sperm production but most of them ultimately cause irreversible infertility. Gossypol, a plant-derived product isolated initially from cotton seed, induces azoospermia or severe oligozoospermia in more than 90% of men. However, its use leads to irreversible infertility in 10–15% of men and is associated, in some cases, with potentially life-threatening hypokalaemia. Development of gossypol for male contraception has been discontinued by most investigators.

Physical agents such as irradiation and ultrasound also inhibit sperm production when used at certain doses but the application of such methods for contraception has not been pursued because of concerns about irreversibility and carcinogenesis.

Local, long-term application of a mild temperature increase (1–2 °C), by bringing the testes closer to the inguinal canal, was thought to have possibilities. A polyester sling worn during waking hours was employed for this purpose and, in a first study, led to azoospermia in all 14 men wearing the sling for 12 months. The inhibitory effect on sperm production was fully reversible within 6 months after stopping use of the sling. However, a subsequent trial could not confirm these findings and the approach appears to have been abandoned.

Affecting sperm maturation. Drugs that affect sperm during storage in the epididymis would act quickly and, after withdrawal of the drug, normal spermatozoa would reappear rapidly in the semen. No compound has yet reached the stage of clinical efficacy testing in men because of toxicological concerns or insufficient efficacy in animal tests.

A traditional Chinese medicine containing extract of the plant *Tripterygium wilfordii* for treatment of psoriasis, rheumatoid arthritis, glomerulonephritis and other autoimmune diseases shows some promise.

Work is under way to isolate and test the active principle, triptolide, of this extract which is thought to act at various levels of sperm cell formation and transit.

Gonadotrophin releasing hormone analogues

The discovery of GnRH, the hypothalamic peptide hormone that induces the pituitary gland to secrete FSH and LH, created great expectations of a novel form of contraception. Many hundreds of analogues – both agonists and antagonists – of GnRH have been synthesized, but the prospects of using these compounds in fertility regulation now look rather poor. They are expensive, short-acting, cannot be given orally and frequently cause local allergic reactions.

Vaccination against GnRH is summarized in the section on antifertility vaccines (p **413–415**).

In female contraception

GnRH and its agonists normally stimulate the secretion of FSH and LH. Paradoxically, ovulation will be inhibited when agonists are given over long periods and in sufficiently high dose. If ovarian activity is completely suppressed, potentially deleterious effects on bone and on the cardiovascular system may occur (similar to changes in the postmenopausal state). The hypo-oestrogenism resulting from complete GnRH agonist-induced ovarian suppression would require replacement therapy with low-dose oestrogen and progestogen. Conversely, incomplete suppression of ovarian activity might result in long periods of unopposed oestrogen, increasing the risk of endometrial carcinoma.

The feasibility of keeping ovulation suppressed in the short term in breast-feeding women by giving the GnRH agonist, buserelin, by nasal spray has been demonstrated. Further development of this approach awaits cheaper agonists that can be more easily administered.

In male contraception

To date, pilot trials in humans and monkeys with combination regimens of GnRH agonists and androgens have not provided adequate suppression of spermatogenesis.

Steroid hormone receptor antagonists

Steroid hormone receptor antagonists bind with receptor sites to prevent the native steroid hormone from occupying the same sites. They are often referred to as antihormones. Anti-androgens (e.g. cyproterone acetate in

Dianette) and anti-oestrogens (e.g. clomiphene) have been in clinical use for some time but agents that block the receptor for progesterone were only discovered in the early 1980s.

Anti-androgens

Cyproterone acetate which has strong progestogenic activity in addition to being a potent anti-androgen has been used in combination with intramuscular testosterone undecanoate for suppression of spermatogenesis. Results of these pilot studies are encouraging but efficacy of the regimen has not yet been tested.

Anti-oestrogens

Many anti-oestrogens, including clomiphene, have proved inactive as contraceptive agents in the human.

A non-steroidal agent, centchroman, which has weak oestrogenic and potent anti-oestrogenic activities, is in use as a once-a-week pill in India only. Thought to exert its contraceptive action by preventing implantation, the compound is given in a dose of 30 mg twice a week for the first 3 months, followed thereafter by 30 mg once a week. A failure rate of 1.8 per 100 woman-years has been reported for this regimen.

Antiprogestogens

Because progesterone is essential for a range of reproductive functions, including the establishment and maintenance of pregnancy, antiprogestogens such as mifepristone offer considerable potential for the regulation of fertility (Van Look and von Hertzen 1995). The use of antiprogestogens, mifepristone in particular, for inducing abortion is described in Chapter 11. A summary of the current state of research in the other possible applications is given below.

Menstrual regulation. The sequential combination regimen of mifepristone and a prostaglandin appears to be an effective method for menstrual regulation (induction of missed menses). In a trial by WHO, a total of 228 women with menstrual delay of up to 11 days was studied. Vaginal bleeding was induced in all of the 193 pregnant women and all but four of them had a complete abortion, giving a success rate of 98%. 35 women were not pregnant.

Although this study showed 'proof of concept', there are legal, political and ethical issues that make it unlikely that this approach would receive widespread acceptance (Baird and Glasier 1999). Also, in the WHO study, there was considerable variation in the timing of onset of the next menses, which would make it difficult for women to decide whether and when to take the pill again in subsequent cycles.

Once-a-month contraception. Antiprogestogens given during the luteal phase of the cycle have a profound effect on the endometrium and hence have been proposed for use as once-a-month contraceptives. Taken in the early luteal phase, they could prevent implantation, while taken in the late luteal phase, they could disrupt it.

Accurate timing of the antiprogestogen administration in the early luteal phase is essential. If the drug is taken too early, ovulation will be suppressed and menses will be delayed. If taken too late, endometrial bleeding may occur but an already implanting embryo may not be dislodged. Thus, the use of an antiprogestogen as a once-a-month contraceptive in the early luteal phase is not likely to be a practical method of family planning until such time that a simple and reliable method to detect ovulation has been discovered.

Trials of mifepristone, when used alone or in combination with the prostaglandin misoprostol, as a *late* luteal, once-a-month contraceptive have been disappointing and this approach is no longer being pursued.

Emergency contraception. Antiprogestogens have been shown to be highly effective for emergency postcoital contraception (Ch. 8).

Once-a-week contraception. A small dose of antiprogestogen given once a week can disturb endometrial development without causing ovarian dysfunction. When such a low dose (5 mg) was tested for contraceptive effectiveness, however, it was found to be not effective. A higher weekly dose might be effective by preventing ovulation but would almost certainly disturb menstrual cyclicity.

Daily use. Studies have shown that a very low daily dose of mifepristone (e.g. 0.5 mg) does not upset ovarian cyclicity, yet profoundly disturbs endometrial development. This finding led to the suggestion that antiprogestogens may represent a new generation of 'minipills', but this expectation was not fulfilled when this dose was tested for contraceptive efficacy. Slightly higher (2–5 mg) daily doses inhibit ovulation and prevent the formation of a secretory endometrium. Oestrogen levels are maintained at those found in the follicular phase of the menstrual cycle and preliminary data suggest that most women are amenorrhoeic (and presumably therefore infertile) while taking the antiprogestogen in such a daily dose.

Cyclical use. An alternative contraceptive strategy would be to use a higher dose of mifepristone (e.g. 5–10 mg) in a sequential regimen with an oral progestogen. This regimen would allow development of a secretory endometrium and the occurrence of timely, well-controlled vaginal bleeding. A related strategy under study is the use of cyclical antiprogestogen to induce monthly withdrawal bleedings in women relying on progestogen-only injectables or implants.

New delivery systems for steroid hormones

Non-oral routes of administering steroid hormones have several advantages.

1. The first pass through the liver is avoided which allows the use of lower doses of hormone and reduces metabolic side effects.
2. It is possible to achieve steady hormone levels and avoid the peaks and troughs that are associated with the oral route of administration and which may be responsible for some of the side effects.

The two new delivery systems discussed below – the hormone-releasing vaginal rings and transdermal systems – have major advantages in having contraceptive actions which can be easily reversed and are entirely under the control of the woman.

Vaginal rings

Most steroid hormones are absorbed efficiently through the vaginal epithelium and can be released from a vaginal ring made out of Silastic. Rings up to 75 mm in diameter usually stay in the vaginal fornix. To achieve release of the steroid at the desired dose and at a constant rate, several designs can be used (Fig. 18.1). The release rate is a function of the surface area of the ring, the solubility of the steroid in the Silastic matrix and the distance the steroid has to diffuse in order to reach the surface of the ring.

Combined oestrogen–progestogen rings. This type of ring is worn for 3 weeks and then removed for 1 week to allow withdrawal bleeding to occur. The '3-week-in/1-week-out' schedule is continued for the lifetime of the ring.

Like COC pills, vaginal rings releasing both oestrogen and progestogen are intended to inhibit ovulation with minimal disturbance of vaginal bleeding patterns. Examples of combined rings that are in final phases of

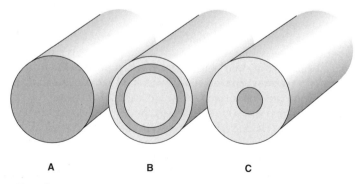

A   **B**   **C**

Figure 18.1   Cross-sectional views of contraceptive rings in which the shaded areas are micronized steroid: (A) homogeneous ring; (B) Shell ring (no longer used); (C) core ring.

clinical development include two rings that release etonorgestrel and ethinyloestradiol (Organon) and a ring that releases norethisterone acetate and ethinyloestradiol (Population Council).

Progestogen-only rings. Depending on the amount of progestogen released, the ring acts either by inhibiting ovulation or in a manner similar to the POP. A ring that is intended to block ovulation would be used in a '3-week-in/1-week-out' schedule to ensure regular withdrawal bleeding. Rings that release a smaller dose of progestogen are worn continuously, although they can be removed for short periods if desired (e.g. for cleaning or during intercourse). Like the POP, the efficacy of rings that are worn continuously depends on a combination of effects, including thickening of cervical mucus, inhibition of ovulation and prevention of implantation. An example of a progestogen-only ring is the ring delivering the progestogen ST 1435, which is inactive when taken orally, and is intended for use by breast-feeding women.

Transdermal systems

The transdermal route of drug administration is an area of growing interest as can be seen by the increasing number of transdermal hormone replacement products. Drug delivery through the skin can be accomplished in two ways:

1. By an aerosol/aeropowder or a semisolid or liquid vehicle that contains the drug.
2. By a drug-delivery patch which ensures fairly constant release rates.

Transdermal delivery of contraceptive steroids is a growing field of interest. Several types of patches are being tested, including combined patches for the delivery of either ethinyloestradiol plus levonorgestrel or ethinyloestradiol plus (17-deacetyl) norgestimate, and a progestogen-only patch releasing ST 1435.

Antifertility vaccines

The aim is to develop a vaccine – for either women or men – that will inhibit reproduction by immunological means and which is safe, effective, reversible and free of endocrine and metabolic side effects.

The first step in this development process is to identify a suitable, reproduction-specific molecule that can be used as an immunogen. A large number of reproduction-specific molecules exists but not all of them represent attractive options since their immunological removal or neutralization could result in endocrine or other side effects. Molecules found in, or produced by, the sperm, egg and the peri-implantation embryo are the most appropriate targets.

Furthest advanced amongst the antifertility vaccines is the one directed against human chorionic gonadotrophin (hCG). Some work is also in progress on the development of vaccines for men against GnRH and FSH.

Anti-human chorionic gonadotrophin vaccines

The main function of hCG, which is produced by the pre-implantation embryo within a few days of fertilization, appears to be the maintenance of the corpus luteum, thus ensuring the continued production of progesterone essential for successful implantation. Immunological inhibition of the production or function of hCG would lead to regression of the corpus luteum, followed by declining progesterone levels and the occurrence of menstrual bleeding at or about the expected time of the next menses.

One of the candidate vaccines being studied consists of a synthetic peptide representing the apparently unique part of the β-subunit of hCG (β-hCG-CTP) linked to an immunogenic carrier molecule such as tetanus or diphtheria toxoid and injected together with adjuvants that further enhance the immune response (Griffin 1991).

A Phase I study conducted by WHO with this vaccine preparation showed that it can induce a level of antibodies high enough to neutralize hCG for a period of some 6 to 12 months. To prolong the antifertility effect, by a similar period of time, booster injections would need to be given.

An alternative approach is the use of the whole β-hCG subunit. In India, an anti-hCG vaccine is under development that consists of the whole β-subunit coupled to the α-subunit of ovine LH and to diphtheria and tetanus toxoid carrier molecules. A phase II clinical trial carried out with this preparation has confirmed its antifertility effect (Talwar et al 1994).

In addition to lack of long-term safety data, one potentially major problem with anti-hCG vaccines is the individual variability in the antibody response. To detect those women who have responded poorly or not at all and to determine when the antifertility effect has worn off, it will probably be necessary to develop a simple, dipstick-type method for assessing the antibody level in blood or saliva following administration of the vaccine.

Antisperm vaccines

A small proportion (about 5%) of male and female patients attending infertility clinics appear to be infertile because they have antibodies against spermatozoa. Auto-antibodies are also found in a substantial percentage of vasectomized men and are thought to be responsible for the low pregnancy rate after vasectomy reversal even in men in whom the re-anastomosis procedure appears to have succeeded.

Since the presence of antisperm antibodies in either men or women seems to cause no ill effects other than infertility, the feasibility of developing a safe and effective antisperm vaccine appears very real. However, difficulty in finding an appropriate sperm antigen for use as the immunogen in the vaccine means that an antisperm vaccine is unlikely to become available within the next 5 to 10 years.

Anti-ovum vaccines

Most of the research directed at developing an anti-ovum vaccine has focused on the zona pellucida (ZP), the outer layer of the ovum. One glycoprotein component, ZP3, is essential for fertilization. Active immunization of animals against ZP3 causes infertility. Unfortunately, the immunized animal eventually loses all the primordial follicles from its ovaries and experiences a premature, irreversible menopause. Research in this area appears to have been largely abandoned.

Other antifertility vaccines

Pilot studies on the feasibility of immunizing men against GnRH have been initiated, but this approach would require hormone substitution therapy and could induce damage to the pituitary. Similar concerns have been voiced about vaccination of men against FSH, which has been tested in India, although no adverse physiological or behavioural effects have been observed in male monkeys actively immunized for periods of more than 10 years.

REFERENCES

Baird DT, Glasier AF 1999 Science, medicine, and the future. British Medical Journal 319: 969–972
Coutinho EM, Mascarenhas I, Mateo de Acosta O, et al 1993 Comparative study on the efficacy, acceptability, and side effects of a contraceptive pill administered by the oral and the vaginal route: an international multicenter clinical trial. Clinical Pharmacology and Therapeutics 54: 540–545
Division of Reproductive Health 1998 Unsafe abortion. Global and regional estimates of incidence of and mortality due to unsafe abortion, with a listing of available country data (document WHO/RHT/MSMS/97.16). World Health Organization, Geneva
Griffin PD 1991 The WHO Task Force on Vaccines for Fertility Regulation. Its formation, objectives and research activities. Human Reproduction 6: 166–172
Guha SK, Singh G, Srivastava A, et al 1998 Two-year clinical efficacy trial with dose variations of a vas deferens injectable contraceptive for the male. Contraception 58: 165–174
Khanna J, Van Look PFA, Benagiano G 1994 Fertility regulation research: the challenges now and ahead. In: Khanna J, Van Look PFA, Griffin PD (eds) Challenges in reproductive health research. World Health Organization, Geneva, p 34–57
Population Division (Department of Economic and Social Affairs, United Nations) 1999a The world at six billion (document ESA/P/WP.154). United Nations, New York

Population Division (Department of Economic and Social Affairs, United Nations) 1999b World contraceptive use in 1998 (document ST/ESA/SER.A/175). United Nations, New York

Talwar GP, Singh O, Pal R, et al 1994 A vaccine that prevents pregnancy in women. Proceedings of the National Academy of Science, USA 91:8532–8536

Van Look PFA, von Hertzen H 1995 Clinical uses of antiprogestogens. Human Reproduction Update 1: 19–34

World Health Organization Task Force on Methods for the Regulation of Male Fertility 1990 Contraceptive efficacy of testosterone-induced azoospermia in normal men. Lancet 336: 955–959

FURTHER READING

Drife JO, Baird DT (eds) 1993 Contraception. British Medical Bulletin 49: 1–258

Henshaw SK, Singh S, Hass T 1999. The incidence of abortion worldwide. International Family Planning Perspectives 25 (Suppl): S30-S38

Sitruk-Ware R, Bardin CW (eds) 1992 Contraception – Newer pharmacological agents, devices and delivery systems. Marcel Dekker, New York

Van Look PFA, Pérez-Palacios G (eds) 1994 Contraceptive research and development 1984 to 1994 – The road from Mexico City to Cairo and Beyond. Oxford University Press, Delhi

World Health Organization 1994 Health, population and development (WHO Position Paper for the International Conference on Population and Development 1994, Cairo; document WHO/FHE/94.1). World Health Organization, Geneva

World Health Organization 1997 Communicating family planning in reproductive health. Key messages for communicators (document WHO/FRH/FPP/97.33). World Health Organization, Geneva

Index

Abbreviations used: COCs, combined oral contraceptives; FP, family planning; HRT, hormone replacement therapy; PID, pelvic inflammatory disease; PMS, premenstrual syndrome; POC, progestogen-only contraception/contraceptive; POP, progestogen-only pill; STIs, sexually-transmitted infections.

A

Ablative methods
  condyloma acuminatum, 300
  PMS, 364
Abortion (spontaneous) *see* Miscarriage
Abortion (therapeutic), 17, 241–242, 249–262
  alternatives, discussing, 252
  assessment, 253
  complaints/litigation, 241–242
  contraception after, 261
    COCs, 51–52
  effectiveness, 6, 17
  follow-up, 260–261
  information/counselling, 251–252,
    263–264
  legal aspects, 250–251
  older women, frequency, 391
  referral for, 253–254
  safety/side-effects of various methods,
    11, 241–242, 255, 256, 259–260
  techniques, 254–259
    early first trimester (up to 9 weeks),
      254–257
    late first trimester (9–14 weeks), 257
    mid-trimester, 258–259
    teenagers, 220–221
  WHO medical eligibility criteria for FP
    methods following, 23
  worldwide patterns, 396–397
Abortion Act (1967), 249, 250–251
Abscess, Bartholin's, 336
Abstinence, periodic *see* Natural FP
Aciclovir, HSV, 297, 298
Acne
  with COCs, 71–72
  with POCs, 86
Actinomycosis and IUDs, 122–123
Acyclovir (aciclovir), HSV, 297, 298
Adenoma, hepatic, POC and, 100
Adenomyosis, 340
  treatment, 99
Adenosis, vaginal, 337

Adherence (compliance)
  in HRT, 388
  IUD, 109–111
Adolescents/teenagers, 215–230, 319–320
  age of consent, 232
  confidentiality, 228–229, 233
  contraception, 225–228, 319–320
    condoms, 98, 215, 226–227
    improving provision, 222
    oral contraceptives, 98, 225–226, 227
    POCs, 98, 227–228
  pregnancy *see* Pregnancy
  reproductive health
    global perspectives, 215–216
    UK perspectives, 216–217
  sexuality, 319–320
  see also Puberty
Adverse effects *see* Safety
Advice *see* Information
Aerosol foams, spermicidal, 150
  instructions, 153
Age
  COC and breast cancer and, 69
  of consent to sex, 232
  death by, causes, 267
  FP methods by
    UK patterns of use, 3
    WHO medical eligibility criteria, 23
  IUD and, 114
  maternal, chromosomal abnormalities
    and, 391
  POC and, 82
Ageing and sexuality, 322–323
  see also Older women; Perimenopause
AIDS *see* HIV
Alcohol, pre-pregnancy counselling, 351
Alimentary system and COCs, 63–65
Allergy condoms, 147
Alternative therapy in PMS, 363
Amenorrhoea, 343–344
  causes, 343
  POCs/POPs, 85, 392
  infertility in, 354
  investigations/treatment, 343–344

Amenorrhoea (*cont.*)
  lactational *see* Lactational amenorrhoea
  in perimenopause, 372
Anal intercourse/sex, 158
  condoms for, 147, 304
  HIV-infected individual, 304
Anger and sexual assault, 317
Antenatal screening, 351
Anterior fornix, diaphragm repeated
      inserted into, 136
Anti-androgens (anti-testosterones), 410
  in COC-related skin disorders, 71–72
  COCs containing *see* Dianette
  in hirsutism, 345
Antibiotics
  bacterial vaginosis, 291
  chlamydial/non-chlamydial non-specific
      urethritis, 289–290
  COCs and, 54, 55
  gonorrhoea, 286–287
    resistance to, 283, 286
  pre-abortion, 253
  trichomoniasis, 293
Antibodies to sperm, 189, 414–415
Anticoagulants and IUDs, 114
Anticonvulsants and COCs, 54
Antidepressants
  in perimenopause, 379
  in PMS, 363
Anti-epileptics (anticonvulsants) and
      COCs, 54
Antifertility vaccines, 413–415
Antifibrinolytics, menorrhagia, 341–342
Antifungals
  candidiasis, 294, 295
  COCs and, 54
Antigestogens *see* Antiprogestogens
Antimetabolites, condyloma acuminatum,
      300
Antimicrobial spermicides, 153, 157, 398,
      405
Antimitotics, condyloma acuminatum, 300
Anti-oestrogens, 410
Antiprogestogens, 410–411
  abortion, 256–257
  contraception, 411
    emergency contraception, 208, 411
  menstrual regulation, 410–411
  see also Mifepristone
Anti-sex education campaigners, 225
Anti-testosterones *see* Anti-androgens
Antivirals
  HIV disease, 304, 307
    in pregnancy, reducing vertical
      transmission, 301, 307
  HSV, 297, 298
Anxiety
  premature ejaculation and, 320–321

sexual interest and, 317–318
Arcing diaphragm, 129
Arousal, sexual, post-orgasmic reduction,
      317
Arrhythmias on IUD insertion, 117–118
Arterial disease (and COC use)
  as COC contraindication, 38, 49
  as COC risk, 44–46, 49
Arthropod infestations, 308–309
Aspirin
  dysmenorrhoea, 346
  menorrhagia, 341
Asthma and COCs, 60
Atrophy (urogenital incl. vaginal atrophy),
      336, 349–350, 375
  treatment, 336, 381–382
Attitudes to/satisfaction with FP methods
      (users')
  back-up methods, 16
  measuring, 13–15
Autoantibodies to sperm, 189, 414–415
Autoimmune disease
  POCs, 100
  vasectomy and, 189
Aylesbury spatula, 277
Azoles
  bacterial vaginosis, 291
  candidiasis, 294
  trichomoniasis, 293

B

Bacterial infections, sexually-transmissible,
      282–283
Bacterial vaginosis *see* Vaginosis
Barrier methods, 127–159
  costs, 20, 21
  discontinuation rates, 13
  emergency contraception after 'accidents'
      with, 205
  HIV-infected persons, 305
  home-made, 146, 405
  menopause and, 393
  new/improved types, 143–144, 403–405
  PMS and, 367
  postpartum, 174–175
  risk vs benefits, 158
  safety/side-effects, 11
  sexual effects, 330–331
  STI protection with, 12
  teenagers, 226–227
  UK use, 3
  worldwide use, 4, 397
  see also specific methods
Bartholinitis, gonococcal, 283
Bartholin's cyst and abscess, 335–336
Basal body temperature, 163

measurement (as FP method), 164–168
  effectiveness, 169–170
  improved methods, 406
  mucus characteristics plus
    see Symptothermal method
  see also Multiple index method
Bellagio guidelines see Lactational
    amenorrhoea
Benzalkonium chloride, 156
Beta-lactamase (penicillinase)-producing
    N. gonorrhoea (PPNG), 283, 286
Biliary disease
  COC-related, 64
  HRT contraindications, 384
  WHO medical eligibility criteria for FP
    methods, 26
Billings method see Mucus
Biochemical tests and POCs, 102
Biodegradable implants, 401
Biopsy, endometrial, in postmenopausal
    bleeding, 343
Bioself-110, 406
Biphasic COCs, 32, 33
  new awaited, 33
Biphosphonates in osteoporosis, 377
Bleeding
  antenatal, early, 351–352
  breakthrough (and spotting), with COCs,
    65–66
  breakthrough (and spotting), with POC,
    84
    management, 86
    prolonged/frequent, 84–85
  dysfunctional (and its management), 341
    postmenopausal, 342–343
  menstrual (menstrual period)
    contraceptives reducing/controlling,
      12–13, 56–57
    IUD increasing/prolonging, 112,
      120–121
    IUD insertion during, 116
    prolonged/heavy see Menorrhagia
    sterilization and, 183–184
    WHO medical eligibility criteria for FP
      methods, 25
  withdrawal (with COCs)
    absence, 66
    changing preparations and, 52
Blood pressure
  measurement, 279
    COC users, 57
  raised see Hypertension
  screening, 279
Bolam principle, 233–234
Bolitho criterion, 234
Bone loss (and mineral density loss)
  with depot medroxyprogesterone acetate,
    93

measurement, 376
  menopausal, 375–377
Bougies for vacuum aspiration, 257
Bowel obstruction and female sterilization,
    184
Bradycardia on IUD insertion, 117–118
Breast(s)
  awareness, 269
    HRT and, 390
  examination
    HRT candidate, 388, 389
    routine, 269
    self, 267–268
Breast cancer/carcinoma, 268–270
  contraindications in
    for HRT, 385
    for POC, 83, 99
  detection, 268–270
  risk of
    COCs and, 68–70, 392–393
    HRT and, 386–387
    injectables and, 93
Breast disease/disorders (in general)
  POC and, 99
  WHO medical eligibility criteria for FP
    methods, 25
  COCs and, 68–70
Breast-feeding
  contraindicated FP methods, 174, 175
  contraindicated in HIV-infected mother,
    305
  emergency contraception and, 176
  fertility and effects of, 171–174
    see also Lactational amenorrhoea
  POC and see Progestogen-only
    contraception
  sexual intercourse and hormonal effects
    of, 322
  WHO medical eligibility criteria for FP
    methods, 23
Bromocriptine in PMS, 364
Bruising, vasectomy, 188
Buserelin, 409

C

CA125 levels, pelvic masses and, 338
Calcium supplements
  in osteoporosis prevention/treatment,
    377
  in PMS, 363
Calendar (rhythm) method, 164
  effectiveness, 169
  worldwide use, 397
  see also Multiple index method
Cancer (predominantly carcinoma)
  breast see Breast cancer

Cancer (predominantly carcinoma) (*cont.*)
  cervical *see* Cervical cancer
  COC-related risk of
    breast cancer, 68–70
    gynaecological cancer, 64–65
    liver cancer, 64
    skin cancer, 72
  endometrial *see* Endometrium, cancer
  HRT contraindications, 384–385
  injectable-related risk, 93–94
  IUD-related risk of, 111
  ovarian *see* Ovaries, cancer
  POC and, 100
    POC contraindications in cancer, 83, 99, 100
    POC-related risk of cancer, 78
  vasectomy-related risk, 189, 198–199
  WHO medical eligibility criteria for FP methods, 25
  see also Pre-malignant disease
Candidiasis, vulvovaginal, 293–295
Cap *see* Cervical cap; Occlusive pessaries
Carbon dioxide laser, tubal division, 179–180
Carcinoma *see* Cancer *and specific sites*
Carcinoma in situ, cervical, 274
Cardiovascular/circulatory disease (men), with vasectomy, 189
Cardiovascular/circulatory disease (women)
  medical eligibility criteria for FP methods, 24–25
    COCs, 24–25, 36–37, 38
    POC, 83, 99
  menopause and, 377–378
  risk
    with COCs, 42–46, 48–49, 59–60
    with HRT, 387
    with POC, 79
    see also Heart disorders/disease; Vascular system
Carpal tunnel syndrome, 70
Caruncle, urethral, 350
CD4 cell count in HIV disease, 302, 303
Centchroman, 410
Central nervous system disorders
  pre-existing, POC and, 100–101
  risk with COCs, 60–63
Cephalosporins in gonorrhoea, 287
Cervical cancer/carcinoma, 272–278
  precursors of/non-invasive, 274
    HPV and, 298
    management, 278
  prevention/detection, 275–277
    screening, 275, 299–300
  risk factors, 273–274
    COCs, 65
    HPV, 274, 299–300

    injectables, 93
Cervical cap, 138–141
  advantages/disadvantages, 139–140
  discontinuation rates, 13, 14
  effectiveness, 9, 138
  indications/contraindications, 139
  mode of action, 138
  new/improved types, 143–144, 404
  safety/side-effects, 11
  selection/fitting, 140
  teaching/instructions, 141
  variations, 138
Cervix
  cancer *see* Cervical cancer
  cervical cap fitted onto, 140
  diaphragm covering, checking, 134, 137
  dilatation (for abortion), 257
    and evacuation, 258
  ectropion/erosion, 337
  in menstrual cycle, 162, 163
  mucus *see* Mucus
  palpation (as FP method), 167–168
  polyp, 337–338
  smears *see* Smears
Chemical agents
  spermicidal *see* Spermicides
  tubal-occluding, 180–182, 400
Children
  gonorrhoea
    clinical features, 286
    diagnosis, 286
    sexual abuse possibility, 287
  of teenage mothers, health concerns, 221
  see also Adolescents; Girls; Infants; Neonates
China
  implants, 401
  injectables, 402
Chinese injectable No. 1, 402
Chlamydia trachomatis, 288
  infertility and, 253
Chloasma
  COCs and, 71
  POCs and, 101
Chlorhexidine, 156
Cholestasis, obstetric, POC and, 100
Cholesterol levels, 272
Cholic acid, 156
Chorea and COCs, 63
Choriocarcinoma and COCs, 65
Chromosomal abnormalities and maternal age, 391
Circulatory disease *see* Cardiovascular disease
Cirrhosis, WHO medical eligibility criteria for FP methods, 26, 37
Clearplan-One Step, 406
Climacteric *see* Perimenopause

Clindamycin, bacterial vaginosis, 291
Clinic(s)
    access to
        FP clinics, 16, 17
        genitourinary medicine clinics, 281–282
        health/sexual health clinics,
            adolescents, 220
        PMS clinic, presentation at, 358
Clinical trials of FP methods, 7–8
Clips (for tubal occlusion), 179, 180
Clonidine, perimenopause, 379
Clotrimazole, candidiasis, 294, 295
Coagulation and POC, 79
    see also Anticoagulants
Coil-spring diaphragm, 128, 129
    fitting/using, 134
Coitus see Intercourse
Coitus interruptus (withdrawal method),
        58–59
    advantages/disadvantages, 158
    age and patterns of use (UK), 3
    effectiveness, 9, 157
    mode of action, 157
    PMS and, 367
    sexual effects, 331
    worldwide use, 4, 397
Collaborative Group on Hormonal Factors
        in Breast Cancer, 68, 69
Combined oestrogen–progestogen
        injectables, 89–90, 400
    WHO medical eligibility criteria, 23–27
Combined oestrogen–progestogen rings,
        412–413
Combined oestrogen–progestogen therapy
        in menopause, 382–383
    continuous, 383
Combined oral contraceptives (COCs),
        29–76, 391–392, 402
    advantages, 41
    in amenorrhoea/oligomenorrhoea, 344
    biphasic see Biphasic COCs
    breaks in pill-taking, 73, 226
    clinical management, 46–58
        choice, 47
        examination, 47
        follow-up, 57–58
        history-taking, 46–47
    complaints/litigation, 243, 244–245
    complications/safety/side-effects (and
        management), 11, 58–72, 73–75, 245,
        391–392
        reducing incidence, 400
    contraindications/eligibility criteria,
        36–41, 49
        breast-feeding, 174, 175
        WHO, 23–27, 36–39
    costs, 20, 21
    disadvantages, 41–46

dose change with breakthrough bleeding,
        66
    in dysmenorrhoea, 346
    effectiveness, 9, 34–35
    in endometriosis, 339
    historical perspectives, 29–30
    HIV-infected persons, 305
    indications/benefits, 35–36, 391
        non-contraceptive, 35–36, 226
    information see Information
    menstrual bleeding controlled with,
        12–13, 56–57
    missed, 52
        emergency contraception, 205
    mode of action, 34
    monophasic see Monophasic COCs
    new, 33, 400
    in PMS
        as contraceptive, 367
        as treatment, 366, 367
    postpartum, 51–52, 175
        contraindicated with breast-feeding,
            174, 175
    pregnancy outcome, 73
    preparations, 30–33
        changing, 52
    prescribing, 34, 48–53
    reversibility, 72
    risks/benefits, 73–75
    sexual effects, 61, 329–330
    starting, 50–52
    stopping, 392
        indications, 58
        at menopause, 392
        pre-pregnancy and, 350
    teenagers, 225–226
    transfer from POP to, 88
    tricycle regimen see Tricycle regimen
    triphasic, 32, 33
Communication, good, 247
Complementary (alternative) therapy in
        PMS, 363
Compliance see Adherence
Conception difficulty see Infertility
Condoms (female) see Female condom
Condoms (male and in general), 146–150,
        331
    adolescents, 98, 215, 226–227
    advantages/disadvantages, 148–149
    for anal intercourse, 148, 304
    discontinuation rates, 14
    effectiveness see Effectiveness
    history, 146–147
    HIV-infected individuals, 304, 305
    indications/contraindications, 148
    instructions, 149
    menopause and, 393
    mode of action, 148

Condoms (male and in general) (*cont.*)
  safety/side-effects, 11
  sexual effects, 331
  types, 147
    new, 147, 403
    worldwide use, 4, 397
      USA, 3–4
Condyloma acuminatum, 298, 299
  treatment, 299, 300
Confidentiality, 232–233
  under-16s/adolescents, 228–229, 233
Congenital vaginal malformations, 337
Conjugated equine oestrogens, 379–380
Consent to sexual relations, age of, 232
Consent to treatment, 234–235, 246
  sterilization
    female, 235
    male, 200
Consultation, FP/well-woman,
      gynaecological disorders revealed,
      335–355
Consumer concerns, injectables, 94
Contact lenses and COCs, 63
Contracap, 404
Contraception
  after abortion *see* Abortion
  in amenorrhoea/oligomenorrhoea, 344
  back-up options, 15–17
  choice, 1–28
  costs *see* Cost
  in early marriage, 321
  effectiveness *see* Effectiveness
  failure rate, perfect-use vs typical use,
      5–6, 9
  HIV-infected individuals, 305–306
  HRT and *see* Hormone replacement
      therapy
  menstrual problems related to *see*
      Menstrual disorders
  new/improved/prospective methods, 33,
      143–144, 207–208, 395–416
    males, 332, 407–409, 409
    need for, 395–398
    public vs private research, 396–397
  non-contraceptive benefits, 12–13, 56–57,
      226
  older women *see* Middle age; Older
      women
  PMS and, 366–367
  postcoital *see* Emergency (postcoital)
      contraception
  postpartum *see* Postpartum period
  safety *see* Safety
  sexual effects, 61, 328–332
  stopping, 88, 102, 391–393
    indications, 58, 102, 350
    at menopause, 391–393
  teenagers *see* Adolescents

user considerations, 13–19
Copper IUDs, 106, 107–108
  choosing, 115
  costs, 20, 21
  effectiveness, 109
  indications, 113
  mode of action, 108–109
  safety/side-effects, 11
    PID risk, 122
  WHO medical eligibility criteria, 23–27
Copper T 380 *see* Ortho-Gynae T 380
Corticosteroids in lichen sclerosus, 336
Cost (economic), 19–21
  IUD, 20, 21, 110
  of unintended pregnancy, 21
  to user, 16, 18, 19–21
Counselling *see* Information
Crab louse, 308–309
Creams, spermicidal, 141, 150
  instructions, 153
Crohn's disease and COCs, 37, 64–65
Culture and fertility, 314–315
Curettage at sterilization, 182
Cutaneous disorders *see* Skin disorders
Cyclo-oxygenase (COX) inhibitors *see* Non-
      steroidal anti-inflammatory drugs
Cyclofem, 402
Cycloprovera, 402
Cyproterone acetate, 410
  COCs containing, 31
    in amenorrhoea/oligomenorrhoea, 344
    in COC-related skin disorders, 71–72
    in hirsutism, 345
Cyst(s)
  Bartholin's, 335–336
  ovarian, 338
    as POC contraindication, 83
    as POC side effect, 85, 86
  vaginal wall, 337
Cystoceles and diaphragms, 134
Cytomegalovirus, 308
  in HIV disease, 306, 308

D

Dalkon shield and PID, 122
Danazol
  emergency contraception, 207
  endometriosis, 339
  PMS, 364, 366
Death
  causes by age and sex, 267
  risk of (with FP methods), 11
    COCs, 11, 46
    vacuum aspiration, 255
Depo-Provera *see*
      Medroxyprogesterone acetate, depot

Depot medroxyprogesterone acetate *see* Medroxyprogesterone acetate
Depression and COCs, 60–61
Dermatological disorders *see* Skin disorders
Desogestrel (DSG) in COCs, 31
  prescribing, 49
  venous thromboembolism risk and, 43
  see also Ethinyloestradiol/desogestrel COC
Developing countries, FP in, 4, 396–397
Diabetes mellitus, 49
  as arterial disease risk factor with COCs, 49
  POC and, 101
  WHO medical eligibility criteria for FP methods, 24
    COCs, 24, 40–41
Dianette, 31, 410
  amenorrhoea/oligomenorrhoea, 344
  COC-related skin disorders, 71–72
  hirsutism, 345
Diaphragm (Dutch cap), 128–138, 330–331, 404
  advantages/disadvantages, 130–131
  care, 136
  discontinuation rates, 14
  effectiveness, 9, 130
  indications/contraindications, 130
  introducer, 134, 137
  menopause and, 393
  mode of action, 129
  new/improved types, 144–145, 404
  removing, 136
  safety/side-effects, 11
  selection and fitting, 132–135
    follow-up after, 137–138
  sexual effects, 330–331
  size
    to be fitted, estimating, 132
    wrong, 134, 135
  teaching and instructions, 134–137
  variations, 128–129
Diarrhoea
  COCs and, 52–53, 65
  POPs and, 88
Diathermy coagulation
  fallopian tubes, 179, 181
  vas deferens, 186
Diet
  breakthrough bleeding with COCs and, 63
  PMS management, 362
  pre-pregnancy, 350–351
Diethylstilboestrol and vaginal adenosis, 337
Digestive system and COCs, 63–65

Dilatation, cervical (for abortion), *see* Cervix
Discontinuation rates, 13–14
Diseases, pre-existing *see* Pre-existing diseases
Diuretics in PMS, 363
DNA detection, chlamydial, 289
Documentation, importance, 247
Domestic violence, 271
Dominance in relationships, 316–317
Double check method *see* Multiple index method
Down's syndrome and maternal age, 391
Drospirenone, 400
Drugs
  adverse/side-effects
    ejaculatory failure, 327–328
    postmenopausal bleeding, 342–343
  interactions
    COCs, 53, 54, 55–56, 65
    emergency contraception, 209
    POC, 79, 101
    WHO medical eligibility criteria for FP methods, 26–27
  nurse prescribing, 235–236
  sperm production-reducing, 408–409
  therapeutic use
    abortion induction *see* Medical abortion
    amenorrhoea/oligomenorrhoea, 344
    atrophic vaginitis, 336, 381–382
    dysmenorrhoea, 346
    endometriosis, 339
    hirsutism, 345–346
    lichen sclerosus, 336
    menopause, 379–390
    menstrual dysfunction, 342–343
    osteoporosis, 377
    PMS, 363–364, 365, 366
  see also Chemical agents *and specific (types of) drugs*
Dual X-ray absorptiometry (DXA), 376
Dutch cap *see* Diaphragm
Duty of care, 233
Dysmenorrhoea (menstrual pain), 346–347
  causes, 346
    IUDs, 120–121, 121
  investigations, 346
  treatment, 346
Dyspareunia, 325–326
Dysrhythmias on IUD insertion, 117–118
Dysuria, 349–350
  causes, 349–350
  management, 349–350
  presenting at FP consultation, 348

E

Econazole, candidiasis, 294
Economic cost *see* Cost
Ectopic pregnancy
history of, emergency contraception and, 206
pregnancy test *see* Pregnancy tests
risk of
IUDs, 109, 111, 123–124
POPs, 88
sterilization, 184
Ectropion, cervical, 337
Education
children and adolescents
global perspectives, 215–216
on sex *see* Sex education
health professionals, on PMS, 368
on specific contraceptive use *see*
Information
Effectiveness (and failure) of FP methods, 4–8, 9
abortion, 6, 17
cervical cap, 9, 138
coitus interruptus/withdrawal, 9, 157
condom
female, 9, 145
male, 9, 148
diaphragm (Dutch cap), 9, 130
emergency contraception, 6–7, 203–204
implants, 9, 96–97
injectables/depot preparations, 9, 90–91, 402
IUDs, 9, 109
measuring, 5–8
natural methods (periodic abstinence), 9, 169–170
oral contraceptives, 9
COCs, 9, 34–35
POPs, 88
spermicides, 9, 151
sponge, 9, 154
sterilization, female, 9, 184, 192, 195
complaints/litigation, 239
sterilization, male, 9, 188, 189–190, 192, 197–198
complaints/litigation, 240
Egg (mature ovum), vaccines, 415
Ejaculation
failure, 327–328
premature/rapid, 326–327
in early marriage, 320–321
Elcometrine (ST1435), 401
Electronic FP devices, 406
Embolism *see* Thromboembolic disease

Emergency (postcoital) contraception, 17, 201–213, 411
adolescents, 228
clinical management, 208–209
complaints/litigation, 245
effectiveness, 6–7, 203–204
follow-up, 210
indications/contraindications, 205–206
information, 209–210, 211, 212
kept at home, 212
methods, 202–203
mode of action, 203
new prospects, 207–208
POP use and, 88
postpartum, 176
safety/side-effects, 11, 207
use and availability, 210–212
Emesis *see* Vomiting
Emmett device, 124
Endocervical brushes, 277
Endocrine changes at menopause, 372
Endocrine disorders
oligomenorrhoea/amenorrhoea with, 343
investigations/treatment, 344
post-vasectomy, 189
see also Psychoneuroendocrine disorder
Endometriosis, 338–339
HRT contraindications, 384
treatment, 99, 339
Endometrium
ablation in PMS, 364
biopsy in postmenopausal bleeding, 343
cancer
COCs and, 64
HRT contraindications, 384
injectables and, 93
oestrogen (unopposed in HRT) and, 382
POC and, 78
polycystic ovarian syndrome and, 344
in menstrual cycle, 162, 163
Enjoyment *see* Pleasure
Enzyme-inducing drugs and COC use, 55, 55–56
tricycle regimen with, 56–57
Epididymitis, chlamydial, 288
Epididymo-orchitis, gonococcal, 283
Epilepsy
COCs and, 63
IUD insertion and, 118
POCs and, 101
Erectile dysfunction, 327
in early marriage, 321
self-esteem and, 316
Ethinyloestradiol (EE) in COCs, 30
dose, 50
monophasic pills, 31
Ethinyloestradiol/desogestrel COC, 32

new, 33
Ethinyloestradiol/gestodene COC
    bi-/triphasic, 32
    monophasic, 32
Ethinyloestradiol/levonorgestrel COC
    bi-/triphasic, 32
    monophasic, 32, 33
    new, 33
Ethinyloestradiol/levonorgestrel
        emergency contraception (Yuzpe
        method; Schering PC4), 202
    breastmilk production and, 176
    contraindications, 206
    effectiveness, 204
    mode of action, 203
    safety/side-effects, 11
Ethinyloestradiol/norethisterone COC
    bi-/triphasic, 32
    monophasic, 32
Ethinyloestradiol/norgestimate COC, 32
Ethynodiol diacetate in COCs, 31
Etonogestrel in implants, 95
Europe, teenager pregnancy statistics, 218
Evacuation, dilatation and, 258
Evening primrose oil in PMS, 362
Expulsion of IUDs, 112, 113
Eye problems and COCs, 63

F

Factor V Leiden, 44
Failure of FP methods *see* Effectiveness
Fallopian tube *see* Tubes
Falope ring, 179, 181
Famciclovir, HSV, 297
Family, influencing teenage pregnancy rate,
        219–220
Family history
    breast cancer, 270
    ovarian cancer, 278, 279
Family planning clinic *see* Clinic
Female(s)
    ageing and sexual interest, 323
    asserting femininity, 316
    death, causes, 267
    sexual exchanges and control issues, 317
    sexual problems, 323, 324–326
    STIs in
        candidiasis, 293
        examination, 282, 311
        genital herpes, 296
        genital warts, 299
        gonorrhoea, 283, 286
        non-specific urethritis, 288
        trichomoniasis, 292
    see also Girls
Female condom, 144–146, 404

adolescents, 227
effectiveness, 9, 146
HIV-infected persons, 305
reversibility, 192–193
Female sterilization (tubal
        block/division/ligation), 177–184,
        399–400
    advantages/disadvantages, 190–191
    age and patterns of use (UK), 3
    clinical management, 182–183
    complaints/litigation, 237–240
    discontinuation rates, 13, 14
    effectiveness/failure, 9, 184, 192, 195
    indications/contraindications, 189–190
    methods, 179–182
        of access, 177–180
        improved, 180–182, 399–400
    PMS and, 367
    postpartum, 176
    safety/side-effects/complications, 11,
        183–184, 195, 238, 239
    sexual effects, 332
    worldwide use, 4, 397
Female sterilization (tubal
        block/division/ligation)/counselling,
        information/advice, 182–183,
        191–192, 195
FemCap, 404
Femidom, 145
    adolescents, 227
Femininity, asserting, 316
Feminist concerns, injectables, 94
Fertility, 314–315
    breast-feeding and *see* Breast-feeding
    future (reversibility), FP method and, 16,
        19
        COCs, 72
        injectables, 91, 102
        IUDs, 111
        POCs, 91, 101–102
    monitoring *see* Ovulation
    older women, 390
    reduced *see* Infertility/subfertility
    regulation methods
        natural *see* Natural FP
        vs strategies, 1–4
Fetus
    effects of exposure
        to COCs, 73
        to emergency contraception, 205–206
        to progestogens, 83, 93, 102
            injectables, 93
    HIV infection, prevention, 301
    residual tissue from, post-abortion, 259
Fibroids (leiomyomas)
    COCs and, 66
    HRT and, 384
    POCs and, 100

FibroPlant-LNG, 403
Films, spermicidal, 151–153
Filshie clip, 179, 180
Flat-spring diaphragm, 128, 129
    fitting/using, 134
Flexi-T 300, 106
Fluconazole, candidiasis, 294, 295
Fluoroquinolones in gonorrhoea, 287
Foam, spermicidal, 150, 151
    instructions, 153
Folate supplements, 351
Follicle(s), ovarian, persistent, with POC,
    85, 86
Follicle-stimulating hormone (FSH), 162,
    163
    in amenorrhoea, measurement, 344
    at menopause, elevated levels, 372
        diagnostic value, 372, 392
    suppressed levels with
        breast-feeding/lactation, 172
    vaccination against, 415
Follicular cysts with POC, 85
Follicular phase of menstrual cycle, 162
Fornix, anterior, diaphragm repeated
    inserted into, 134
Fourex, 148
Fractures, osteoporotic, 376
    prevention, 377
Frameless IUDs, 107–108, 403
Frequency dysuria syndrome (FDS), 349,
    350
Fungal infections, 293–295
    drug therapy see Antifungals

G

Gallbladder disease, HRT contraindications,
    384
Gallstones
    COCs and, 64
    HRT and, 384
    POCs and, 100
Gastrointestinal system and COCs, 63–65
Gels, spermicidal, 150, 152
    instructions, 153
Gender identity, 316
    see also Sex (biological)
Genetic counselling, 351
Genital herpes see Herpes simplex infection
Genital system/tract disorders see
        Gynaecological disorders
Genital warts see Condyloma acuminatum
Genitourinary medicine clinics, 281–282
Gestation, stage, determination, 253
Gestational trophoblast disease see
        Trophoblastic disease

Gestodene (GSD) in COCs, 31
    prescribing, 49
    venous thromboembolism risk and, 43
    see also Ethinyloestradiol/gestodene COC
Gestrinone in endometriosis, 339
Gillick competence, 232
Girls
    prepubertal, gonorrhoea
        clinical features, 286
        diagnosis, 286
        sexual abuse possibility, 287
    pubertal see Adolescents
Global perspectives
    adolescent reproductive health, 215–216
    patterns of FP, 2–4, 395–397
Gonadotrophin see Follicle-stimulating
        hormone; Luteinising hormone
Gonadotrophin-releasing hormone (GnRH)
    lactational infertility and, 172
    vaccination against, 415
Gonadotrophin-releasing hormone
        analogues (agonists/antagonists)
    as contraceptives, 409
    endometriosis, 339
    PMS, 364, 366
Gonorrhoea (*N. gonorrhoea* infection),
        282–287
    clinical features, 283–286
    diagnosis, 286
    transport medium for *N. gonorrhoea*, 311
    treatment, 286–287
Gossypol, 405, 408
Gramicidin, 156
Granulomas, sperm, 188, 198
Greasy skin and COCs, 71–72
Gynaecological disorders (incl. genital
        tract/system), 335–355
    COC-related, 65–67
    FP consultation revealing, 335–355
    IUD benefits, 110–111
    pre-existing, POC use and, 99–100
GyneFix, 106, 107, 403
    insertion, 117

H

Haematoma with vasectomy, 188
Haemorrhagic stroke risk, COCs, 45–46
Hamou tubal plug, 399
Headaches, 61–62
    with COCs, 59, 61–62
        as contraindication, 61–62
    WHO medical eligibility criteria for FP
        methods, 25
    see also Migraine
Health clinic see Clinic
Health personnel/professionals

HIV infection precautions, 304
PMS education, 368
Health promotion, 265–280
Healthcare system, user interaction with, 16, 17–18
Heart disorders/disease
  arrhythmias on IUD insertion, 117–118
  valvular *see* Valvular heart disease
  WHO medical eligibility criteria for FP methods, 25, 37
  see also Cardiovascular disease
Hepatitis
  POC exacerbating, 100
  viral, 307–308
    hepatitis B, 307
    hepatitis C, 307–308
    WHO medical eligibility criteria for FP methods, 26, 37
Hepatocellular carcinoma and COCs, 64
Herpes simplex infection (genital herpes), 295–298
  clinical features, 296
  diagnosis, 297
  natural history, 295–296
  in pregnancy, 298
  recurrent, 296
  treatment, 297–298
Heterosexuals, HIV infection, 301
Hirsutism, 345–346
  causes, 345
    progestogens, 71–72
  clinical management, 345–346
HIV/AIDS, 300–307
  clinical features, 301–302
  contraception, 305–306
  diagnosis, 303–304
    assessment following, 306–307
  epidemiology, 300–301
  health personnel precautions, 304
  management, 304–307
  natural history, 302–303
  spermicides preventing HIV infection, 151, 156, 305
  WHO medical eligibility criteria for FP methods, 26
Homosexuals
  condoms for anal intercourse, 147, 304
  HIV infection risk, 301
Hormonal contraceptives (in general)
  after abortion, 261
  complaints/litigation, 243–246
  emergency use, 202, 212, 411
    side-effects, 207
  historical perspectives, 29–30
  HIV-infected persons, 305
  menstrual bleeding controlled by, 12–13, 56–57
  mode of action, 34

new/improved, 33, 207–208, 400–403, 409–413
  men, 407–408
  sexual effects, 61, 329–330
  worldwide use, 4
  see also specific methods
Hormonal therapy, PMS, 363–364
Hormone(s)
  changes in/disorders of *see* Endocrine changes; Endocrine disorders
  sex steroid *see* Sex hormones
Hormone-releasing IUD (progestogen/levonorgestrel-impregnated), 78, 98, 108
  costs, 110
  effectiveness, 109
  gynaecological benefit, 110–111
  indications, 113
    PMS, 366, 368
  mode of action, 109
  new/improved, 403
  WHO medical eligibility criteria, 23–27
Hormone replacement therapy (HRT), 371–372, 379–390
  adherence, 388
  complications, 385–386
  contraception and, 393–394
    complaints over HRT use as contraceptive, 245–246
  contraindications, 384–385
  duration of use, 390
  in endometriosis treatment, 339
  'no period' HRT, 383
  PMS induced by, 367–368
  preventive/protective effects, 377
    cardiovascular disease, 378
    osteoporosis, 377
  routes, 379, 380
  special considerations, 386–388
Hostility and sexual assault, 317
Hot flushes, 373
HPV *see* Human papilloma virus
Hulka–Clemens clip, 179, 180
Human chorionic gonadotrophin (hCG)
  pregnancy testing *see* Pregnancy tests
  vaccination against, 414
Human papilloma virus (HPV), 298–300
  cancer/precancer and, 298
    cervical, 274, 298, 299–300
  clinical features, 298–299
  management, 299–300
Hydrogel plug, 399
5-Hydroxytryptamine (5-HT) *see* Serotonin
Hypercholesterolaemia, 272

Hypericum (St Johns Wort) in PMS, 363
Hyperprolactinaemia *see* Prolactin
Hypertension
    COC users, 58
        as arterial disease risk factor, 49, 59–60
    HRT contraindications, 384
    in POC users, 84, 99
        risk of, 79
    WHO medical eligibility criteria for FP methods, 24
Hysterectomy
    in PMS, 364, 368
    sterilization and risk of, 184
    as sterilization method, safety/ side-effects, 11

I

Imidazoles, candidiasis, 294
Immune system in HIV disease/AIDS, 302–303
Immunization *see* Vaccines
Immunological tests in HIV infection, 306
Immunomodulatory agents, condyloma acuminatum, 300
Immunosuppressive drugs and IUDs, 114
Implanon, 81, 95, 96
    administration, 96–97
    complaints/litigation, 244
    effectiveness, 97
    specific attributes, 95
Implants, subcutaneous/subdermal oestrogen, 381
Implants, subcutaneous/subdermal progestogen, 14, 78, 94–96
    administration, 95, 96–97
    adolescents, 228
    choice, 81
    complaints/litigation, 243, 244
    costs, 20, 21
    effectiveness, 9, 96–97
    improvements, 401
    indications/contraindications, 97
    safety/side-effects, 11, 97
        controversies/medicolegal aspects, 97–98
    specific attributes, 94–95
    WHO medical eligibility criteria, 23–27
    worldwide use, 4, 397
Incontinence, urinary, 272
    causes, 348
Infants
    HIV-infected, 301
    newborn *see* Neonates
Infections, 281–311

in abortion, 260
    pre-treatment assessment for, 253
with COCs, 72
    urinary tract, 65
with diaphragms, urinary tract, 131
in HIV, opportunistic, 308
    serological tests, 306
with IUDs, 121–123
    history of, 114
    risk of, 112, 114, 121–123
sexually-transmitted *see* Sexually-transmitted infections
with sterilization
    females, 183
    males, 188
in surgical abortion, 242
urinary tract *see* Urinary tract infections
Infertility/subfertility, 352–354
    abortion causing, 260
    C. trachomatis causing, 253
    clinical management, 352–354
    IUD use and, 105
    lactational *see* Breast-feeding; Lactational amenorrhoea
Inflammatory bowel disease and COCs, 37, 64–65
Inflammatory disorders and COCs, 72
Information/advice/instructions/teaching and counselling (on contraceptive use), 15
    abortion, 251–252, 263–264
    cervical cap use, 141–142
    COC use, 50
        inadequate, 244
    condom use
        female, 146
        male, 149
    diaphragm use, 134–137
    emergency contraception, 209–210, 211, 212
    HIV, 304–305
        pre-test counselling, 303
    injectables, 245
    IUDs, 119
        deficient, 242, 243
    natural FP, 171
    pre-pregnancy, 350–351
    sexual problems, 333
        premature ejaculation, 326
    smoking cessation, 272
    spermicides, 153
    sponges, 155–156
    sterilization, 191–192
        deficient, 238–239, 240
        female, 182–183, 191–192, 195
        male *see* Vasectomy
        on reversal, 192

vault cap use, 142
vimule use, 143
Injectables, 78, 89–94
adolescents, 227
complaints/litigation, 245
contraindications, 83, 91
breast-feeding, 174
costs, 21
discontinuation rates, 14
effectiveness, 9, 90–91, 402
improvements, 401–403
indications, 91
male, 408
return to fertility after, 19
safety/side-effects, 11, 91–94
controversies and medicolegal issues,
92–94
specific attributes, 89–90
stopping at menopause, 392
WHO medical eligibility criteria,
23–27
worldwide use, 4, 397
Instructions *see* Information
Intercourse, sexual
adaptations
as contraceptive method, 158–159
non-vaginal *see* Anal intercourse; Oral
sex
bleeding after, 341
FP method and frequency of, 16, 19
interrupted *see* Coitus interruptus
older women, frequency, 390
pain on, 325–326
postnatal, 321–322
International perspectives *see* Global
perspectives
Intestinal obstruction and female
sterilization, 184
Intimacy, sexual, fostering, 315–316
Intimate partner *see* Partner
Intracranial hypertension, benign, COCs
and, 63
Intraepithelial neoplasia
cervical, 274
HPV and, 298
management, 278
penile, HPV and, 298
vulval, HPV and, 298
Intrauterine device *see* IU(C)D
Introducer, diaphragm, 134, 137
Ischaemic stroke risk, COCs, 45
Itraconazole, candidiasis, 294
IU(C)D (intrauterine contraceptive device),
105–126, 202, 242–243, 330, 393
adolescents, 228
advantages, 109–111
assessment for use, 115–120
changing/replacing, 120

complaints/litigation, 242–243
costs, 20, 21, 110
disadvantages, 112
discontinuation rates, 13, 14
effectiveness, 9, 109
HIV-infected persons, 305
improvements, 107–108, 403
indications/contraindications,
113–114
information *see* Information
insertion, 115–119, 209
failure, 119
follow-up, 119
post-abortion, 261
postcoital *see subheading below*
lost, 125–126
at menopause, 393
mode of action, 108–109
PMS and, 367
postcoital insertion (as emergency
contraception), 202
effectiveness, 204
mode of action, 203
side-effects, 207
postpartum use, 175
pregnancy, 109, 111, 123–124
removal, 119–120
at menopause, criteria, 393
safety/side-effects/complications, 11,
105, 120–126, 207, 242
sexual effects, 330
sterilization and, 182
threads *see* Threads
types, 106–108, 115
copper-bearing *see* Copper IUDs
hormone-releasing *see*
Hormone-releasing IUD
inert/non-medicated types,
106–107
selection, 115
UK use, 3
WHO medical eligibility criteria, 23–27
worldwide use, 4

J

Jadelle (Norplant-11)
administration, 96
effectiveness, 97
specific attributes, 95
Jaundice with COCs, 64

K

3-Keto-desogestrel in implants, 95
KoCap, 404

L

Laboratory tests and POCs, 102
Lactational amenorrhoea (FP method; Bellagio guidelines), 172–174
effectiveness, 9
Laparoscopy
diagnostic, in pelvic pain, 347
female sterilization via, 177–178, 195
complaints/litigation, 237–238
Laparotomy *see* Mini-laparotomy
Laser vaporization, tubal division via, 179–180
Latex rubber for condoms, 147
alternatives to, 147, 403
Law *see* Medicolegal issues
Lea's shield, 143–144, 404
Leg pains/cramps and COCs, 70–71
Legal issues *see* Medicolegal issues
Leiomyomas *see* Fibroids
Levonelle-2, 202
Levonorgestrel (LNG)
in COCs, 31
prescribing, 48, 49
see also
Ethinyloestradiol/levonorgestrel COC
in emergency contraception, alone, 202, 212
effectiveness, 204
mode of action, 203
in emergency contraception, with ethinyloestradiol *see* Ethinyloestradiol/levonorgestrel emergency contraception
in implants, 94, 95
IUD impregnated with *see* Hormone-releasing IUD
Levonorgestrel butanoate, 403
Levonova (Mirena), 81, 108
Libido *see* Sexual desire
Lice, crab/pubic, 308–309
Lichen sclerosus, 336
Lifecycle approach to contraception, 2
Lifestyle, sexual *see* Sexual behaviour
Life-table techniques (measuring FP method effectiveness), 7–8
Lipid profile, HRT (oestrogen) effects, 378
Litigation, 231, 237–247
reducing risk, 246–247
Liver
disease
neoplastic *see* Tumours
POC users, 84, 100
WHO medical eligibility criteria for FP methods, 26, 37

inflammation of covering (perihepatitis), 288
metabolism of COCs, 42
Louse, crab, 308–309
Lubricants
oil-based *see* Oil-based lubricants
postpartum use, 174–175
Lunelle, 402
Luteal phase of menstrual cycle, 162
Luteinising hormone (LH), 162, 163
breast-feeding/lactation and levels of, 172
measurement
for contraception, 169, 406
for increasing conception chances, 354
menopause and levels of, 372
Lymphadenopathy, persistent generalized, 301

M

Magnesium supplements in PMS, 363
Males
asserting masculinity, 316
bolstering self-esteem, 316
causes of death, 267
new contraceptive methods, 332, 407–409, 409
sexual problems, 323, 326–327
sterilization *see* Vasectomy
STIs in
candidiasis, 293
genital herpes, 296
genital warts, 299
gonorrhoea, 283, 286
non-specific urethritis, 288
trichomoniasis, 292
Malignancy *see* Cancer
Mammography, 269–270
Marriage
bartering over sex, 318
early, 320–321
see also Parenthood; Partner
Masculinity, asserting, 316
Masculinization of female fetus, injectables, 93
Material gain, sex for, 318
Medical abortion
early first trimester, 256
contraindications, 256
side-effects, 256
mid-trimester, 258–259
patient information sheet, 263
Medical eligibility criteria for FP, WHO *see* WHO
Medicolegal issues, 231–248

abortion, 250–251
injectables, 92–94
POPs, 89
Medroxyprogesterone acetate, depot
    (DMPA; marketed as Depo-Provera)
    administration, 90
    adolescents, 227
    complaints/litigation, 245
    contraindications, 83, 91
    effectiveness, 9, 90
    fertility return after, 19, 102
    HIV-infected persons, 305
    indications, 82, 91
        sickle cell disease, 101
    in PMS, 366, 367
    sexual lifestyle and, 18
    side-effects/complications, 91
        controversies and medicolegal issues,
        92, 93, 94
        specific attributes, 90
    stopping at menopause, 392
    WHO medical eligibility criteria, 23–27
Mefenamic acid, menorrhagia, 341
Melanoma and COCs, 72
Melasma and COCs, 71
Men see Males
Menopause, 371–394
    consequences/symptoms of (ovarian
        failure at), 373–378
    defined, 371
    diagnosis, 372–373
    endocrine changes, 372
    management, 378–390
    sexuality and, 323
    see also Perimenopause; Postmenopausal
        women
Menorrhagia, 340
    with IUDs, 121
    treatment, 341–342
Menstrual cycle, 162–164
    antiprogestogens in regulation of,
        410–411
    COCs manipulating, 12–13, 56–57
    fertile period, detection
        for contraception see Natural FP
        to increasing conception chances, 354
    hormones of, 162, 163
    IUD insertion and, 116
    POC-related disturbances, 84–85
        POPs, 89
    pregnancy risk related to, 201
    sexual interest and, 324
Menstrual disorders/disturbances, 340–342,
        343–344, 346–347
    with contraceptives, 340
        with emergency contraception, 207
        with IUDs, 112, 120–121
    IUD benefits in, 111

management/treatment, 341–342
    POCs contraindicated, 83
Menstrual extraction technique/kit, 255
Menstruation (menstrual period)
    irregularity, 340–341
    migraine during, 348
    painful see Dysmenorrhoea
    prolonged/heavy see Menorrhagia
    see also Bleeding, menstrual
Mental illness see Psychiatric disorders
Mesigyna, 402
Mestranol/norethisterone COC, 32
Metabolic effects
    COCs, 42
    POC, 79
Metronidazole
    bacterial vaginosis, 291
    trichomoniasis, 293
Miconazole, candidiasis, 294
Microbicidal spermicides, 153, 157,
        398, 405
Micturition
    painful see Dysuria
    urgent/frequent
        causes, 348
        management, 349
Middle age
    contraception, 323
    sexuality, 322–323
    see also Older women
Mifepristone (RU 486), 410–411
    abortion, 11
        adverse/side-effects, 11
        early first trimester, 256–257
        late first trimester, 257
        mid-trimester, 259
    contraception, 411
        emergency, 208, 411
    menstrual regulation with, 410–411
Migraine
    and COC use
        occurrence as arterial disease risk, 49,
            61–62
        use contraindicated, 61–62
    menstrual, 348
Mineral supplements in PMS, 363
Mini-laparotomy (approach to sterilization),
        178–179
    postpartum, 176, 178
    wound healing, 183
Mirena (Levonova), 81, 108
Miscarriage (spontaneous abortion)
    COCs after, 51–52
    older women, 391
    recurrent, 352
Misoprostol for IUD removal, 120
Mittelschmerz, 163
Molluscum contagiosum, 308

Monophasic COCs, 31–33
  new awaited, 33
  postponing period, 56
  in tricycle regimen (enzyme-inducing
      drug users), 56–57
Mood state and sexual interest, 317–318
  perimenstrual, 324
Moral issues in sex education, 224, 225
Mortality see Death
Mucus, cervical
  hormonal contraceptives altering, 34
  measurements (=Billings or ovulation
      method), 166–167
    effectiveness, 170
    improved methods, 406
    temperature measurement plus see
        Symptothermal method
    see also Multiple index method
Multiload Cu250, 106
Multiload Cu375, 106
Multiple index method, 168
  effectiveness, 170
Musculoskeletal disorders and
    COCs, 70–71
Mycoplasma genitalium, 288
Myocardial infarction
  previous
    HRT, 384
    POC and, 99
  risk with COCs, 44–45

N

Natural FP (periodic abstinence), 161–176,
    331–332
  advantages/disadvantages, 170–171
  age and patterns of use (UK), 3
  biological basis, 162–164
  costs, 20
  discontinuation rates, 13, 14
  effectiveness, 9, 169–170
  indications, 170
  menopause and, 393
  methods, 164–169
  new/improved methods, 405–407
  PMS and, 367
  sexual effects, 331–332
  teaching, 171
Natural steroids, injectable, 402
Nausea with emergency contraception, 207
Needs, user's, assessing, 15
Negligence, 233–234
Neisseria gonorrhoea see Gonorrhoea
Neodymium:YAG laser, tubal division, 180
Neonates
  exposure to injectables, 93
  HIV infection and its prevention, 301, 307

Neoplasms see Tumours
Nestorone, 401
Neural tube defects and folate, 351
Neurological disorders
  pre-existing, POC and, 100–101
  risk with COC, 60–63
Neurotransmitters and PMS, 361
Night sweats, 373
No-scalpel vasectomy, 186, 398
Nomogestrol acetate in implants, 95
Nonoxynol-9
  preparations containing, 151
    films, 151
    sponges, 154
  STIs and effects of, 151, 305
Nonoxynol-11 containing preparations,
    152
Non-specific urethritis, 288–290
Non-steroidal anti-inflammatory drugs
    (COX inhibitors; prostaglandin
    synthase inhibitors)
  dysmenorrhoea, 346
  menorrhagia, 341
  PMS, 363
Norethisterone (NET; norethisterone
    acetate)
  in COCs, 31
    prescribing, 48, 49
  menorrhagia therapy, 342
  see also Ethinyloestradiol/norethisterone
      COC; Mestranol/norethisterone
      COC
Norethisterone enanthate (NET-EN)
    injectables
  administration, 90
  effectiveness, 91
  indications, 91
  return to fertility after, 19
  side-effects/complications, 91
  specific attributes, 90
  WHO medical eligibility criteria, 23–27
Norgestimate in COCs, 31
  see also Ethinyloestradiol/norgestimate
      COC
Norplant (and Norplant-2), 94, 244
  administration, 95
  adolescents, 228
  complaints/litigation, 243, 244
  effectiveness, 9, 96
  side-effects/controversies/medicolegal
      issues, 97–98
  specific attributes, 94
  WHO medical eligibility criteria, 23–27
Norplant-11 see Jadelle
Nova-T 380, 106, 107
  levonorgestrel-impregnated (Mirena),
      81, 108
Nulliparity and IUD, 114

Nurses' extended role, 235–236
  prescribing, 235–236, 246
Nutrition *see* Diet
Nystatin, candidiasis, 294

O

Obesity *see* Overweight
Occlusive pessaries (caps), 127–144
  damage, 144
  historical aspects, 127–128
  new types, 143–144, 404
  see also specific types
Occlusive plugs *see* Plugs
Ocular problems and COCs, 63
Oestrogen(s)
  in COCs, 30–31, 32
    dose, 50
    dose, and thromboembolic disease risk,
      42–43
    new, 400
  deficiency, 336
    dysuria in, 349–350
  in emergency contraception, 202
    contraindications, 206
    high-dose, 203
  in menopause, 379–382
    atrophic change improved with, 336,
      381–382
    in cardiovascular disease prevention,
      378
    in diagnosis, 373
    in HRT, side-effects, 385
    in osteoporosis treatment/prevention,
      376–377
    routes of administration, 379, 380
  in menstrual cycle, 162, 163
  plant-derived, 379
  in PMS therapy, 364, 366, 368
  see also Hormone replacement therapy
    and specific oestrogens
Oestrogen–progestogen combined
  preparations *see entries under*
  Combined
Oestrogen receptor modulators, selective
  (SERMs)
  in menopause, 383
    in osteoporosis, 377
  in PMS, 368, 369
Oestrone-3-glucuronide (E3G), dipstick
  measurement, 169
Oil-based lubricants causing damage
  to condoms, 149
  to occlusive pessaries, 144
Older women
  contraception, 390–391
    COC and breast cancer, 69

POC, 82, 98
  fertility, 390
  pregnancy, 390–391
  see also Ageing; Middle age;
    Perimenopause
Oligomenorrhoea, 343–344
  infertility, 354
Oophorectomy in PMS, 364
Open-ended vasectomy, 186
Ophthalmological problems and COCs, 63
Oral contraceptives (pill), 29–103, 391–392
  adolescents, 98, 225–226, 227
  combined *see* Combined oral
    contraceptives
  complaints/litigation, 243, 244–245
  costs, 20, 21
  discontinuation rates, 14
  effectiveness *see* Effectiveness
  male, 407
  missed, 52, 88
    emergency contraception, 88, 205
  new/improved, 33, 400
  in PMS
    as contraceptive, 367
    as treatment, 364, 366, 367
  progestogen-only *see* Progestogen-only
    pill
  safety/side-effects, 11
  sexual effects, 61, 329–330
  stopping, 88, 102, 392
    indications, 58, 102
    at menopause, 392
  UK use, 3
  WHO medical eligibility criteria, 23–27,
    36–39
  worldwide use, 4, 397
Oral manifestation of HIV disease, 302
Oral oestrogens in HRT, 380
Oral sex, 158
Orgasm
  arousal reduced after, 317
  female dysfunction, 325
Ortho-Gynae T 380 (Copper T 380), 107
  380A, 106
  380S, 106
  choosing, 115
Osteoporosis, 375–377
  management, 376, 377
  risk factors, 376
    depot medroxyprogesterone acetate as,
      93
Ovabloc, 399
Ovarian failure, consequences, 373–378
Ovariectomy (oophorectomy) in PMS, 364
Ovaries
  cancer/carcinoma, 278–279
    COCs and, 64
    detection, 278–279

Ovaries (*cont.*)
    injectables and, 93
    sterilization and, 184
    cysts *see* Cysts
    functional elimination in PMS therapy,
        365
    hormones, in menstrual cycle, 162, 163
    POC actions, 80
    POC pathological effects, 85
        management, 86
    polycystic *see* Polycystic ovarian
        syndrome
    removal (oophorectomy) in PMS, 364
Overdosage, POP, 80
Overweight and obesity, 270–271
    with COCs
        as arterial disease risk factor, 49
        caused by COCs, 64
    HRT and, 389–390
    with injectables, 91–92
    as POC contraindication, 83
Oves cap, 144
Ovulation
    breakthrough, missed pills and, 52
    inhibition by hormonal contraceptives, 34
    monitor device for contraception, 406
        personal *see* Persona
    monitor device for increasing conception
        chances, 354
    mucus method of detection,
        see Mucus
Ovum, vaccines, 415
Ovutest, 406

P

P-block, 399
Pain
    leg, with COCs, 70–71
    menstrual *see* Dysmenorrhoea
    at ovulation time (mittelschmerz), 162
    pelvic, 347
    post-vasectomy, chronic, 188
    in sexual intercourse, 325–326
    on urination *see* Dysuria
Pair-bonding, 315–316
Paraurethral glands, gonococcal infection,
    283
Parenthood, early, 321–322
Parity and IUD, 114
Partner, sexual/intimate
    role in FP, 16, 18–19
    sexual problems involving both, 328
    violence, 271
    see also Marriage
Patches, steroid hormone, 413
Pearl index, 7

Pelvic congestion, 347
Pelvic examination
    before emergency contraception,
        209
    before female sterilization, 182
    before HRT, 388, 389
    dysmenorrhoea, 346
    endometriosis, 339
    ovarian cancer detection, 279
    postmenopausal bleeding, 343
Pelvic inflammatory disease (PID)
    chlamydial, 288
        treatment, 290
    diaphragms and risk of, 131
    emergency contraception and, 206
    gonococcal, 283
    IUDs
        PID as contraindication, 114
        risk of PID, 112, 122
    WHO medical eligibility criteria for FP
        methods, 25–26
Pelvic masses, 338
Pelvic pain, 347
Penicillins in gonorrhoea, 287
    resistance (penicillinase-producing
        organisms; PPNG), 283, 286
Penis
    erectile dysfunction *see* Erectile
        dysfunction
    intraepithelial neoplasia, HPV and, 298
Percutaneous non-surgical vas occlusion,
    186, 398
Perihepatitis, 288
Perimenopause (climacteric)
    changes in, 372
    defined, 371
    non-hormonal treatment, 379
    POC, 82, 98
    sexuality, 323
Periodic abstinence *see* Natural FP
Perlutal, 402
Persona (personal fertility monitor), 168,
    406
    costs, 20, 21
    effectiveness, 170
Pessaries (vaginal)
    occlusive *see* Occlusive pessaries
    spermicidal, 150, 151
        instructions, 153
pH
    vaginal, at menopause, 375
    vaginal discharge, measurement, 291
Pharyngeal gonorrhoea, 283
    treatment, 286–287
Photosensitivity and COCs, 71
Phthiriasis, 308–309
Phyto-oestrogens, menopause, 379
Pill *see* Oral contraceptives

Pill-free interval
  changing preparations and, 52
  missed pills and, 52
Pituitary hormones and menstrual cycle, 162, 163
Placental residual tissue, post-abortion, 259
Plastic condoms, 148, 403
Pleasure/enjoyment, sexual, 315
  loss by woman, 324
Pleurisy risk, COCs, 60
Plugs, occlusive
  fallopian tubes, 399–400
  vas deferens, 399
Podophyllin resin, 300
Podophyllotoxin, 300
Political issues in sex education, 224, 225
Polycystic ovarian syndrome
  amenorrhoea/oligomenorrhoea in, 344
  endometrial cancer risk, 344
Polymerase chain reaction, HIV RNA detection, 303
Polyp, cervical, 337–338
Polyurethane condoms, 148
Porphyria and POC, 100
Postcoital bleeding, 341
Postcoital contraception see Emergency contraception
Postmenopausal women, pelvic masses, 338
Postpartum/postnatal period
  contraception, 174–176
    COCs see Combined oral contraceptives
    POC see Progestogen-only contraception
    sterilization, 176, 178
    WHO medical eligibility criteria for various methods, 23
  sexual adjustment, 321–322
Post-tubal sterilization syndrome, 184
Post-vasectomy syndrome, 188
Poverty and teenage pregnancy, 219, 221–222
Power in relationships, 316–317
Precancers see Pre-malignant disease
Pre-conception procedures see Pre-pregnancy
Pre-existing diseases
  and medical eligibility criteria for FP methods, 24–27
  POCs and, 82, 98–101
    POPs exacerbating disease, 89
Pregnancy
  after abortion, complications, 260
  bleeding in early stages, 351–352
  COC users, outcome, 73
  ectopic see Ectopic pregnancy

fetal effects of exposure to hormonal contraceptives see Fetus
HIV infection, 304
  vertical transmission (and its prevention), 301, 307
HSV infection, 298
older women, 390–391
risk related to cycle, 201
suspected, emergency contraception and, 205
teenage, 217–222
  causes, 219–220
  intended, 220
  outcome, 220–221
  reduction strategies, 221–225
  statistics, 217–218
  termination (medical/surgical) see Abortion (therapeutic)
unintended
  cost, 21
  counselling, 251–252
  with IUDs, 109, 111, 123–124
  worldwide patterns, 396–397
  see also Effectiveness
Pregnancy mask and COCs, 71
Pregnancy tests (hCG levels), 352
  abortion candidate, 253
  ectopic pregnancy, 352
  IUD user, 123–124
Pre-malignant disease
  cervical see Cervical cancer, precursors
  diaphragms and, 131
  vulvovaginal, 298, 336, 337
Premature ejaculation see Ejaculation
Premenstrual syndrome (PMS), 357–369
  aetiology, 361
    HRT-related, 367–368
  consequences, 359
  contraception and, 366–367
  definitions, 357
  diagnosis, 358
  management, 362–369
    evidence-based approach, 362
  prevalence, 359
  quantifying, 358
  seriousness, acceptance, 357, 369
  symptoms, 357, 358–359
    character, 358
    timing, 358–359
  treatment related to, 365
Prenatal screening, 351
Prentif cavity-rim cap, 138
Pre-pregnancy counselling, 350–351
Pre-pregnancy screening, 279
Prescribing
  of COCs, 34, 48–53
  by nurse, 235–236, 246
Privacy, 16, 19

Proctitis
  chlamydial, 288
  gonococcal, 283
Progesterone
  measurements in infertility, 354
  therapeutic use in PMS, 363–364, 366
Progestogen(s)
  in COCs, 31, 32
    new, 400
    thromboembolic disease risk and type
      of, 43
    see also Combined oral contraceptives
  in HRT
    licensed types/dosages, 382
    as PMS-inducing agents, 367, 368
    side-effects, 385–386
    see also Combined
      oestrogen–progestogen therapy
  in implants, 94, 95
    see also Combined
      oestrogen–progestogen injectables
  IUD impregnated with see
      Hormone-releasing IUD
  male contraception, 408
  menorrhagia therapy, 342
  PMS therapy, 363–364, 366
  in POPs, 87
Progestogen-only contraception (POC) in
      general, 77–103, 392, 400, 403
  adolescents, 98, 227–228
  advantages (non-contraceptive), 78–80
  assessment for use, 81
  choice of method, 81
  complaints/litigation, 244, 245
  contraindications, 82–84
  delivery systems, choices, 78
  disadvantages, 80
  drug interactions, 79, 101
  HIV-infected persons, 305
  improvements, 400–401, 402
  indications, 82
  individual methods, 87–98
  migraine sufferers, 62
  modes of action, 80–81
  postpartum/in breast-feeding, 79, 93, 174
    contraindications, 84
  sexual effects, 329, 330
  side-effects see Safety
  special considerations, 98–102
  stopping, 88, 102, 392
    indications, 102
    at menopause, 392
Progestogen-only pill/oral contraceptives
      (POPs), 78, 87–89, 392
  administration, 87–88
  adolescents, 98, 227
  choice/preparations, 81, 86, 87
  controversies and medicolegal issues, 89

effectiveness, 9, 88
  HIV-infected persons, 305
  HRT and, 393–394
  improvements, 400
  indications/contraindications, 89
  missed, 88
    emergency contraception, 88, 205
  PMS and, 367
  safety/side-effects, 11, 89, 392
  specific attributes, 87
  starting, 87–88
  stopping, 88
    at menopause, 392
  WHO medical eligibility criteria, 23–27
Progestogen-only rings, 78, 400, 413
Progestogen-only therapy at menopause,
      379
ProgestURINE RAMP, 406
Prolactin, elevated levels (incl.
      hyperprolactinaemia), 344
  with breast-feeding/lactation, 172
Propranolol as spermicide, 156
Prostaglandin(s) (PGs), in abortion, 11
  for cervical dilatation, 257
  mid-trimester, 258, 259
  in persistence of placental/fetal tissue,
      260
Prostaglandin synthase inhibitors see
      Non-steroidal anti-inflammatory
      drugs
Prostate cancer and vasectomy, 189,
      98–99
Prostitution, 318
Protein C, activated, resistance, 44
Protozoal infestation, 292–293
Psychiatric/mental disorders
  abortion and, 260
  COC risk of, 60–61
Psychological dimensions
  abortion, 260
  COC use, 61, 329
  menopause, 374
  pelvic pain, 347
  PMS, 358
  sexual problems
    adolescents, 319
    early parenthood, 322
    men, 327, 328
    middle age, 322
    women, 61, 322, 324–325
Psychoneuroendocrine disorder, PMS as,
      361
Psychotherapy in PMS, 363
Psychotropic drugs in PMS, 363
Pthirus pubis (phthiriasis), 308–309
Puberty, 319
  hirsutism, 345
  see also Adolescents

Pubic (crab) louse, 308–309
Pulmonary disease risk with COCs, 60

Q

Quinacrine, tubal occlusion, 181–182, 400

R

Raloxifene
  in menopause, 383
  in PMS, 368, 369
Rape and hostility, 317
Records/documentation, importance, 247
Rectal infection
  chlamydial, 288
  gonococcal, 283
Referral
  abortion, 253–254
  bleeding in early pregnancy, 352
  infertility, 353, 354
Relationships
  power and dominance in, 316–317
  sexual, evolving of, 318–323
Religion and sex and fertility, 314–315, 331
Reproductive health promotion, 265–280
Reproductive system disorders *see*
      Gynaecological disorders
Research, contraceptive, public vs private,
      396–397
Respiratory disease risk with COCs, 60
Resuscitation and IUD insertion, 118
Retrievette, 124
Rhesus isoimmunization in abortion, 253
Rhythm method *see* Calendar method
Rifamycins and COCs, 54, 55
Rings
  falope, 179, 181
  vaginal, 78, 400, 412–413
Risk/benefit
  barrier methods, 158
  COCS, 73–75
  sterilization, 193
Risk-taking, sexual, 318
RNA detection, HIV, 303, 306
Roman Catholicism and sex, 315, 331
RU 486 *see* Mifepristone
Rubber, latex *see* Latex
Rubella screening, 279, 351

S

Safety/side-effects/complications (FP
      methods), 8–12
  abortion, 11, 241–242, 255, 256, 259–260

COCs *see* Combined oral contraceptives
  emergency contraception, 11, 207
  implants *see* Implants
  injectables, 11, 91–94
  IUDs, 11, 105, 120–126, 207, 242
  POC, 80, 84–87, 392
    management, 86–87
    POPs, 11, 89, 392
  spermicides, 11, 154
  sterilization
    female, 11, 183–184, 195, 238, 239
    male, 11, 187, 188–189, 198–199, 240
Safety/side-effects/complications (HRT),
      385–386
St Johns Wort in PMS, 363
Sarcoptes scabiei var. *hominis*, 309
Satisfaction, user *see* Attitudes
Scabies, 309
Schering PC4 *see*
          Ethinyloestradiol/levonorgestrel
          emergency contraception
Sclerosants, tubal-occluding, 181–182, 400
Scotland
  abortion
    legal aspects, 251
    rate, 249, 250
  birth rate, 250
  teenager pregnancy rates, 218, 219
Screening, 265–266
  antenatal, 351
  cancer
    breast, 269–270
    cervical, 275, 299–300
    ovarian, 278–279
  cholesterol, 272
  domestic violence, 271
  STIs, 271
  other screening procedures, 279
Scrotal bruising or haematoma with
      vasectomy, 188
Second preparation (Perlutal etc.), 402
Selective oestrogen receptor modulators *see*
      Oestrogen receptor modulators,
      selective
Selective serotonin reuptake inhibitors *see*
      Serotonin reuptake inhibitors,
      selective
Self-esteem, bolstering, 316
Self-examination, breast, 268–269
Serological tests
  HIV, 303, 304
  HIV-related opportunistic infections,
      306
Serotonin (5-HT), deficiency in PMS, 361
Serotonin reuptake inhibitors, selective
  ejaculatory failure caused by, 327–328
  in PMS, 363, 365, 366, 368, 369
  in premature ejaculation, 326

Sex (biological), cause of death by, 267
  see also Female; Gender; Girl; Male
Sex (sexual relations), 314–318
  age of consent, 232
  avoidance/aversion in women, 325
  functions, 314–318
  'normal' vs 'abnormal', concepts of, 333
  see also Intercourse
Sex education, 222–225
  content, 223–224
  increasing, 222
  opposition to, 225
  teacher training, 224
Sex hormones/steroids
  antagonists (antihormones), 409–411
    see also Anti-androgens; Anti-
      oestrogens; Antiprogestogens
  history of conditions affected by, 38
  menstrual cycle, 162, 163
  natural, injectable, 402
  new delivery systems, 412–413
  *see also specific (types of) steroids and entries
    under* Hormone; Hormonal
Sexual abuse, gonorrhoea, 287
Sexual assault and hostility, 317
Sexual behaviour/lifestyle
  adolescents (UK), changing patterns, 217
  FP methods and, 16, 19
  IUDs and, 114
Sexual desire/interest (libido)
  men losing, 328
  women gaining, COC use and, 61
  women losing, 324
    COC use and, 61, 329–330
Sexual health services *see* Clinic
Sexual intercourse *see* Intercourse
Sexual partner *see* Partner
Sexual problems/dysfunction/difficulties,
    323–328, 333
  adolescent, 319
  early marriage, 320–321
  management, 333
  middle age, 322–323
  postnatal, 322
Sexual relations *see* Sex
Sexual relationships, evolving of, 318–323
  see also Marriage
Sexuality, 318–323
  contraceptives affecting, 71, 328–332
  development, 318–323
  education, 223–224
Sexually transmitted infections (STIs), 271,
    281–311
  clinics for, 281–282
  examination (female), 282
    suggested routine, 311
  prevalence, 281
  protection (with contraceptives) from, 12

choice/needs relating to, 1, 2, 15
  HIV infection, 151, 156, 305
  spermicides giving, 151, 156, 398, 405
Sheep's intestine, condoms, 147
Sickle cell disease
  COCs and, 40
  POCs and, 101
Side-effects *see* Safety
Sildenafil, 327
Sino-plant, 401
Skin disorders
  with COCs, 71–72
  with HIV infection, 301
  menopausal, 375
  with POCs, 101
    exacerbated, 86
Smears, cervical, 276–278
  abnormal, management, 277–278
  in postmenopausal bleeding, 343
  screening programme, 275
  taking, 276–277
Smoking, 272
  as arterial disease risk factor with COCs,
    49
  POCs for smokers, 82
  stopping, 268, 272
    pre-pregnancy counselling, 351
  WHO medical eligibility criteria for FP
    methods, 23
'Sniff test', 291
Social factors in pelvic pain, 347
Society and fertility, 314–315
Socio-economic deprivation and teenage
    pregnancy, 219, 221–222
Spatula, smear-taking, 276, 277
Specialist, referral to *see* Referral
Sperm
  autoantibodies, 189, 414–415
  production and maturation, agents
    affecting, 332, 408–409, 409
  vaccination against, 414–415
Sperm banking, 193
Sperm granulomas, 188, 198
Spermatogenesis, suppression, 332,
    408–409, 409
Spermicides, 150–156, 405
  advantages, 151–153
  cervical caps and, 141
  costs, 21
  diaphragm used continuously without,
    404
  diaphragm used with, 136
  disadvantages, 153
    side–effects, 11, 153
  discontinuation rates, 13, 14
  effectiveness, 9, 154
  HIV infection prevented by, 153, 156, 305
  indications/contraindications, 151

instructions, 153
mode of action, 151
new/alternative agents, 156, 398, 405
postpartum use, 174–175
types, 150–156
  commonly used, 152
vault caps and, 142
vimules and, 143
Spinnbarkheit, 166
Spironolactone in COC-related skin
  disorders, 345–346
Sponge, vaginal (incl. Today sponge),
  153–156, 405
advantages/disadvantages, 154–156
discontinuation rates, 14
effectiveness, 9, 154
improvements, 405
indications/contraindications, 154
instructions, 155–156
mode of action, 154
safety/side-effects, 11
ST1435, 401
Standard Days method, 407
Sterilization, 177–200, 332
advantages/disadvantages, 190–191
complaints/litigation, 237–240
consent see Consent
effectiveness see Effectiveness
female see Female sterilization
HIV-infected persons, 306
improved techniques, 398–399
indications/contraindications, 189–190
information see Information
male see Vasectomy
postpartum, 176, 178
reversibility, 192–193
risk/benefits, 193
  see also Safety
sexual effects, 332
UK use, 3
worldwide use, 4, 397
Steroids see Corticosteroids; Sex hormones
STOP, 400
Stress incontinence
causes, 348
management, 349
Stroke risk, COCs, 45–46
Subcutaneous/subdermal implants see
  Implants
Subfertility see Infertility
Surgery
COC stopped before, 58
in PMS, 364, 368
POC continuation with, 80
preoperative assessment, importance, 246
see also specific procedures
Symptothermal method, 165, 168
effectiveness, 170

Syncope on IUD insertion, 117
Syphilis, 287

T

Tablets, foaming spermicidal, 150
instructions, 153
Tactylon, 403
Tamoxifen, 383
Teacher training in sex education, 224
Teaching on specific contraceptive use see
  Information
Teamwork, 246
Teenagers see Adolescents
Temperature
basal body see Basal body temperature
testicular, raising, 408
Testicles/testes
cancer, vasectomy and, 189, 199
suppression function, 332, 407–408
temperature, raising, 408
Testosterone enanthate injections, 408
Tetracyclines
chlamydial/non-chlamydial non-specific
  urethritis, 289, 290
COCs and, 55
Threads of IUD, 117
lost/missing (and their location), 124
pelvic infection and, 122
on removal
  broken, 120
  visible, 120
retrieval devices, 124
Thromboembolic disease (embolism and
  deep venous thrombosis)
HRT contraindications, 384
risk with COCs, 42, 48, 71
  asthma patients, 60
  prescribing and, 48, 49
risk with emergency contraception, 206
risk with HRT, 387
risk with sterilization, 183
WHO medical eligibility criteria for FP
  methods relating to, 24, 36–37
  COCs, 24, 36–37
Thrombophilias and COC
congenital, COC increasing
  predisposition to, 44
as contraindication for COC, 36–37
Tibolone, 383
Today sponge see Sponge
Toxic shock syndrome and sponges, 156
Toxicity see Safety
Toxoplasmosis in HIV disease, 306
Training of sex education teachers, 224
Tranexamic acid, menorrhagia, 341–342
Tranquillizers in menopause, 379

Transdermal contraception, 413
Transdermal oestrogens in HRT,
    381–382
Treponema pallidum, 287
Trials, clinical, FP methods, 7–8
Triazoles, candidiasis, 294
Trichomoniasis, 292–293
Tricycle regimen, 56–57
    headaches and, 62
Triphasic COCs, 32, 33
Tripterygium wilfordii, 408–409
Trophoblastic disease
    COCs and, 67
    IUDs and, 114
    WHO medical eligibility criteria for FP
        methods, 23
Trophoblastic residual tissue, post-abortion,
    259
Tube(s), fallopian
    hormonal contraceptive effects, 34
    surgical occlusion/ligation *see* Female
        sterilization
Tuberculosis
    drugs treating, COCs and, 54, 55
    WHO medical eligibility criteria for FP
        methods, 27
Tumours, liver
    COC risk of, 64
    POC and previous history of, 100
    WHO medical eligibility criteria for FP
        methods, 64
TwoDay method, 407

U

UK
    abortion
        legal aspects, 250–251
        rate, 249, 250
    adolescent/teenagers
        pregnancy, 217–219
        reproductive health, 216–217
    FP use patterns, 2–3
Ulcerative colitis and COCs, 37
Ultrasound
    pelvic, in pelvic pain, 347
    vaginal, in postmenopausal bleeding, 343
Uniplant, specific attributes, 95
United Kingdom *see* UK
United States, FP use patterns, 3–4
Ureaplasma urealyticum, 288
Urethral gonorrhoea, 283
Urethral prolapse/caruncle, 350
Urethral syndrome (frequency dysuria
    syndrome; FDS), 349, 350
Urethritis, non-specific, 288–290
Urinary problems, 348–350

incontinence *see* Incontinence
    menopausal, 375
Urinary tract infections (UTIs), 349
    with COCs, 65
    with diaphragms, 131
    recurrent, prevention, 350
Urination *see* Micturition
USA, FP use patterns, 3–4
Uterotubal junction cautery, 399
Uterus
    fibroids *see* Fibroids
    perforation
        by IUD, 112, 118–119, 125–126
        by surgical abortion, 241
    removal *see* Hysterectomy

V

Vaccines
    antifertility, 413–415
    hepatitis B, 307
Vacuum aspiration
    complications, 259
    early first trimester, 255
    late first trimester, 257
    patient information sheet, 263
Vagina
    adenosis, 337
    congenital malformations, 337
    cysts in wall, 337
    discharge
        COCs and, 66
        investigation algorithm, 284–285
        IUDs and, 121–122
        pH measurement, 291
    dyspareunia and, 325–326
    oestrogen application in atrophic change,
        336, 381–382
    pH at menopause, 375
Vaginal pessaries *see* Pessaries
Vaginal rings, 78, 400, 412–413
Vaginal sponge *see* Sponge
Vaginal ultrasound in postmenopausal
    bleeding, 343
Vaginismus, 325
    in early marriage/sexual relationships,
        321, 325
Vaginitis, atrophic *see* Atrophy
Vaginosis, bacterial, 290–291
    clinical features, 291
    diagnosis, 291
    with IUDs, 121–122
    treatment, 291
Valaciclovir, HSV, 297
Valves, vas-occluding, 399
Valvular heart disease
    IUDs and, 114

WHO medical eligibility criteria for FP
methods, 25
Vas deferens occlusion/division
percutaneous non-surgical occlusion, 186,
398
surgical *see* Vasectomy
Vascular system, HRT (oestrogen) effects,
378
Vasectomy (male sterilization; vas deferens
division/occlusion), 184–192,
398–399
advantages/disadvantages, 190–191
age and patterns of use (UK), 3
clinical management, 186–188
complaints/litigation, 240
discontinuation rates, 13, 14
effectiveness/failure *see* Effectiveness
indications/contraindications, 189–190
information/advice/counselling,
187–188, 192, 197–200
inadequate, 240
postnatal, 176
reversibility, 193, 199
safety/side-effects, 11, 187, 188–189,
198–199, 240
sexual effects, 332
techniques, 184–186
improved, 186, 398–399
worldwide use, 4, 397
Vasomotor symptoms, menopausal,
373–374
therapy, 379
Vasovagal syncope on IUD insertion, 117
Vault cap, 141–142
variation (vimule), 142–143
Venous disease
as COC contraindication, 38
as COC risk, 42–43
Venous thrombosis *see* Thromboembolic
disease
Viagra, 327
Vimule, 142–143
Violence, domestic, 271
Viral infections, 295–308
spermicides preventing, 153, 157, 398
Visual disturbances and COCs, 63
Vitamin B6 in PMS, 362
Vitamin D in osteoporosis
prevention/treatment, 377
Vomiting

with COCs, 63
conception risk, 52–53
as side-effect, 63, 65
with emergency contraception, 207
with POPs, conception risk, 88
Vulva
intraepithelial neoplasia, HPV and,
298
lichen sclerosus, 336
Vulvovaginitis
candidal, 293–295
gonococcal, 286
other causes, 286

W

Warfarin and IUDs, 114
Warts, genital *see* Condyloma
acuminatum
Weight (COC users)
excess/increased *see* Overweight
measuring, 57
WHO (on FP methods)
medical eligibility criteria (incl.
contraindications), 23–28
safety, 10
Withdrawal method *see* Coitus
interruptus
Women *see* Female; Female condom; Female
sterilization
World Health Organization *see* WHO
Worldwide perspectives *see* Global
perspectives

Y

Yuzpe method *see*
Ethinyloestradiol/levonorgestrel
emergency contraception

Z

Zidovudine in pregnancy, reducing vertical
transmission, 301, 307
Zona pellucidum, vaccination
against, 415